S0-CEZ-706

THE TIME-CRUNCHED CYCLIST

3rd Edition

THE TIME-CRUNCHED CYCLIST

Race-Winning Fitness in 6 Hours a Week

CHRIS CARMICHAEL and JIM RUTBERG

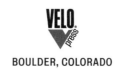

BOULDER, COLORADO

The Time-Crunched Cyclist, 3rd edition, is part of THE TIME-CRUNCHED ATHLETE™ series.

▼velopress®

3002 Sterling Circle, Suite 100
Boulder, CO 80301–2338 USA

VeloPress is the leading publisher of books on endurance sports. Focused on cycling, triathlon, running, swimming, and nutrition/diet, VeloPress books help athletes achieve their goals of going faster and farther. Preview books and contact us at velopress.com.

Distributed in the United States and Canada by Ingram Publisher Services

Library of Congress Cataloging-in-Publication Data
Names: Carmichael, Chris, 1960- author. | Rutberg, Jim, author.
Title: The time-crunched cyclist: race-winning fitness in 6 hours a week / Chris Carmichael and Jim Rutberg.
Description: 3rd edition. | Boulder, Colorado: VeloPress, 2017. | Includes bibliographical references and index.
Identifiers: LCCN 2016055402 (print) | LCCN 2016059236 (ebook) | ISBN 9781937715502 (pbk.: alk. paper) | ISBN 9781937716837 (ebook)
Subjects: LCSH: Cycling—Training. | Cyclists—Time management. | Endurance sports—Training.
Classification: LCC GV1048 .C38 2009 (print) | LCC GV1048 (ebook) | DDC 796.6—dc23
LC record available at https://lccn.loc.gov/2016055402

This paper meets the requirements of ANSI/NISO Z39.48-1992 (Permanence of Paper).

Art direction by Vicki Hopewell
Cover design by Andy Omel; cover photography by Philip Beckman
Interior design by Erin Farrell / Factor E Creative
Illustrations by Charlie Layton

Text set in Minion Pro

17   18   /   10   9   8   7   6   5   4   3   2   1

CONTENTS

FOREWORD

The 2011 Leadville 100 was an event I'll never forget, full of exhilarating moments, unexpected challenges, and an inordinate amount of dust. You might expect someone who co-founded Strava, the social network for athletes, to feel at home in a race like this, but I had no business whatsoever at the Leadville starting line. I had never competed in a bicycle race before, and just a few years earlier I had a crash that cost me eleven surgeries. I avoided road riding like the plague, and my mountain biking was pretty tentative. Most of my friends thought I was crazy to be back on a bike at all, let alone training for a race like Leadville.

But I had committed to this race, with a goal of finishing in under nine hours. Thankfully, I found Carmichael Training Systems. I befriended a coach there named Jason Siegle, and we chased this goal together.

When I began working with Jason, it was clear that my lifestyle was going to present a challenge. Constantly changing schedule. Unexpected travel. Prone to injury and prone to bailing on workouts when time got tight. Talk about time-crunched. I was the living embodiment.

Thankfully, Jason tossed everything I thought I knew about training out the window. Using the precepts of the Time-Crunched Training Program, he taught me the value of efficiency, rest, and proper nutrition. We experimented with hydration, saddle height, and tubeless tires. And I learned the importance of measuring performance based on power and heart rate.

This training coincided with some of the early days of Strava. Jason and I explored ways to leverage the Strava experience for communication, inspiration, and entertainment. He reviewed my activities and adjusted my workouts on the fly. We scoured Strava for the perfect route and longest climbs, constantly looking for local challenges similar to the Leadville course. And we evaluated my weekly performances together, looking for clues within the analytics.

It worked. Despite the unexpected race-day challenges (like my front derailleur imploding at mile 25!), my Leadville experience was as near a "sure thing" as one could hope. The months of training, designed and implemented by the crew at CTS, proved the perfect combination for achieving what had long been one of my bucket list events. I did not break nine hours (9:37 was my official time), but I could not have been happier with my day.

Best of all were the memories formed in the preceding months that included countless weekends in the saddle, searching for hills that would approximate the infamous Leadville Powerline climb. The training experience taught me the value of being smart, listening to my body, staying positive, and getting motivation and inspiration from other athletes. Quite simply, enjoying the journey.

In my role at Strava I get to see firsthand the impact that technology, data, and education can have on human performance. For the vast majority of us it's no longer about the number of training hours we put in—it's the quality of the training itself that makes all the difference.

And that's a good thing. Because I am the definition of a "time-crunched cyclist." As a single father of twin boys and with an office an hour from home, workouts are often the first victims of my lifestyle.

This is why when Chris and Jim reached out to me for a few good words on the latest edition of *The Time-Crunched Cyclist*, I jumped at the chance to contribute. And I am confident you too will benefit from the insights and perspective shared by these masters.

—Mark Gainey

Co-founder and CEO, Strava

INTRODUCTION

One of the first judgments I make about a book is based on how it feels in my hand. I want it to be substantial and have some weight. And therein lay the challenge of writing a book called *The Time-Crunched Cyclist*. This is a book for people who lead busy lives, people who wake up early and hit the ground running, juggle one or more jobs while raising one or more kids. Time is in short supply, and the whole point of this program is to get more from less. So why is this book so thick?

To be fair, the first edition was a quicker read. When we released it, I was concerned that we skipped a few topics, but I expected that readers would likely have a few other books on their shelves that covered the basics of cycling. Not wanting to be redundant, I kept it short and focused on new training concepts specific to time-crunched cyclists. Athletes loved the book and achieved great progress, and at their request I added more programs to the second edition (which of course made it thicker). This revised and expanded third edition is longer still because I've added material to address readers' requests and to include new areas of sports science and nutrition that impact a time-crunched cyclist's performance.

To help you move through the content more quickly, the book is divided into four parts. Part I talks about the program's origin, the science that backs it up, and how to measure training intensity. If you decide to skim through some of that material, pay attention to Chapter 3 where you'll learn about the opportunities and limitations of training as a Time-Crunched Cyclist.

Part II starts with an overview of the workouts you'll find in the training programs, which you'll need for reference material. After that you can read about all the training plans or just skip directly to the one you want to use.

Part III is where you will find information on sports nutrition, shortcuts for the grocery store and kitchen, and recipes from renowned chefs Michael Chiarello and Matthew Accarrino. If you're short on time, head to Chapter 10 which focuses on modifying how we eat more than what we eat. Chapter 13, on Hydration and Heat-Stress Management, is important too; it describes how heat is the real enemy of performance and how hydration status and other choices can help you or hurt you.

My favorite portion of Part IV is Chapter 15, Making the Most of Your Fitness. You'll find practical and proven tips to help you leverage your time-crunched fitness into great performances on the bike.

Until we developed the Time-Crunched Training Program, superior performance in cycling and other endurance sports was out of reach for time-crunched athletes. The old model of endurance training only works if you have more than 10 hours a week to spend on your bike. I don't have that kind of time anymore, and neither do a lot of the athletes who come to CTS. But the Time-Crunched solution leverages the potential of high-intensity interval workouts to make high-performance cycling accessible to you. The program is backed by science, has been proven effective by tens of thousands of real athletes, and is your ticket to achieving the fitness necessary to obtain the results you desire.

The program described in this book breaks some of the "rules" of traditional endurance training. The workouts are hard, but the rewards are great, even if they are relatively brief. Yes, the program has limitations in the length of time that you'll be able to maintain top fitness, but it also offers unbeatable opportunities for getting the most out of your limited training time.

In short, the Time-Crunched Training Program will put you back at the front of the pack, where you belong. So let's get started.

PART I

The Time-Crunched Advantage

The first notion we have to dispel is that being a Time-Crunched Athlete is a disadvantage. It is not. You can achieve a high level of fitness, compete or participate in the events you choose, and ride with power and confidence using this high-intensity, low-volume training plan. You can have fun on the group ride, push the pace, get in the breakaway, and sprint for the finish.

In Chapter 1 I'll take you through the genesis of the Time-Crunched Cyclist Program and show you why it's the best program for athletes who have limited time to train. In Chapter 2 we'll take a closer look at the science behind the program, which has been validated by a growing number of studies since the first edition of this book was released.

Chapter 3 is one of the most important in the entire book, because it outlines the terms and conditions for time-crunched training. My promise is that time-crunched training will make you fit and fast, but the caveat is that to be at your best for a certain range of activities you also need to accept that you won't be at your best for others. I think you'll find that the value proposition in Chapter 3 is a good deal, especially since the programs prepare athletes for exactly the types of events and goals that fit into a time-crunched athlete's schedule. In the final chapter of Part I we'll take a look at how you can use technology to accurately measure your workload, track your progress, and save time.

1

THE NEW PARADIGM FOR ENDURANCE TRAINING

I'M A CYCLIST AT MY CORE, but these days my life doesn't revolve around my bike the way it did when I was 20. I'm a cyclist, but I also have a family and own a business. I don't have endless hours to spend building up the massive endurance base that characterizes so many classic training programs. I don't have time to be the cyclist I was decades ago, and to be honest, I don't have any desire to be that guy again. My life is fuller—and more fulfilling—than it has ever been, so while being a fast and competitive cyclist is still important to me, I'm equally glad those goals rank behind my family and business in terms of priority.

My current relationship with cycling is not unique; there are tens of thousands of cyclists in the United States who still love to ride but used to ride a lot more than they do now. Almost every cyclist over the age of 30 has some version of the same story. They all used to go out on epic 4-hour-plus rides on weekends and put in 15 to 20 hours of training on a weekly basis. Many raced, and some even claim to have kicked butt. Then they got a real job, fell in love, bought a house, had kids, and so on. Cycling is still their passion and still takes up significant space in the garage, but now the car is worth more than the bike

3

on the roof (instead of the other way around), and the kids' soccer games and recitals take precedence over a long training ride or driving 3 hours each way to race a 1-hour criterium.

Our relationship with our sport may have changed, but our desire to be fit, fast, and powerful hasn't diminished. I hate being slow, especially because I know what it feels like to be fast. I hate getting dropped, because I know what it feels like to drive the pace and make others suffer. And I hate to see riders soft-pedaling ahead of me at the tops of rolling hills, because I used to be the one politely slowing down so my friends could keep up.

I love the feeling of being on top of the gear, spinning along effortlessly in a fast-moving pack. I love knowing I have the power to accelerate up a small hill, jump out of a corner, bridge a gap, or take a good pull through a strong headwind. I love how it feels to look around and know I have more left in the tank than some of the other riders, and that they're closer to their limits than I am to mine. I like being fit, fast, and powerful on the bike, and after talking to thousands of cyclists on my travels around the world, I know you do, too.

For the majority of working cyclists, your training program is the only thing stopping you from enjoying cycling the way you used to. Why? Because most cyclists are still training with 30-year-old science. Yes, we have dramatically improved the precision of training with power meters, heart rate monitors, and global positioning system (GPS) units, but the fundamental infrastructure of training hasn't changed in a long time. As athletes, our lifestyles have changed dramatically, but our approach to training has remained essentially the same.

The Time-Crunched Training Program (TCTP) is not a shortcut to fitness; there's no such thing. Instead, this program is a new approach to training that takes a different path to endurance fitness. It works around busy schedules by systematically applying greater intensities to achieve bigger gains with fewer and shorter rides. The workouts are strenuous and the workload is high.

Because of that, the benefits match and sometimes exceed those achieved through programs that call for twice the weekly training hours.

If your ambition is to race at a high level, either again or for the first time, the TCTP will make you competitive in local and regional races. If you just want to improve your strength and stamina on the bike, it will give you the fitness you need to push the pace at the local group ride and enjoy challenging rides. If you want to achieve high-performance fitness in the limited time you have available for training, it's time to embrace a new approach to endurance training.

• • •

CASE STUDY
THE DECLINE OF STERLING SWAIM

The limitations of the classic endurance training model, and the benefits of the time-crunched model my coaching staff and I have developed, are clearly illustrated through the experiences of three CTS athletes. Sterling Swaim, Taylor Carrington, and John Fallon could fit right in at any group ride across the country. They're not pros or former pros, they're not freakishly gifted in terms of VO_2max (maximum aerobic capacity), and they probably wouldn't be the strongest or the weakest riders in your local ride. In other words, they're a good representation of the modern American cyclist. We'll start with Sterling.

Sterling has lived in Winston-Salem, North Carolina, pretty much all his life, and he's been racing since he was 13 years old. As a young man he raced the junior version of Paris–Roubaix and rode the United States Cycling Federation (USCF) National Road and Criterium Championships as a junior and senior rider. Throughout his 20s he raced as a Category (Cat.) III in criteriums and road races up and down the eastern seaboard and as far west as the Mississippi River. For years his brother (a Cat. I) and other racing buddies urged him to devote more time to training and move up to the Cat. II or Cat. I level, but Sterling had other priorities. He built a lucrative car-detailing business in his driveway to raise tuition money so he could attend the University of

North Carolina–Greensboro at night and earned a degree in business administration. All the while, he continued training about 14 to 16 hours a week and went racing on weekends.

After graduation Sterling gave his car-detailing business to his brother, Ben, and went to work as an investment broker. Though the work was less backbreaking, the hours were longer, and he cut his training back to about 10 to 12 hours a week. Falling in love, getting married, buying a house, and having two daughters all followed in short order, and soon after Sterling was struggling to find 10 hours a week for training.

With his years of experience, Sterling had become accustomed to placing in the top 10 on a consistent basis in Cat. III criteriums and road races in the Southeast. But as his training time fell below 10 hours, racing became more difficult. He found himself in the middle of the pack, then the back. Where he used to push at the front on group rides, he now followed wheels. He started opting out of most of the long loops he used to enjoy with his brother and friends because he didn't want to deal with struggling to keep up or being the "slow guy." Cycling rapidly lost its appeal, his fitness declined, his weight went up, and his bikes started collecting more dust than miles.

THE PROMISE OF A NEW PARADIGM

Sterling's case is remarkably common. Here's a guy who loves cycling, is pretty good at it, has been doing it for years, and would genuinely like to continue doing it for years to come. But being slow and out of shape isn't much fun, and cycling is too difficult a sport to bother with when it's not fun.

I can't change the reality of Sterling's life to magically create more time for him to use for training. I can't—or at least I never would—ask him to give up time reading to his daughter so he can put in more time on the bike and race for $50 primes and $200 purses at regional criteriums. The value proposition (trade-off) there doesn't make any sense (rightfully so, I might add). Yet cycling will not regain its appeal for Sterling, or for thousands of cyclists facing similar value propositions, unless he's able to perform at a level that's worth the effort of training.

The classic endurance training model won't work for Sterling because he doesn't have enough time to go through the slow and gradual buildup of deep aerobic fitness. He has 6 hours a week—8 if he's lucky—and that's it. Under the old training paradigm, there is no way for him to be competitive in Cat. III criteriums.

The reason this section refers to a new paradigm and not just a new training program is that the changes I'm going to ask you to make go way beyond adding a new interval workout to your routine. For this to work—and it will—you have to be willing to rethink your overall approach to endurance training. When CTS coach Jim Rutberg suggested the TCTP to his longtime friend and former teammate, Sterling thought he was nuts. For someone who had been a bike racer for more than 15 years, the time-crunched program Rutberg wanted to put Sterling on didn't look like anything he'd done before. Though he was an investment broker, he had read numerous cycling training books and had subscriptions to *Bicycling* and *VeloNews*, and Rutberg was suggesting he train in ways those trusted publications told him not to! Then again, Sterling missed being a strong cyclist and wasn't very happy being mediocre, so what did he have to lose?

Cyclists in the Carolinas are fortunate to have two significant blocks of criterium racing each year, one from May to June and the other from September to October. In the spring the traveling circus that is professional cycling swings through the Southeast for races such as the Hanes Park Classic, the Dilworth Criterium, and the Athens Twilight Criterium. Then in the fall there are a bunch of local criteriums, leading up to the Carolina Classic in Greensboro, North Carolina, and the Greenville Cycling Classic near George Hincapie's adopted hometown of Greenville, South Carolina. There is some racing at other times in the year, but not as much, and nothing that attracts such large and strong fields of pros and amateurs.

Rutberg put Sterling on the TCTP six weeks before the start of the spring races in the Carolinas. Sterling rode four times a week, never more than 7 hours total, raced four times in 8 weeks, and finished fourth, eighth, first, and third. In the only race he had entered the previous fall, he hadn't even finished.

Purists will tell you the TCTP won't work, and some will even tell you it's dangerous. Well, I'm telling you it does work, I'll show you exactly how and why it works, and I guarantee it's no more dangerous than being a cyclist in the first place. What's more, it's based on sound science, has been proven effective by real athletes, and offers the opportunity of high-speed, high-power, full-throttle fun for cyclists who can't get there using antiquated training methods.

"I am a physician assistant and married and have to make the most of every hour I have on the bike. The time-crunched cycling programs have made me a stronger cyclist. I have used the programs in the book to train for a specific event, such as the Solvang Century, and sometimes just as a training block for developing fitness. It is by far the best cycling training book on the market."

A BRIEF HISTORY OF TRAINING

Even though we can trace some theories of athletic training, such as periodization, back to the ancient Greeks, the level of sophistication in training was very low until the middle of the 20th century. That's not to diminish the abilities or accomplishments of athletes such as Major Taylor, Jesse Owens, Babe Ruth, and Jim Thorpe. They were great athletes in their time and would be great champions today as well. But early Olympians and professional athletes rose above their competitors based largely on natural talent and their ability to endure great punishment. Some trained for their sports, a few trained maniacally, and the best athletes were those who managed to survive and adapt to brutal training regimens that destroyed everyone else.

With relatively little scientific knowledge of how and why the training worked, training methods came and went as athletes observed and copied the workouts used by each new champion. Coaches saw this and theorized that improvement was based on the load an athlete could handle (recovery was largely ignored), and subsequently they based the process of athlete recruitment on pushing relative beginners harder and harder, until only a handful were left standing.

Structured interval training started appearing in the 1930s, when German scientist Woldemar Gerschler refined the less formal but highly effective practices already used by the Swedes and Finns (inventors of "Fartlek" running, which used natural terrain to interject periods of intensity and recovery into long runs; Fartlek means "speed play" in Swedish). Gerschler made intervals more intense, kept the recovery periods short, and even used heart rate to govern the intensity of efforts. If you're interested in reading more about training during this period, I recommend *The Perfect Mile*, by Neal Bascomb, which describes the training methods used by elite runners as they sought to become the first to run a mile in less than 4 minutes.

The science of training took significant steps forward after World War II, largely because of the cold war. Even though the basic idea of periodization— systematically changing the focus and workload of training to maximize the positive impact of overload and recovery on training adaptations—had been around in various forms for thousands of years, it gained more widespread acceptance after Tudor Bompa and other Eastern Bloc coaches started creating detailed systems for improving athletic performance and winning medals by the truckload.

With the world's greatest armies in a perpetual standoff, the Olympics became both a real and a symbolic battleground between East and West. Right along with the arms race and the space race was an ongoing battle to see who could win more Olympic medals—the sports race. From 1945 to 1989 the space and arms races pushed technology ahead faster than at any previous period in human history, and the cold war fight for athletic supremacy also led to giant advances in sports science. As a result, by 1990 our understanding of the athlete's response to exercise, altitude, hydration, nutrition, and recovery had never been greater. There was still plenty left to learn, and there still is, but we know more about how the body adapts to training than ever before.

For most amateur athletes in the postwar period, however, the training methods in use were relatively primitive. When I started training seriously in the 1970s, we had a basic understanding of interval training, but all we did was break down the different aspects of bike racing and train them individually. Monday was a rest day, Tuesday was sprinting, Wednesday was endurance, Thursday was climbing or a training race, Friday was a short spin, and then you raced on the weekend. If a race was particularly important, you rested a little more than usual during the preceding week. In the winter you used smaller gears and focused more on endurance, and maybe did some cyclo-cross racing. As amateurs, we did exactly what the pros did, but we rode fewer hours and did fewer intervals.

In the 1980s we started doing more lab testing. We were poked and prodded and informed of our VO_2max and lactate threshold values, but those numbers were largely useless outside the lab. By the mid-1980s you could use a heart rate monitor during your rides (although they were huge and not very accurate). Dr. Edmund Burke, a physiologist with the US Cycling Team who later became a great mentor and friend of mine, was one of the first scientists to realize that endurance athletes could use heart rate ranges to target specific training adaptations. It was a big step forward because it allowed athletes to establish personal training intensities instead of relying on pace and perceived effort.

In the early 1990s, as heart rate monitors became widely available and heart rate training gained widespread acceptance, a new technology was being developed that would greatly increase the effectiveness and precision of cycling training. I think I first saw an SRM power meter in 1990 at the world championships in Japan, on the Germans' team time trial bikes. In 1993, working with a team that included US Olympic Committee biomechanist Jeff Broker and sports scientists Ed Burke and Jay T. Kearney, we mounted a prototype wheel-based power meter from Look to evaluate the aerodynamic advantages of different time trial positions. The next year, Dean Golich, who worked for me at USA Cycling and is now a CTS Premier coach, mounted SRMs on the bikes of US National Team riders to study the power output of individual cyclists during the Tour DuPont.

Power meters finally provided the ability to take the power numbers derived from VO_2max and lactate threshold tests and apply them to everyday training out on the road. We developed individual power ranges to target specific training adaptations, then developed field tests to monitor and evaluate athletes' progress without having to go back into the lab. The science and technology were later pushed even further by Hunter Allen and Andrew Coggan when they developed TrainingPeaks software, which dramatically improved the ability to analyze the data from power files.

Despite the distance that training and technology have come since the end of World War II, however, the training programs used by most modern cyclists still don't meet their needs. That is because there's a fundamental problem with the classic training model for endurance cycling (including criteriums, cyclocross, mountain biking, and road racing).

THE CLASSIC ENDURANCE TRAINING MODEL

The classic endurance training model has always taken a top-down approach, meaning we have taken principles proven at the elite level and modified them to the needs and constraints of average and novice athletes. This is where we got the idea of long-term base training, or foundation training as it is also known. For decades, pro athletes have spent a significant portion of the fall and winter engaged in high-volume, low- to moderate-intensity training. This was followed by a gradual increase in intensity and the inclusion of some longer intervals at intensities around lactate threshold. Hard intervals and training races were then thrown into the mix in the four to eight weeks prior to racing.

Once the racing season started, training volume and intensity varied according to the athlete's racing schedule, but racing itself provided a significant amount of the overall training stimulus. During the season, athletes cycled through a series of race-and-recover periods in which there was very little actual training on the days between competitions. Because alternating between high-intensity racing and easy recovery days can only sustain competitive fitness for about six to eight weeks, athletes would shift to a lighter racing schedule—or a series of second-tier events they were doing for training rather than results—while devoting more attention to endurance and lactate threshold training. Then it was back to the race-and-recover cycle for several weeks in an effort to get results, earn some prize money, and keep their jobs.

And so it went from March to October. After the final race of the season, we were all so tired that we tossed the bike into the garage and slept for a month. Then the process started all over again, and we were ready to race by March. It was like that in the 1970s, and it's like that today for many young men and women trying to make a living as bike racers.

THE IMPACT OF POWER ON THE CLASSIC ENDURANCE TRAINING MODEL

Although power meters had been around since the very early 1990s, it took several years to get them on enough bikes and gather enough data to see how power could transform training. The same is true with newer technologies today. There are now monitors that can provide real-time blood lactate and oxygen saturation values, and there's even a running power meter that could finally measure the true workload of running. But just because you can measure something doesn't mean you can improve performance with the data. The key with these technologies, as it was with power meters, will be to determine the best way to apply the data to improve training results.

With the advent of the power meter, we could finally measure workload accurately. Initially, that information didn't change the way I trained athletes with the US National Team. I still took an old-school approach; I pushed my athletes to their limits, and those who could adapt and grow stronger were the ones who stayed on the team, went to Europe, became Olympians, and then pros. Basically, I coached the way I had been coached, but with the benefit of hindsight it's clear there were major flaws in that method.

I changed my coaching methods when data from power meters showed there was more benefit from performing longer efforts at a more sustainable intensity level, particularly just below lactate threshold power. A rider's lactate threshold marks his or her maximum sustainable effort level. You can complete efforts above this power output, but only for a limited time before you're forced to slow down.

Perhaps even more important, power data clearly showed the critical importance of adequate recovery between workouts. Instead of crushing athletes equally and seeing who could handle the stress, power meters enabled greater precision and personalization of training, and power data was crucial to determining how much recovery athletes needed before they were ready for more high-quality work.

Longer, submaximal efforts at power outputs just below lactate threshold elicited similar increases in lactate threshold power, and because the training intensity was lower, athletes could do more of this targeted training in a given week or month compared with the older, harder method. Going a little bit easier actually made them stronger and faster.

I explained these concepts in detail in *The Ultimate Ride*, and they are widely used by novice, amateur, and professional athletes and their coaches to this day. Now, lest you think I'm arrogant enough to believe I'm the only one to figure out the value of this approach, many of the same concepts—especially the importance of submaximal efforts in improving sustainable power at lactate threshold—were discussed in books such as *The Cyclist's Training Bible* by Joe Friel, *Serious Training for Endurance Athletes* by Rob Sleamaker and Ray Browning, *Serious Cycling* by Ed Burke, *High Performance Cycling* by Asker Jeukendrup, and more recently in *Training and Racing with a Power Meter* by Hunter Allen and Andrew Coggan.

During the same time frame, a transition was happening in the way professional racers competed throughout the year. In my opinion, Eddy Merckx will forever be regarded as the greatest cyclist who ever raced a bike. He won just about every race there was, more than once in many cases, and he won races from the earliest part of the spring to the latest events in the fall. His commitment to racing and winning throughout the season was shared by all professional cyclists of the time, and indeed by most riders well into the 1990s. Riders focused a bit more on particular races they wanted to win, but for the most part they raced full bore from Milan–San Remo in March through the Giro di Lombardia in October. That started to change in the 1990s when athletes began focusing on being their absolute best for shorter periods within the long season.

Instead of racing week in and week out through the spring, riders preparing specifically for the Tour de France focused on training first and using select races for training. There's no way to completely replicate the physical and psychological demands of racing in training, so difficult races such as Paris–Nice and the Dauphiné Libéré were typically included in Tour de France preparation. However, compared with riders from previous generations, Grand Tour contenders now had fewer days of racing in their legs before starting the Tour in July. Similarly, once the Tour de France was over, those same riders allowed themselves a substantial break from racing. It was an enormously successful strategy, and it has completely changed the way pro riders specialize in different portions of the season—the spring classics, the grand tours, the fall classics and world championships, and so on.

ADAPTING PRO-LEVEL TRAINING FOR AMATEURS

As I mentioned previously, I launched CTS to deliver world-class coaching to athletes of all abilities. I was frustrated by the gap between the level of expertise available to elite athletes and the relatively archaic training methods that were being used by novice cyclists and amateur racers. Over the next 10 years

I coached, taught other coaches new training methods, hosted camps and clinics, wrote books and countless articles, and built a successful coaching business. Along the way, CTS raised awareness about the benefits of coaching and helped give rise to an industry. In 2000 there were fewer than 200 licensed USA Cycling coaches. As demand grew from the cycling community, so did the number of coaches, and by the end of 2014 there were more than 1,500.

There are dozens of reasons why the coaching industry thrived and grew, and I believe the subtle shift to submaximal training intensities was an important factor. It made training easier and therefore more pleasant, yet it still prepared athletes for great personal performances. Initially it was pretty simple for my coaches and me to adapt the principles I'd been using with pros to athletes who were training for one-third to one-half of the pros' weekly training hours. If pros were riding 24 hours a week and completing four 30-minute climbing efforts, then it was absolutely reasonable to prescribe three 15-minute climbing efforts to a Cat. III rider training 12 hours a week. The relative intensities were the same, expressed as an identical percentage of each rider's lactate threshold power output (if the rider had access to a lab) or average power from the CTS Field Test (the performance test used for the workouts and training programs in this book; see Chapter 4). Although heart rate intensities are less accurate than power measurements, we also derived them for athletes who did not have access to power meters.

Effective training comes down to applying a workload to an athlete that is both specific to his or her activity and appropriate for that person's current levels of fitness and fatigue. The load has to be enough to stimulate a training response from the body, but not so great that it creates more fatigue than the body can cope with. And you have to give the body enough recovery time to replenish energy stores and adapt to the applied stress. Physically, the principal differences between training an elite athlete and an amateur are the workloads necessary to cause positive adaptations, the workloads the athletes can handle, and the time the athletes have available to train.

CTS coaches have worked with more than 17,000 cyclists, and more than 95 percent of them are novices, recreational riders, and amateur competitors. In the early years, the average CTS athlete was training about 10 to 12 hours a week. The riders who raced Cat. II or Cat. III or fast masters categories were closer to 12 to 16 hours a week, and some of the recreational riders and century riders were at about 8 to 10 hours a week. They were all being coached using the same method I was using with pro athletes, essentially an updated version of the classic endurance training model. It worked beautifully, and amateur athletes experienced incredible gains in their sustainable power outputs and race performances. They were finishing centuries faster than ever before, winning criteriums and road races left and right, leaving their riding buddies behind on climbs, and having more fun on their bikes than they had in years.

The biggest complaint we heard in those days was that the training was too easy. We had to have the same conversation with almost every athlete who signed up for coaching. My coaches would build the first few weeks of the athlete's schedule, then the athlete would log onto our web site to see it and immediately call to let the coach know he or she could handle more. The intensity was too low, the intervals weren't long enough, the rides weren't long enough, and there were far too many rest days in the week. Yes, we'd say, we know it looks different than what you've done for the past 5 years (which was based on 30-year-old science), but try this for 6 weeks and then tell us if you want to go back to the way you trained before.

With rare exceptions, the coaching program adapted straight from what I was doing with pros worked for novices, recreational riders, and amateur racers, and our athletes were ecstatic about the results. As time went on, however, I started hearing about athletes for whom the program wasn't working. At first they were few and far between, and it was tempting to dismiss them as "uncoachable" (a term I despise, and a circumstance I don't believe in) or just within that small percentage of people you can never satisfy. But if that were true, I reasoned, the number—or at least percentage—of those athletes should remain somewhat constant. If my coaching methodology worked 95 percent of the time, it should always work 95 percent of the time.

In the mid-2000s, however, I started to see an increase in the percentage of athletes who were achieving results that were below my expectations. Many of the athletes were perfectly happy with their results, but their coaches expressed concern about what they saw as diminishing returns. The athletes were still making progress, but not as much, and the gains were more difficult to come by.

It took some digging to find the common link among these athletes, but as it turned out, it was remarkably simple. The problem was time.

ENDURANCE TRAINING AT THE CROSSROADS

The common factor shared by athletes who were experiencing subpar results from their coaching programs was a lack of training time. In almost every case I examined, the athletes in question were training fewer than 8 hours a week, some as few as 5. Many had training schedules that called for 10 to 12 hours, but they weren't able to complete all the training sessions because of their hectic work and family schedules. Others had worked with their coaches to build 6- or 8-hour schedules and were following their programs to the letter but were still not seeing results.

Time and intensity add up to workload, and all other things being equal, too little training time means there's an insufficient training stimulus. That's when it hit me. We had found the point at which the classic endurance training model breaks down. Once you get below 8 hours of training a week, the old tried-and-true methods derived from pro-level athletes no longer work. With the kind of workouts and interval intensities typically used in classically based programs, there's simply not enough time to generate the workload necessary to overload the body's systems and force them to adapt and grow stronger. Athletes stop improving and stagnate instead. And after a few months of training at a level that's insufficient to move them forward, they get frustrated, lose their motivation, complete halfhearted workouts, and subsequently experience a decline in fitness and performance.

We were seeing an increase in the percentage of people struggling to make progress, because in those years the popularity of cycling and coaching was increasing, and a growing number of the athletes signing up for coaching were leading extremely busy lives. At the same time, athletes who had been working with CTS coaches for two or three years were experiencing changes in their lifestyles: marriage, kids, promotions, mortgages, and so on.

As I saw it, there were two choices: Write off a highly motivated population of athletes because they weren't able to commit enough time to fit into the classic endurance training model, or change the model. Since the only time I ever encouraged athletes to stop exercising was when their physicians said their sport or activity level might kill them, I chose to change the model.

THE TIME-CRUNCHED SUCCESS STORY

What I love most about coaching is helping athletes achieve more than they thought they were capable of. Training plans and data files can give athletes the tools to improve, but inspiration is what enables them to outperform the sum of their data. That was my goal with the previous editions of this book, and it is still my goal with this edition.

The training plans here will work, of this I am certain. My bigger goal is to inspire you to use the concepts in this book to push the boundaries of what you think is possible on your limited training time. Tens of thousands of athletes have already done just that and are racing and performing at levels they thought they'd never reach or never regain. Throughout the book you'll find snippets of just some of the messages I've received over the years about the Time-Crunched Training Program. Here are a few:

"I've been following the Experienced Century workouts with four colleagues from work. Two of the guys lost 30 lbs. each, and all improved power outputs significantly. Really happy with the results—thank you for writing the book!" —THOMAS T.

"After picking up road cycling 3 years ago after many years of casual mountain biking, my intensity and volume of training peaked this year. However, my fitness seemed to plateau until I discovered The Time-Crunched Cyclist. *Since using the program, my more structured, higher-intensity sessions have pushed me further and faster than I ever thought I could go. As a dad with two young kids and a wife to keep happy, thanks!"* —RICHARD C.

"I've been following your commuter program for the last 9 weeks in an effort to improve my fitness and race performances. I'm pleased to report that the program definitely seems to work for me as I had my first win in a local race I participated in on Sunday. Now everyone wants to know what I've been doing for the last 9 weeks!" —PHIL C.

"I'm currently using the Time-Crunched Cycling Program on a stationary exercise bike in Afghanistan. The workouts are the highlight of my day. Even had my wife ship my shoes, pedals, and wrench here." —MIKE M. (US ARMY)

OVERVIEW OF THE TIME-CRUNCHED TRAINING PROGRAM

Before stepping through the details and the science of how it works, I want to give you a broad overview of the Time-Crunched Training Program.

The TCTP consists of a maximum of 4 workouts per week. There's some latitude in terms of scheduling, but generally it comes down to a combination of the following:

- Two to three weekday workouts, each lasting 60 to 90 minutes
- One to two weekend rides, each lasting 1 to 3 hours

Three-hour rides are rare in the program, and there's nothing longer than that. Weekly training volume will be 6 hours, with the option to increase workout duration and accumulate up to 8 hours. The exceptions to these rules will be in the Ultraendurance and Commuting chapters. The Ultraendurance training program features more volume on the weekends while maintaining shorter interval workouts during the workweek, and there are a few weeks of that schedule that feature a fifth workout day. The Commuter training plans assume that you're commuting to and from work 4 to 5 days a week, although the actual weekday workouts stick with the 60- to 90-minute range.

In the absence of time, intensity is the key to performance. Remember, workload is a product of time and intensity, so if you want to keep the workload constant as time decreases, then intensity must increase. For a training program to work on fewer than 8 hours a week, you pretty much have to focus entirely on intensity. Make no mistake: The workouts in this program are hard. Very hard. You will be performing some efforts just below your lactate threshold power output and some right at it, but many efforts will be much more difficult, at maximum intensity.

The TCTP is a high-intensity, low-volume training program that produces the fitness and power necessary to push the pace in local group rides and to be competitive in local and regional criteriums, cross-country and short-track mountain bike races, and cyclocross races. If you're not a competitive cyclist but want to be stronger than you are right now, this program will give you the fitness to fully enjoy weekend rides, bike tours, and cycling camps.

However, there are limits to what you're going to be able to accomplish on fewer than 8 hours of training per week. For instance, with this program you can prepare to have a good day on a century ride, but it's not likely to be the fastest 100 miles you've ever ridden. And although the program lets Sterling race for the win, in the same way that we've seen the pros prioritizing a specific portion of the season, there's a reason Sterling is focusing on the spring and fall series instead of trying to win races throughout the entire season.

The TCTP will not be the perfect solution for every cyclist, and I have included Chapter 3, called "Terms and Conditions," to help you decide whether this program is for you.

Placing your family and career ahead of your cycling goals is a wise choice for pretty much anyone who has either a real career or a family, and pretty much the only choice if you have both. But focusing on your career and your family doesn't change the fact that you're a cyclist, nor does it invalidate your desire to be fit, fast, and powerful.

Simply put, a reduction in training time doesn't automatically doom you to back-of-the-pack finishes or another season of fruitless suffering. If you're willing to work hard with the limited time you have, and if you're ready to let go of antiquated training methods and try something new, then it's time to get off your butt and retake your rightful place at the front of the pack.

2

THE SCIENCE OF THE TIME-CRUNCHED TRAINING PROGRAM

WHETHER YOU HAVE UNLIMITED TIME TO TRAIN or only a few hours a week, your performance depends on developing three fundamental energy systems. These energy systems power all activities, and the goal of performance training is to get all three working at optimum levels. The systems are:

- Immediate energy, which involves the adenosine triphosphate (ATP) and creatine phosphate (CP) systems
- Aerobic system, which is the body's preferred energy system
- Glycolytic system, which the body uses to meet the demands of relatively short, high intensity efforts

The end product of all three systems is ATP, which releases energy when one of its three phosphate bonds is broken. The resulting adenosine diphosphate is then resynthesized to ATP so it can be broken again, and again, and again. The best way to think of these three energy pathways is from the viewpoint of demand.

THE IMMEDIATE ENERGY SYSTEM: DO OR DIE

The ATP/CP system supports high-power efforts that last fewer than about 10 seconds. You use it when you have to jump out of the way of a speeding bus, and from an athletic standpoint it's most important in power sports such as football. As a cyclist, you mostly use this system for a powerful standing start or when you almost rip the cranks off trying to avoid getting run over by a car. During those few seconds, you demand energy faster than either the glycolytic or aerobic energy system can deliver it. The ATP/CP system is immediate because the ATP part is the energy-yielding molecule produced by the other systems. The very limited supply of ATP that is stored in your muscles can provide energy without the more than 20 steps required to produce ATP through the aerobic system. However, because endurance cycling doesn't rely heavily on this energy system, cyclists have little reason to focus on it during training.

THE AEROBIC ENGINE: ALL-DAY ENERGY

The aerobic system is the body's primary source of energy, and it's an utterly amazing machine. It can burn carbohydrate, fat, and protein simultaneously and can regulate the mixture it burns based on fuel availability and energy demand. It's a flex-fuel engine that's remarkably clean and efficient; when the aerobic system is done with a molecule of sugar, the only waste products are water and carbon dioxide. In comparison, the glycolytic system (discussed below) produces energy faster, but it can only use carbohydrate, produces less ATP from every molecule of sugar it processes, and produces lactate as a by-product (more on this later).

The rock stars of the aerobic system are little things called mitochondria. These organelles are a muscle cell's power plants: Fuel and oxygen go in, and energy comes out. For an endurance athlete, the primary goal of training is to increase the amount of oxygen your body can absorb, deliver, and process. One of the biggest keys to building this oxygen-processing capacity is increasing mitochondrial density, or the size and number of mitochondria in muscle cells. As you ride, having more and bigger power plants running at full capacity gives you the ability to produce more energy aerobically every minute.

THE GLYCOLYTIC ENERGY SYSTEM: BUYING WITH CREDIT

When training increases the power you can produce aerobically, you can go harder before reaching the point where you're demanding energy faster than the aerobic engine can deliver it, a point known as lactate threshold. But increasing your power at lactate threshold is only part of the equation. With specific training at intensities near your lactate threshold power output, you can also increase the amount of time you will be able to ride at and slightly above threshold.

There's been a lot of confusion about the glycolytic system, mainly because of semantics. This is the system people often refer to as anaerobic, which literally means "without oxygen." The terminology causes confusion because it implies that the body has stopped using oxygen to produce energy, which is not the case. As exercise intensity increases, you reach a point at which your demand for energy matches your aerobic engine's ability to produce it in working muscles. Then you decide to push a little harder, or you hit a hill or a headwind, or your buddy attacks and you have to respond. Your energy demand increases, and in order for your mitochondria to continue producing enough energy, your body uses a metabolic shortcut called anaerobic glycolysis. Although the actual process involves many chemical reactions, glycolysis—to put it in its simplest terms—rapidly delivers the ATP necessary to meet your increased energy demand by converting glucose (sugar) into lactate in order to keep other energy-producing reactions moving.

Lactate is a partially used carbohydrate that leads to trouble when it builds up in your muscles. The molecule is created as a normal step of aerobic metabolism, and lactate is constantly being recycled back into usable energy. The problem isn't that more lactate is being produced; instead, as exercise intensity increases, you reach a point where lactate removal or processing can no longer keep up with production. A disproportionate amount of lactate builds up in the muscle and blood, and this accumulation is what we look for when we're determining an athlete's lactate threshold.

What ultimately happens to these lactate leftovers? Lactate has gotten a bad rap for years. It has been blamed for the burning sensation in your muscles when you surge above your sustainable pace. It has been blamed for delayed-onset muscle soreness. People have tried to massage it away, flush it out, and buffer it. But the best way to get rid of lactate is to reintegrate it back into the normal aerobic metabolism to complete the process of breaking it down into energy, water, and carbon dioxide.

One of the key adaptations you're seeking as an endurance athlete is an improvement in your ability to get that lactate integrated back into the normal process of aerobic energy production so it can be oxidized completely. The faster you can process lactate, the more work you can perform before lactate levels in your muscles and blood start to rise, and the faster you can recover from hard efforts.

There's a difference between talking about energy systems and effort levels. The glycolytic system produces energy, but lactate threshold is an effort level that correlates to a shift in energy production. Similarly, there's an effort level that correlates with the greatest amount of oxygen your body can take in and process, and that's called VO_2max. We'll cover it next.

MAXING OUT: VO_2MAX

Lactate threshold is the point at which your demand for energy outstrips the aerobic system's ability to deliver it, but lactate threshold doesn't define the maximum amount of oxygen your body can use. When your exercise intensity reaches its absolute peak, and your body is pulling in and using as much oxygen as it possibly can, you're at VO_2max. This is your maximum aerobic capacity, and it is one of the most important indicators of your potential as an endurance athlete.

An exceedingly high VO_2max doesn't automatically guarantee you'll become a cycling champion; it just means you have a big engine. To make a comparison to car engines, some people are born with eight cylinders, whereas others have four (and extremely gifted athletes are born with twelve). A finely tuned four-cylinder Acura can go faster than a poorly maintained V8 Corvette, and twelve-cylinder supercars can beat everything, but they can be finicky and difficult to control. You have to have a big engine to be a pro, but no matter what size engine you start with, you can optimize your performance with effective training.

It takes a great effort to reach intensities near your VO_2max, and during VO_2max-specific workouts you generate an enormous amount of lactate and burn calories tremendously fast. But the reward is worth the effort, because increasing your power at VO_2max gives you the tools to launch and respond to attacks. We all know cyclists who can ride at a hard and steady pace all day but can't accelerate to save their lives. They're the guys you love to have around in a breakaway, because they'll pull all day long, and then you can ditch them with one or two strong accelerations in the final mile. Their training gives them tremendous power at lactate threshold but fails to develop the ability to handle repeated maximal efforts.

Not only does increasing your power at VO_2max, and the amount of time you can sustain that power, give you the ability to accelerate hard during an attack, but the training further improves your ability to tolerate lactate threshold intensity. As such, VO_2max training complements the interval work you're doing at or near lactate threshold intensity. In the end, this means you'll be able to better handle the inevitable surges and pace changes that push you over your lactate threshold power during everything from criteriums to training races, centuries, and local group rides.

THE ENDURANCE STRING THEORY

Sports scientists and coaches, myself included, have told you that training at 86 to 90 percent of your maximum sustainable power output will target your glycolytic energy system and increase your power at lactate threshold. And although this is true, the glycolytic system isn't the only one doing the work at that intensity, nor is it the only one that will reap a training benefit.

You are always producing energy through all possible pathways, but your demand for energy determines the relative contribution from each. At low to moderate intensities, the vast majority of your energy comes from the aerobic engine (mitochondria breaking down primarily fat and carbohydrate). As your intensity level rises above about 60 percent of VO_2max, the contribution from the glycolytic system starts to increase, and then it really ramps up quickly once you reach lactate threshold. Because glycolysis only burns carbohydrate, the overall percentage of energy coming from carbohydrate increases dramatically as your intensity increases from lactate threshold to VO_2max. You're still burning a lot of fat, however, because your mitochondria are also still chugging along as fast as they can.

Rather than seeing your various energy pathways as separate and distinct, it's better to think of them as segments of one continuous string, arranged based on the amount of energy derived from each. At one end is a large segment representing the aerobic system, which theoretically could power your muscles at a moderate intensity level forever if it had sufficient oxygen and fuel. After that is the glycolytic system, which can do a lot of work but can run at full tilt for a limited time before you will have to reduce your exercise intensity.

Finally, there is the segment for VO_2max, which is the maximum amount of work you can do but represents an intensity that is sustainable for only a few minutes. We can put the small but powerful contribution from the immediate energy system (ATP/CP) in this region, too, since it powers maximal efforts that are only a few seconds long.

Improving fitness in one system is like lifting the string in that region—all other areas of the string rise, too. The extents of these ancillary improvements vary, based on the system you initially targeted. For instance, targeting VO_2max has a greater lifting effect on lactate threshold fitness and aerobic metabolism than training at aerobic intensities has on lifting lactate threshold or VO_2max. All the systems are interconnected, and how you focus your training affects the amount of work you can do not only with the system you're focusing on but with all the others as well.

THE SCIENCE OF HIGH-INTENSITY TRAINING

When you view the energy systems as interconnected parts of the same string, it starts to make sense that when training pulls up on the VO_2max end of the string, you'll see a subsequent increase in performance from the aerobic and glycolytic systems. To use an old phrase, a rising tide lifts all boats.

High-intensity training has been extensively studied, and the basic premise of a training program that utilizes intervals at and near an athlete's VO_2max is that efforts at this intensity level lead to many of the same physiological adaptations that result from more traditional endurance training models. In fact, Burgomaster et al. (2005) found that high-intensity interval training doubled an athlete's time to exhaustion on a ride performed at 80 percent of peak VO_2. This is appealing to the time-crunched athlete because the efforts required are up to five times shorter than the traditional intervals used to target power at lactate threshold. I know a lot of athletes are genuinely interested in the science of performance, so let's take a closer look at the science that supports a high-intensity, low-volume training program.

What Constitutes Improvement?

At the end of the day, improvement can be measured by whether you can produce more power at the same relative effort level as before and/or whether you can sustain that power output longer than you could before. After training, if you can go faster from point A to point B (in similar conditions), then you have made progress. But many factors are involved in getting from A to B more quickly, including a learning curve that helps athletes become faster over familiar territory even when they have made no improvement in fitness. So how do you know whether an athlete's improved performance is due to physiological changes or the fact he or she has learned how to perform better when tested? You look inside the muscles.

Having more mitochondria in muscle cells allows you to oxidize more fat and carbohydrate through aerobic metabolism. For a long time we thought the most effective way to increase mitochondrial density was to perform long rides at moderate intensities. And although there's still debate about the exact mechanism at work, evidence suggests that the depletion of ATP in muscle cells, which happens when intense exercise leads you to consume ATP faster than it can be produced, may kick-start a cascade of biochemical processes that ends with increased production of mitochondria (Willett 2006).

Studies examining the effectiveness of short high-intensity intervals for improving aerobic performance have shown an increase in muscles' oxidative capacity (the maximum amount of oxygen a muscle can utilize) and in levels of key enzymes used in the process of aerobic metabolism. In 1982 Dudley et al. reported that intensities of 95 percent and above throughout a 20-minute maximum power output are required to create the largest concentration of mitochondrial enzymes. Conversely, they also reported that there is no increase in muscle enzyme density after 60 minutes of continuous work.

Although the original research was completed using rat muscle fiber, the study has been frequently cited in later research performed on athletes. It has been suggested that the lack of increased muscle enzyme activity after 60 minutes of continuous work (such as during a long, moderate-intensity endurance ride) may occur because the increased exercise duration lowers the athlete's power output below what is needed to stimulate up-regulation of enzymes.

You can also measure an athlete's VO_2max to determine whether a training program has improved his or her capacity to utilize oxygen. In 1986 Dempsey found a 19 percent increase in VO_2max (from 50 to 61) using a 12-week program of 4 workouts a week, featuring 3-minute intervals at VO_2max and 2-minute recovery periods between efforts. Rodas et al. (2000)

were able to take the research a step further because of advances in power meter technology; they reported a 30-watt increase in maximal load and an increase in VO_2max from 57.3 to 63.8 in their high-intensity interval training research. Barnett et al. (2004) found a 7.1 percent increase in mean power output and an 8 percent increase in peak VO_2. Their research also showed a 17 percent increase in resting intramuscular glycogen content; an increase in the amount of carbohydrate fuel a muscle can store is another indicator of improved aerobic conditioning.

Many of the studies looking at high-intensity interval training focus on sprint efforts, particularly 30-second all-out sprints on a Wingate exercise bike. Over the past 10 years, studies have continued to show that short, high-intensity sprint efforts yield physiological adaptations similar to those expected from traditional endurance training (Cochran et al. 2014; Gillen and Gibala 2014; Lundby and Jacobs 2015; Ronnestad 2015; Sloth 2013).

Realizing that 30-second efforts on a Wingate isn't a realistic training methodology for real-world athletes, researchers started looking at longer intervals, particularly those between 1 and 4 minutes. These are still very difficult and elicit peak power at VO_2max, but they are more readily achievable using a regular bicycle in a real-world environment. Little et al. (2010) showed that even 2 weeks (6 sessions) of 8–12 very hard 1-minute intervals improved time to completion of a 750-kilojoule time trial (about an hour-long effort) by 9 percent. They also reported increased muscle oxidative capacity, and markers for mitochondrial growth. The effectiveness of this type of modification to the 30-second sprint tests was confirmed by similar findings from Bayati et al. (2011).

I'd be the first to tell you that riders who look great in the lab are sometimes the first to be shot out the back in real races. A few studies have included actual cycling time trials in their protocols; Laursen and Shing et al. (2002) found that it took only 4 high-intensity training sessions to bring about a 4.4 to 5.8 percent improvement in 40-km time trial performance. Hawley et al. (1997)

found that after only 4 to 6 interval sessions performed over 2 to 3 weeks, peak power output was increased by 15 to 20 watts, which can translate to riding 1.5 to 2 km/hr. faster in a 40-km time trial, or a 90- to 120-second improvement.

These findings support the notion that after training with high-intensity intervals, athletes are able to sustain work at a higher percentage of their peak VO_2 (90 percent versus 86 percent in the latter study). Hawley et al. stated that this improvement is likely due to an increased efficiency in fatty acid metabolism and a "decreased reliance on carbohydrate as a fuel source" due to an increased density of mitochondria in muscle cells.

Similarly, Brooks and Mercier (1994) reported a reduction in carbohydrate oxidation and lactate accumulation following high-intensity interval training when subjects were asked to perform at the same absolute work rate as they had at the beginning of the study. This is crucial for understanding how high-intensity training ends up increasing endurance performance. After the high-intensity training, when athletes ride at higher power outputs, they will be less reliant on the glycolytic system and derive a higher percentage of energy from the aerobic system. As a result, they will use more fat for energy and produce less lactate. Harmer et al. (2000) also found a reduction in glycogen utilization and lactate accumulation following a high-intensity training protocol.

Does It Matter How Strong You Are Now?

Research has shown that if an athlete has a VO_2max over 60 ml/kg/min., endurance performance will not improve without high-intensity interval training (Londeree 1997). Londeree also found that even with a VO_2max lower than 60 ml/kg/min., after 3 weeks of training there will be very few positive training adaptations unless there is an increase in training stimulus. As a matter of perspective, a moderately trained cyclist will have a VO_2max of about 50 to 55, a well-trained cyclist (Cat. III to IV or good in fast group rides) will likely be between 55 and 65, and a high-level amateur or domestic pro is likely to have a VO_2max above 70 ml/kg/min. Laursen et al. (2002), who defined "moderately trained" athletes as having a VO_2max less than 60 ml/kg/min., provided a very useful summary of relevant research. They defined high-intensity training as an interval of 30 seconds to 5 minutes at intensities above lactate threshold, and they looked at a wide range of markers to identify improvement in aerobic metabolism, including changes in muscle fibers and the small blood vessels (capillaries) that deliver oxygenated blood to muscle tissue:

> High-intensity training in sedentary and recreationally active individuals improves endurance performance to a greater extent than does continuous submaximal training alone. This improvement appears due, in part, to an up-regulated contribution of both aerobic and anaerobic metabolism to the energy demand, which enhances the availability of ATP and improves the energy status in working muscle. An improved capacity for aerobic metabolism, as evidenced by an increased expression of Type I fibers [otherwise known as slow-twitch muscle fibers and in contrast to Type II, or fast-twitch muscle fibers], capillarization and oxidative enzyme activity is the most common response to high-intensity training in untrained or moderately active individuals. (Laursen and Jenkins 2002)

Although far less research has been conducted on professional-level cyclists (it's difficult to get them to participate in a study that requires them to try something different), Laursen and Jenkins put together a table that summarizes the results of research into the effectiveness of high-intensity training for highly trained endurance athletes (see Table 2.1).

TABLE 2.1

Summary of Findings in High-Intensity Interval Training (HIIT) Studies in Highly Trained Cyclists[a]

REFERENCE	N	HIIT SESSIONS	REPS	INTENSITY (% P_{PEAK})
Lindsay et al.	8	6	6–8	80
Weston et al.	6	6	6–8	80
Westgarth-Taylor et al.	8	12	6–9	80
Stepto et al.	4	6	4	80
Stepto et al.	4	6	8	85
Stepto et al.	4	6	12	90
Laursen et al.	7	4	20	100
Stepto et al.	3	6	12	100
Stepto et al.	4	6	12	175

[a] Changes indicated based on statistical significance at the p < 0.05 level.
3-HCoA: 3-hydroxyacyl coenzyme A dehydrogenase activity; **CHO$_{OX}$:** carbohydrate oxidation rates; **CS:** citrate synthase activity; **HK:** hexokinase activity; **n:** number of participants; **PFK:** phosphofructokinase activity; **P$_{peak}$:** peak aerobic power output; **Reps:** repetitions; **TF$_{100}$:** time to fatigue at 100%; **TF$_{150}$:** time to fatigue at 150% of P$_{peak}$; **TT$_{40}$:** 40km time-trial performance; **T$_{vent}$:** ventilatory threshold; **ß:** buffering capacity; ↓: decrease; ↑: increase; ↔: no change.

How High Is High Intensity?

Now we're getting to the really important part of this discussion of the science behind the Time-Crunched Training Program. Sports scientists have shown that high-intensity intervals improve an athlete's ability to perform at workloads below and above lactate threshold, but their research has included efforts that range from 15 seconds to more than 5 minutes, and intensities ranging from 95 percent of 20-minute maximum power to well above 120 percent of VO$_2$max power. For instance, Burgomaster et al. (2005) found that 6 sessions of 30-second all-out sprint intervals over 2 weeks doubled athletes' time to exhaustion (from 26 to 51 minutes) at a sustained intensity of 80 percent of peak VO$_2$. Their results prompted Dr. Ed Coyle, a prominent researcher from the University of Texas, to submit an invited editorial to the *Journal of Applied Physiology* in which he wrote, "It is likely that if an experienced runner or bicyclist had only two weeks and very limited time to prepare

WORK DURATION	REST DURATION	HIIT DURATION (WK)	RESULTS
5 min.	60 sec.	4	$\uparrow P_{peak}$, $\uparrow TF_{150}$, $\uparrow TT_{40}$
5 min.	60 sec.	4	$\uparrow P_{peak}$, $\uparrow TF_{150}$, $\uparrow TT_{40}$, $\uparrow \beta$, $\leftrightarrow HK$, $\leftrightarrow PFK$, $\leftrightarrow CS$, $\leftrightarrow 3\text{-HCoA}$
5 min.	60 sec.	6	$\uparrow P_{peak}$, $\uparrow TT_{40}$, $\downarrow CHO_{ox}$
8 min.	1 min.	3	$\leftrightarrow$
4 min.	1.5 min.	3	$\uparrow P_{peak}$, $\uparrow TT_{40}$
2 min.	3 min.	3	$\leftrightarrow$
1 min.	2 min.	2	$\uparrow P_{peak}$, $\uparrow T_{vent}$, $\uparrow TF_{100}$
1 min.	4 min.	3	$\leftrightarrow$
30 sec.	4.5 min.	3	$\uparrow P_{peak}$, $\uparrow TT_{40}$

for a race of about 30 minutes' duration, that sprint interval training would become a mainstay of their preparation."

Now, even though you may not have a ton of time available for training, 6 to 8 hours a week is a lot more time than the subjects in many of the extremely short-interval (15 to 30 seconds) studies. You also have more than 2 weeks to prepare for your next cycling goal, and most likely achieving that goal is going to take longer than 30 minutes. That's why I prefer to limit the most difficult intervals in the TCTP to about 1 to 4 minutes, at intensities that generally will be "as hard as you can sustain for the whole interval." I discuss this more in Chapter 3, but for now suffice it to say that you'll be working at intensities between lactate threshold and VO_2max, and sometimes at VO_2max. You will also be performing longer intervals (6 to 10 minutes) at slightly lower intensities, closer to your lactate threshold power output.

In high-intensity training programs, the recovery times between intervals are just as important as what's referred to as the "work time." If you're doing a set of intervals in which each effort is 2 minutes of work time, there's a big difference between taking 1, 2, and 5 minutes of easy spinning recovery between efforts. Though you will get some additional recovery time in the early portions of the TCTP, once you're into the heart of it, many of the interval workouts will use recovery ratios (work time:recovery time) of 1:1 and 1:0.5. In other words, you'll see interval sets of 2 minutes "on" and 2 minutes "off," or even 2 minutes "on" and 1 minute "off." You won't be completely recovered from one effort before it's time to begin the next, and that's the point. The efforts will generate a lot of lactate, and your body will be working to process it, but starting your next high-power effort while your lactate levels are still elevated helps drive the necessary adaptations that will make you a faster, stronger cyclist.

THINGS YOU CAN'T CUT OUT

Even though the scientific literature and our experiences with real-world athletes show that you can perform well as an endurance athlete even when you cut out a great deal of the volume typically found in endurance training programs, there are some essential principles and components of training that cannot be eliminated.

Principles of Training

One of the first books I wrote, *The Ultimate Ride*, described the five principles of training and the five major components of a productive workout. Those training philosophies are still valid, and my coaches and I use them every day with athletes who have more than 8 hours a week to commit to training. Yet even though I needed to make dramatic changes to the classic endurance training model to optimize performance for time-crunched athletes, this new paradigm is still governed by the same principles and workout components as that model. Rather than reinvent the wheel here, I have revisited some of the material from *The Ultimate Ride* and updated it to reflect the unique demands of the TCTP.

When you distill the world's most successful training programs, across all sports, you arrive at five distinct principles of training:

- Overload and recovery
- Individuality
- Specificity
- Progression
- Systematic approach

Overload and Recovery Principle

The human body is designed to respond to overload, and as long as you overload a system in the body properly and allow it time to adapt, that system will grow stronger and be ready for the same stress in the future. All forms of physical training are based on the body's ability to adapt to stress (or overload).

To achieve positive training effects, this principle must be applied to individual training sessions as well as to entire periods of your training. For instance, a lactate threshold interval workout must be difficult enough and long enough to stress your glycolytic energy system, but lactate threshold workouts must also be scheduled into a block of training so that the training loads from individual workouts accumulate and lead to more significant adaptations.

To benefit from overloading an energy system, you have to give that system time to rest. When you are out on the road and you've got the hammer down in the middle of a PowerInterval (a maximum-intensity interval workout), you are not improving your fitness; you are applying stress. Later, when you are home reading bedtime stories to your kids, then you are improving your fitness. Gains are made when you allow enough time for your body to recover and adapt to the stresses you have applied. This is why I don't separate recovery from training. Recovery is part of your training, and thinking of it that way helps you remain as committed to recovering as you are to working out.

Table 2.2 shows general guidelines for recovery following specific amounts of time at given intensities. Remember that these are only guidelines. Recovery from training varies among individuals.

TABLE 2.2

Guidelines for Recovery

VOLUME OF INTENSITY	SUGGESTED TIME NEEDED FOR RECOVERY (HOURS)
0–6 hrs. at aerobic endurance intensity	8
30–60 min. at tempo intensity	8–10
75–120 min. at tempo intensity	24–36
15–45 min. at lactate threshold	24
60–90 min. at lactate threshold	24–36
10–30 min. above lactate threshold	24–36
45 min. or more above lactate threshold	36–48

Adapting the Overload and Recovery Principle for Time-Crunched Cyclists

Athletes who train 10, 12, or more hours a week tend to have no problem achieving the overload portion of the equation. If anything, they have more trouble setting aside as much time as they need for optimal recovery. For time-crunched cyclists, the opposite is true. With only 6 to 8 hours available for training, recovery is less of a problem because your relative lack of training time means there's plenty of downtime built into your week. The challenge is to accumulate the workload necessary to cause an overload.

Fortunately, the relationship between volume and intensity is not linear. Training workload is the product of volume and intensity, but compared with the effect of increasing volume, increasing intensity results in an exponential increase in workload. As a result, high-intensity training programs can generate great workloads despite very low training volumes.

Some athletes and coaches initially fear that the TCTP will lead to overtraining—which is perhaps more accurately termed "under-recovery"—because it includes so much intensity. Their fear is based on the fact that classic endurance training programs typically only include very high-intensity intervals in the final weeks leading up to big competitions. In those training programs, you couldn't add harder intervals any earlier because the training volume was so high. There's a limit to the total workload an athlete can handle in a week, and in classic programs the volume takes up such a large percentage of that workload that you can't add more high-intensity intervals to it without compromising the athlete's ability to recover and adapt. The workouts and training programs in this book start out with hard intervals and progress to really difficult ones within only a few weeks. This works because your low training volume gives you the opportunity to use high-intensity intervals in ways high-volume trainers cannot.

Individuality Principle

I have always been surprised by how many athletes ignore the individuality principle. The training program that works for you, right down to the individual workouts and interval intensities, has to be based on your physiological and personal needs. Training is not a one-size-fits-all product. All parts of your program—the total mileage, the number and type of intervals, and even the terrain and cadence—must be personalized. That doesn't mean you can't train with your friends or training partners; it just means that while you're with them you have to stay true to your own training program.

Individuality is rarely a problem for time-crunched athletes, because your busy schedule already means training at different times and with different workouts than your friends who have more free time on their hands. Once you start on the TCTP, your training is going to be extremely different from what they're doing, so much so that they may question the wisdom of your choices. But don't give in to peer pressure telling you to revert back to a training model that's no longer relevant for you. Let them tell you this is crazy; the best way to convince them that the TCTP works is to do the program and then ride them off your wheel in a group ride or race.

"About three weeks into the program, I was out on the road doing maximum-intensity PowerIntervals when some of my cycling buddies came rolling by," Sterling Swaim remembers. "They asked what I was doing and nodded politely as I told them, but I could tell they thought I was insane. That night I got a call from a guy I'd been riding with and racing against for 10 years, because he was 'concerned' I was going to ruin my season. A few months later, after I'd killed him in the spring race series, he approached me at a barbeque and asked if I'd let him see my 'radical' new training program."

It may seem paradoxical to talk about the individuality principle and then include a series of training programs in this book. Ideally, every cyclist would work with a coach and get a training program built from scratch, but I understand that personal coaching is not an option for everyone. The workouts and training programs in this book are rooted in the principles my coaches and I use to create custom schedules for our athletes, and you'll be able to apply the individuality principle to them when you establish your personal intensity ranges and fit the workouts into your busy work and family schedules.

Specificity Principle

Your training must resemble the activity you want to perform. In a broad sense, this means that if you want to be a road cyclist, you should spend the vast majority of your training time on two wheels. In a narrower sense, it means you have to determine the exact demands of the activity you wish to perform and tailor your training to address them. Conversely, it also means that your training is going to prepare you optimally for specific events and activities.

The specificity principle is especially important for the time-crunched cyclist. Traditionally we talk about narrowing the focus of a broad endurance training program to enhance the specific skills and power outputs that will lead to success in goal events. But you don't have the time to build broad endurance fitness in the first place, so you need to look at specificity from the opposite direction. With very limited time available for training, the fitness you're going to develop with the TCTP will be best applied to a specific set of events and goals. You will have many opportunities for success (probably more than you have right now), but as I explain in more detail in the next chapter, there are some inescapable consequences to having fewer than 8 hours a week to train for an endurance sport.

Progression Principle

Training must progressively move forward. To enjoy continued gains in performance, you have to increase training loads as you adapt. Time and intensity are the two most significant variables you can use to adjust your workload. For instance, you can increase the number of hours you devote to training, increase the overall intensity of your rides, include more intervals, make the intervals more intense, make the intervals longer, or shorten the recovery periods between the intervals.

You can use the two variables of time and intensity to manipulate training a hundred different ways, but the end result must be that you're generating a training stimulus great enough to make your muscles and aerobic engine adapt. Just as important, once you adapt and grow stronger, you have to manipulate the time and intensity variables again so you further increase the workload to generate another training stimulus.

Interestingly, some of the most compelling evidence supporting the effectiveness of high-intensity interval training relates to the principle of progression. Neither training time nor intensity is limitless, even for professional cyclists. There are only 24 hours in the day, and the human body can only be pushed so hard. Professional racing cyclists are pretty much maxed out in terms of the annual hours and mileage they can accumulate while still performing at a high level. Indeed, studies have shown that for highly trained athletes, even if they could add more training volume, it wouldn't lead to additional improvements in VO_2max, power at lactate threshold, or mitochondrial density (Laursen and Jenkins 2002). With volume effectively maxed out and therefore not a limiting factor for improvement, you can observe the impact of increasing an athlete's workload with high-intensity intervals. Professional cycling has advanced so far that no amount of moderate-intensity training volume will be enough to generate the speed and power necessary to keep up, let alone win. To make the additional progress that's required for success at the highest levels of the sport, pros have to incorporate high-intensity intervals—on top of the intensity they get in races—into their training programs.

Time-crunched athletes aren't maxed out in terms of training volume, but you are maxed out in terms of the amount of time you can devote to training. Even though there are advantages to training more than 6 hours a week, the other commitments in your life mean you have to do what you can in that time. To achieve progression without adding hours, the TCTP manipulates the type and number of intervals, their length, and the recovery periods between them.

Progression is fast in this program, and by the end of 11 weeks the workouts you thought were challenging at the beginning will look like child's play. But around the same time you'll also notice that you're pushing the pace at the front of the group ride or sprinting for the win in a criterium instead of suffering like a dog at the back.

Systematic Approach

For novices, even a haphazard training schedule produces results. Just the act of getting on the bike, or throwing in a few intervals here and there, is enough to develop fitness. Pretty soon, however, that progress plateaus. Just as an architect creates a step-by-step blueprint when designing a house, training must take a systematic approach. A successful training program must be well thought out and organized so your body advances through a planned series of training and recovery periods. If you wake up each day and simply flip a coin to determine your daily workout, you will soon find you are making little progress in your training. This is especially true for athletes who have limited training time. As you embark on the TCTP, remember that with limited training time, every hour and every interval counts.

THE FIVE WORKOUT COMPONENTS

When you throw your leg over your saddle and head out on the road, you can use the following five variables to address the five principles of training discussed in the previous section:

1. Intensity
2. Volume
3. Frequency and repetition
4. Terrain
5. Cadence

You can completely change the goal of a workout by changing one of its components. For instance, climbing intervals that are 10 minutes long can target two completely different energy systems if you simply change the cadence. Climbing at a cadence of 70 revolutions per minute (rpm) will tend to push an athlete to his or her climbing lactate threshold, which is slightly higher than the flat-ground lactate threshold due to an increase in muscle recruitment. I prescribe such workouts to develop an athlete's ability to sustain prolonged climbing efforts in races. But if the same climbing workout is done at a cadence of 50 rpm, the tension applied to the leg muscles increases greatly, and the stress on the cardiovascular system decreases. I use slow cadence climbing efforts to increase muscle fiber recruitment and muscular power development. In this case, varying the cadence of an effort transforms a lactate threshold workout into a neuromuscular workout.

Intensity

Intensity is a measure of how hard you are working, and it should be clear by now that you will be working quite hard in this training program. Because you don't have the time to ride moderately hard for 2 hours, you'll have to achieve the necessary training stimulus in 1 hour. The impact of a workout is directly related to the intensity at which you are working, and over the years we have become increasingly precise in the methods we use to measure intensity.

Precision is important for success with the TCTP, so I strongly encourage you to use a power meter, or at the very least a heart-rate monitor that records average heart rates for individual intervals. Training with power and heart rate is covered in more detail in Chapter 4.

Volume

Volume is the total amount of exercise you're doing in a single workout, a week of training, a month, a year, or a career. By definition, *time-crunched* means low volume, at least in terms of the hours you spend training. But there's another concept here that makes up for some of that reduction in volume, called volume-at-intensity. Classic endurance training programs contain a lot of hours riding at moderate intensity but relatively little time training at higher intensity. The TCTP strips out most of the moderate-intensity volume of those programs but retains—and may even increase—the volume-at-intensity, especially volume-at-high-intensity. In a given week in this program, you're most likely going to spend more time riding at and above your lactate threshold power output than you have during any portion of your previous training programs.

Frequency and Repetition

Frequency is the number of times a workout is performed in a given period of training, whereas *repetition* is the number of times an exercise is repeated in a single session. Riding 3 PowerInterval workouts in a week is frequency; riding 12 PowerIntervals in a single workout is repetition.

Frequency and repetition are used to ensure the quality of your training sessions. In the TCTP your goal is to accumulate time at high workloads, because that's the driving force behind the adaptations you're seeking. PowerIntervals are maximum-intensity intervals, and their effectiveness is based on sustaining your highest possible power output for a given period of time.

Let's say you have a lactate threshold power of 250 watts and can sustain that output for 20 minutes. You might be able to average 300 watts for 3 minutes during a PowerInterval. There's no point in trying to complete a 20-minute PowerInterval, because your output will fall so dramatically after the first 3 to 5 minutes that the rest of the effort will no longer be useful as a PowerInterval. It would feel ridiculously hard, and your heart rate would stay elevated, but once your power output drops that effort is no longer addressing the goal of a PowerInterval. On the other hand, if you do seven 3-minute PowerIntervals at 300 watts each, separated by recovery periods, you'll accumulate 21 minutes at 300 watts. That's why interval training is so effective for improving performance (and burning calories) compared to exercising at a steady pace or level of effort.

Frequency gives you another way to accumulate workload, by repeating individual interval sessions during a given week, month, or even year. For instance, a week with two PowerInterval workouts like the one just mentioned means 42 minutes at 300 watts. The harder the intervals, the more recovery you need before you'll be ready to complete another high-quality training session. Fortunately, this works in favor of the time-crunched cyclist, because your relative lack of training time leaves plenty of time for recovery during the week.

This program has 4 workouts per week, and ideally you'll be able to complete them on the days and in the order they are prescribed. However, because the workouts are so short and the overall volume is so low, you have a lot of latitude to move the workouts around without much risk of diminishing the quality of your training. In other words, if you have to pile 3 hard days of intervals back-to-back in 1 week, that's not ideal, but it's probably better than skipping them because you couldn't do them on the days they were originally planned.

Terrain

As I discuss more in the section about training with power, workload is most accurately expressed as the number of kilojoules—the amount of mechanical work—you produce during a training session. (How rapidly you produce those kilojoules determines your power output.) You can use terrain to manipulate your workload, and this is especially useful for time-crunched athletes, who need to get as much as possible done in 60 to 90 minutes. Riding uphill and performing efforts on hills can significantly increase the overall workload for your intervals, even though it can sometimes decrease the overall workload for the session (depending on the difference between the time spent at higher power outputs going uphill and the time spent going downhill at much lower power outputs).

Intervals on hills can also be useful for overcoming lagging motivation. Sometimes it can be difficult to push yourself through maximum-intensity intervals on flat ground, but a hill adds resistance and a visible challenge, and sometimes that's the little something extra you need to make your workout more effective.

Of course, training on hills is important from a specificity standpoint. If you want to go faster on climbs, it helps to train on them. But if you live in Kansas or some other pancake-flat location, increasing your sustainable power at lactate threshold is the number-one thing you can do to help you go faster uphill (when you finally encounter one). Riding into the wind can be a useful strategy for flatlanders who are training for hills; your power output and effort level will be high as you push against a significant resistance, which will likely bring your cadence down to the sort of levels you would use on a climb (80 to 85 rpm instead of 90 to 100).

Cadence

I have long been a proponent of high-cadence cycling because it improves your ability to maintain high-power efforts longer by pedaling faster in a lighter gear. You can produce 250 watts at 80 rpm or 100 rpm, but your leg muscles will fatigue faster riding a bigger gear at 80 rpm than a lower gear at 100 rpm, even though the power output (wattage) is the same.

Power is a measure of how rapidly you can do work. Think in terms of moving a pile of 250 bricks in a minute. When you divide the work into smaller portions but get it done in the same amount of time, each load is lighter and you can move faster. If you double the number of bricks you carry in each load, you'll move the pile in half as many loads, but you'll have to work harder to move each load, and each trip will take longer.

As an endurance athlete, your training optimizes your muscles' ability to work continuously and contract frequently. High-cadence cycling takes advantage of the adaptations already provided by aerobic training—not only muscular adaptations but also cardiovascular ones. Your heart and lungs don't fatigue the same way skeletal muscles do, and maintaining higher cadences helps shift stress from easily fatigued skeletal muscles to the fatigue-resistant cardiovascular system.

Learning to produce a lot of power while pedaling fast is also helpful when it's time to accelerate. The workouts in the TCTP are high-intensity, high-power efforts, and I encourage you to keep your cadence above 90 rpm for maximal efforts like PowerIntervals. You'll improve in aerobic power, power at lactate threshold, and power at VO_2max from the intensity of the efforts. Maintaining a higher cadence during the efforts will also give you the snap necessary to accelerate hard when it's time to attack, cover an attack, bridge a gap, or just lift out of the saddle to get over a small climb with the group.

Keep in mind, however, that there's no magical cadence everyone should shoot for. Rather than aim for a specific number, I recommend athletes try to increase their normal cruising cadence and climbing cadence by 10 percent in a year (with the understanding that very few cyclists can ride effectively at sustained cadences above 120 to 125 rpm on flat ground).

COACHING AND SCIENCE

Typically, when you have a new problem to solve in training, you start by examining the demands of the goal event. After that you determine the opportunities for improvement, you prioritize them, and then you determine the ways you can manipulate training components and principles to create the workload necessary to achieve the adaptations you want.

With that as context, you could say the TCTP was reverse engineered, because the problem we were trying to solve was directly related to the components and principles of training rather than a change in the demands of the sport. Limited available training time meant finding new solutions to prepare athletes for the well-known demands of cycling events. As you can now see, sports science supports the fundamental principle that low-volume, high-intensity training is effective for improving endurance athletic performance. Additionally, the variables that need to be manipulated to build low-volume, high-intensity training plans are all contained within the same principles and workout components that govern all endurance training. That means the TCTP works, but it also means the fitness you develop is specific to the way you develop it. Time-crunched training creates time-crunched fitness, and it comes with a special set of terms and conditions. We'll cover that next.

3

TERMS AND CONDITIONS

IF YOU HAVE ONLY 6 HOURS AVAILABLE FOR TRAINING each week, the Time-Crunched Training Program is your best option for developing the fitness and power necessary to ride at the front of the group, push the pace, and sprint for the win. It's your best option for building the fitness you need for an enjoyable century or cycling tour, or for feeling strong at your local Tuesday Night World Championship.

The TCTP is designed to maximize the effectiveness of the training you can complete in the limited time you have available. When you complete this program, you'll be more fit, more powerful, and faster than you would otherwise have been on so few training hours.

On the flip side, I can't tell you that you'll be able to do everything that riders who train 16 to 20 hours a week can do. The TCTP would not prepare European or American pros for the rigors of their long seasons. The classic endurance training model works great for pros and athletes who have more than 10 to 12 hours a week to devote to training, and my coaches and I still use that model with elite athletes and many of our amateur racers and cycling enthusiasts. In fact, if you have the time to commit more than 10 hours to training each week, a more traditional endurance training program may serve you better than the one in this book, because you have the time to reap the benefits that additional training volume provides.

If you have fewer than 10 hours for training each week, however, you're at the low end of what I consider to be enough time to make the classic endurance training model work. If your performance is neither stellar nor terrible right now, I encourage you to give the TCTP a try. Based on my coaches' experiences with CTS athletes in similar circumstances, you're far more likely to see significant improvements than appreciable drops in your performance.

The information in this chapter is vital to your success. There are some inescapable consequences to having only 6 hours a week to train for an endurance sport, and there are limitations on the types and lengths of events you'll be optimally prepared for. It is also true that the TCTP may not work for everyone. I can't sugarcoat the realities that time-crunched cyclists face: There are terms and conditions you need to accept if you want to reap the rewards of this training program.

THE 3-HOUR LIMIT

The reason training volume is so beneficial is that it enables you to build the aerobic endurance you need to ride all day. More than that, high-volume training that incorporates high-intensity intervals prepares athletes to ride aggressively all day. As you can imagine, this is crucial for success in pro events, which range from 100-km criteriums to epic mountain stages in the grand tours and 250-km classics such as the Tour of Flanders. Pros have to be able to attack, chase, and sustain tremendous power outputs at the end of long races, sometimes after 5, 6, or even more hours in the saddle. With only 6 hours available to train each week, you can still ride all day when you get the chance, but your best performances will come in rides and events that are 3 hours or shorter.

Before you scoff indignantly at the notion that your best performances may be limited to events that are shorter than 3 hours, take a good look at the events you actually participate in. An informal survey of CTS athletes and coaches, coupled with common sense, suggests that the vast majority of 30- to 50-year-old cyclists regularly compete in or participate in events that last between 45 and 90 minutes. If you want to ride the local criterium series, a bunch of cyclocross races in the fall, or even a regional cross-country mountain bike series, you need the fitness to be fast and powerful for less than 2 hours. Yes, this means you might struggle in 100-mile road races, but how many of those do you enter in a year? For amateurs, most road races—even races that are 60 to 70 miles long—typically take less than 3 hours to complete.

Here's the bottom line: Do you want to be mediocre at every distance, or is it OK to be strong enough to be really good at a smaller selection of the distances and disciplines in cycling? A 3-hour limit covers a large percentage of the events most amateur cyclists participate in, and I'm betting that you don't like being mediocre at anything. That's why I regard the 3-hour limit in a positive light: By accepting that you may not be optimally prepared for every event on two wheels, the TCTP gives you the opportunity to excel in the events you most frequently participate in anyway.

But haven't I been saying this program could be used to prepare for a century? Aren't there Gran Fondo and Ultraendurance MTB programs in this book? All of those events take more than 3 hours, so how do they fit into the 3-hour limit? Well, as you'll see later when we get to the workouts and training programs, there are separate programs for shorter and longer events. The differences are in the interval intensities. The competition programs focus more on developing power for repeatable efforts at VO_2max, and the longer endurance programs focus more on developing sustainable power at lactate threshold. But regardless of which program you use, you're still going to see a change in your performance at about the 3-hour mark of your long rides.

The 3-hour limit was derived purely from anecdotal evidence. My coaches and I noticed that athletes on the TCTP experienced a significant change in their performance about 3 hours into long rides. They got noticeably tired, stopped talking, started skipping pulls, and struggled on climbs. A high-intensity, low-volume training program delivers many of the same physiological adaptations we see in higher-volume training programs, but it stands to reason that there are some adaptations that actually require more time in the saddle.

Epic rides are a defining benchmark for every cyclist. Even if you only get one or two chances a year to get out there for 5, 6, or 7 hours with a couple of buddies or for a long day of wondrous solitude, those rides are part of the very essence of being a cyclist. For beginners, your first ride longer than 5 hours is a rite of passage, and I suspect that many cyclists cling to their antiquated training programs because they fear losing the ability to complete those long days. They view that as an unacceptable step backward.

But being undertrained because you're a low-volume rider on a high-volume training program means you'll suffer from start to finish the next time you get the chance to escape the clutches of normal life and go out for an all-day ride. The 3-hour limit doesn't mean you aren't allowed to go out for epic rides; it just means your best performances will be in rides and events shorter than 3 hours. You can still take advantage of that weekend when your spouse takes the kids and goes to Grandma's house; in fact, I encourage you to. Using the TCTP, you'll feel better for the first half of the ride, and if you use your fitness wisely you can stretch your range and have a good ride all the way to the finish. In Chapter 15 I cover the details of adjusting your habits, from the way you ride to the way you eat and the role you play in the group, so you can effectively extend your range.

TIME-CRUNCHED TRAINING LEADS TO TIME-CRUNCHED FITNESS

The TCTP is a limited-time offer. You will gain fitness and power rapidly, and you will be able to have a lot of fun with it while it lasts, but 10 to 12 weeks after you start the program, you'll have to back off and recover. This program can be used two or three times in a 12-month period, but you should not run through the 11 weeks and then immediately start over at week 1.

To understand why it's necessary to restrict the TCTP to 12 to 16 weeks (the training programs are 11 weeks, but some athletes will be able to stretch the fitness for up to an additional month), we have to refer back to the classic endurance training model. In that model, we built a huge foundation of aerobic fitness with months of long, moderate-intensity training. That aerobic fitness supported the more intense intervals that followed, allowing athletes to handle the workload of repeated interval workouts at or near lactate threshold. By the time these athletes reached the point where they were using high-intensity intervals near VO_2max, their efforts were being supported by a huge aerobic engine and thoroughly built glycolytic system.

Having deeper aerobic fitness means that the aerobic engine is capable of handling a relatively large percentage of the workload even when you're working above lactate threshold. That's important, because the glycolytic system burns through your carbohydrate stores very rapidly, whereas a highly trained aerobic system can burn more fat than carbohydrate (a moderately trained athlete burns about a 50–50 mixture of fat and carbohydrate riding at sub-threshold intensities). With a stronger aerobic system, you can sustain higher power outputs before you reach the intensity at which you start eating into your limited carbohydrate reserves.

The high-intensity intervals in the TCTP build high-end fitness. Your power at VO_2max will increase, and so will your power at lactate threshold. Your glycolytic system will get stronger because of intervals performed at or near lactate threshold, and your body will learn to process and tolerate lactate better as well. At the same time, however, these high-intensity intervals will lead to greater mitochondrial density and improve your ability to produce power with your aerobic system. Just like athletes on traditional high-volume training plans, athletes who perform lactate threshold tests after training on the TCTP have lower blood lactate levels during the early stages of the test, compared to their early-stage blood lactate levels from previous lactate threshold tests. Once the body has produced more and bigger mitochondria, you can process more fat and carbohydrate aerobically, which means you can produce less energy from glycolysis and hence produce less lactate.

The more you rely on high intensity, the faster you'll fatigue. This not only applies to individual efforts and training sessions but also means that your body has to work harder to perform and recover as the weeks of high-intensity training build up. Deeper aerobic fitness derived from high-volume training helps those athletes recover more quickly (and they often have less acute fatigue to recover from after individual workouts), which means they can go longer (like the entire summer) before having to take an extended recovery period. Without that massive endurance base, you're on a much shorter timeline.

I'm not kidding about the timeline, either. Your relative lack of training time allows you to take advantage of a high-intensity training program, but the workouts in this program generate a lot of fatigue. You don't have the aerobic system to support that fatigue forever; your fitness is essentially top-heavy and will collapse under its own weight if you stretch the program too far.

How can you tell when it's time to back off? If you're using a power meter, you'll notice that your average power output for maximum-intensity intervals starts to drop, and that you have trouble completing interval workouts without a dramatic decline in your power outputs during the final set. Quite simply, you'll know because you're really tired, and your performance on the bike is going to decline rapidly and noticeably.

The impact of overextending the TCTP is more dramatic than when you overextend a peak as a high-volume trainer. For high-volume cyclists, the decline in performance is relatively slow when they try to perform past peak fitness, again because of the depth of their aerobic foundation. With far less of a foundation supporting your fitness, performance falls fast when you overdo it. If anything, this reduces the chances you'll end up over-trained, under-recovered, or injured, because the TCTP is more self-limiting than a high-volume training program. Your body will tell you, much more clearly than if you were riding 12 to 16 hours a week, that you're done and it's time to rest.

Initially I had a lot of trouble with the relatively short-term nature of the fitness gained using this program. Coming from the old-school mindset of endurance training, I struggled with the idea of a top-heavy training program that built high-end power without the deep aerobic fitness necessary to support it long-term. But for athletes with limited time to train, the alternative is sticking with old programs that can't possibly generate the fitness necessary to be a successful cyclist. Again and again I kept going back to the value proposition: Would you want to be really good for about 2 months at a time, even if it meant having to back off for 4 to 6 weeks before starting again? Or put another way: Do you want to be really good a couple of times a year, or mediocre all year long?

Another reason I was won over by this program was that because the high-intensity intervals build aerobic fitness as well as power at lactate threshold and VO_2max, many athletes who use the TCTP two or three times in a 12-month period get incrementally stronger each time. In other words, an athlete who starts the program in the spring may average 250 watts during the CTS Field Test (used to establish training intensities for workouts; see Chapter 4). If he or she reduces the training workload to an endurance or maintenance level for 4 to 6 weeks after finishing the program, and then decides to use it again to prepare for a series of late-summer races, he or she will perform another CTS Field Test, and this time the average power output is likely to be higher than 250 watts. So although the TCTP is a relatively short-term, high-intensity, low-volume training program, it produces lasting performance gains and gives athletes the opportunity to continue growing stronger season after season.

• • •

CASE STUDY
THE RESURGENCE OF TAYLOR CARRINGTON

Taylor Carrington is another of CTS coach Jim Rutberg's longtime friends. The two met as students at Wake Forest University, where Rutberg was majoring in sports science and was president of the school's two-man collegiate cycling team. Carrington was a former soccer player who had discovered mountain biking in the summer between high school and college. Being the only two competitive cyclists on campus (after the team's third rider graduated), they trained and traveled to races together, and even worked together as mechanics at the same off-campus bike shop.

After college, Rutberg and Carrington packed their belongings into their cars and split up to travel the country and race their bikes full-time for a few years. They were moderately successful. Rutberg upgraded his way to Cat. I on the road, and Carrington raced as a semipro mountain biker, but by their own admission they were fighting for top-10 finishes in regional events and just hoping to finish in the money at national events. After a few years it was time to put those Wake Forest degrees to work, and both settled into careers out West, Rutberg as my editorial director at CTS, and Carrington as a financial adviser in Denver, Colorado.

A few years later, after both had married, bought and sold their first homes, and had their first children (it's kind of scary how parallel their lives were in those years), Carrington decided he wanted one more shot at elite-level racing before he put it behind him. He and Rutberg talked about it during a mountain bike ride in Crested Butte, Colorado. Taylor wanted to race US Cyclocross National Championships. More than that, he wanted to do well, which meant traveling to races throughout the fall to earn UCI points (points earned by good finishes in races sanctioned by cycling's top governing body, the Union Cycliste International) so he could get a decent starting position for nationals.

As he had with their mutual friend Sterling Swaim, Rutberg described the TCTP, including its terms and conditions. Taylor, who hadn't trained in a structured program for nearly 4 years and had only entered a few races a year for the fun of it, was a perfect candidate for the program. He was married, working a high-stress job more than 50 hours a week, and paying a hefty mortgage to own a modest home in downtown Denver, and he and his wife were doing their best to share the work of caring for their daughter, Sally. His wife, Megan (an accomplished endurance athlete in her own right), supported his goal, especially because most of the required travel coincided with trips he had to take for work anyway.

The only caveat was that because some portion of the time he was going to spend training, traveling, and racing was time she would have to cover for him around the house, she figured she had some ownership of how he spent "her" time. In other words, she told him, "If you're going to do this, do it right and kick some butt."

I think a lot of cyclists face similar expectations. Even in a low-volume training program, we spend a considerable amount of our "free" time on our bikes. Our spouses, significant others, and kids don't necessarily suffer, but there's no denying that time spent training is time you're not spending fixing the windows or cooking Saturday-morning breakfast for the family. For the most part, families figure out the balance that works for them, but I think it's a lot easier for your family to understand and accept your time commitment when spending that time away from them makes you really happy. I don't know too many athletes who enjoy back-of-the-pack finishes or riding home alone after being dropped from the group ride, and I've found that coming home frustrated by your performance makes it more difficult for your family to understand your desire to go in the first place.

Cyclocross is a great place to apply the TCTP, because it's extremely difficult and both the races and the season are very short. Elite races are only an hour long (sometimes shorter). Other categories can be as short as 20 minutes, and the season generally runs from October to December. Taylor did what he could to stay in reasonable shape throughout the summer and then started the TCTP in October. Before daylight saving time ended, he did the workouts outdoors because he was out of work by about 4:00 p.m. (Like many in the financial industry, his hours are based on Wall Street's, which means he starts work at 5:30 a.m. in Denver.) As the days got shorter, he moved his training indoors. Fortunately the workouts in the TCTP are well suited to indoor trainers, and the relatively short high-intensity efforts make the time pass quickly.

Because he had to start racing soon after he started the program, Taylor struggled in his first few events. He and Rutberg knew that would be the case, and they focused those races on honing Taylor's handling skills and equipment choices. Within a few weeks, though, Taylor's power came up to the point where he was competitive in Colorado cyclocross races, even hanging with and finishing with guys who regularly finish in the top 20 at nationals. He traveled and earned his UCI points and even won a minor race in St. Louis before traveling to Providence, Rhode Island, for the US National Championships.

His UCI points earned Taylor a spot in the third row of the starting grid, and after about 62 minutes of battling the pros, he finished 17th out of 90 finishers. Rutberg and Carrington had talked about a top-30 finish as a realistic goal, but within the top 20 was beyond their expectations. Fellow CTS athlete Ryan Trebon won the US National Championship that year, and most of the names between Trebon and Carrington on the result sheet were pedigreed pros. He was beaten by the best in the United States, but he finished in the top 20 at Elite Cyclocross National Championships on only 6 hours of training per week. Six hours a week!

The unexpectedly good result from a relatively small investment of time convinced Taylor that he could do it again. Fortunately his wife was still supportive as well. The following year, having barely ridden his bike during the spring and summer, and using roughly the same program he had used the year before, Carrington drove to Kansas City for much muddier US National Cyclocross Championships. Proving that his past result wasn't a fluke, he finished 20th out of 99 starters, and unlike nearly everyone in front of him, he did so without a pit crew to hand him a clean bike every few laps.

Taylor didn't win at the national championships, but his performances in back-to-back Elite National Championships were comparable to 1999's, when he was training and racing full-time. More than simply achieving his personal goals, Taylor's results showed him that he didn't have to turn his back completely on high-performance goals. Many athletes look back longingly at the days when they felt fit, fast, and powerful. Taylor successfully recaptured that fitness after 7 years of focusing on other important aspects of his life, and he did it without sacrificing the career or family he'd spent so much time and effort building. The TCTP isn't about reclaiming your youth so much as it is about reclaiming your identity. Being a cyclist is an important part of who you are, and it's a lot easier to proudly identify yourself as a cyclist when you're good at it.

SHORT, INTENSE WORKOUTS = LONG-TERM BENEFITS

As the first edition of *The Time-Crunched Cyclist* was being written in the winter of 2009, researchers were demonstrating that the same high-intensity workouts prescribed in this book produced many of the same physical benefits found in a cyclist following a traditional high-volume endurance-training plan. Even more remarkable, the research discovered how dramatically little training (in volume) is necessary to spark the body's ability to process more fuel aerobically before switching to anaerobic systems.

A study with cyclists in Canada (Burgomaster et al. 2008) compared the effects of training 3 days a week for 6 weeks doing four to six 30-second all-out sprints to the effects of training 5 days a week for 40 to 60 minutes at a comfortable aerobic pace. At the end of 6 weeks, the scientists found no difference in the improved metabolic adaptations between the test groups. In other words, the group who trained for 90 minutes a week saw the same energy processing benefits as the group who spun through 5 hours of aerobic training.

If you've been training for any appreciable time, you're likely to be surprised by those study results—not because you think the intervals are too short, but because they were being compared to riding at a comfortable aerobic pace. But isn't accumulating time at a comfortable aerobic pace exactly what cyclists have been doing when they ride "base miles" for several weeks or months?

Time-crunched cyclists don't have time to build a giant aerobic base, and what the research is showing is that the sprinting/interval group did a grand total of 10 minutes of hard, all-out effort per week. That's it. The other 80 minutes were devoted to spinning easily through a warm-up, a recovery from each sprint, and a cool-down. And in return they accomplished the same metabolic adaptations as the other group.

Along the same lines of these 2008 findings, a 2010 study in the *Journal of Physiology* (Little et al.) tested the effects of lactate threshold (LT) intervals (which are somewhat easier than all-out max efforts) on cyclists and found the same biological adaptations as those found in cyclists who follow large-volume endurance training plans. The length and number of these intervals were doubled compared to the 2008 study, but that still only totaled roughly 40 minutes of high-intensity work per week spread over 2.5 hours of riding. As you'll see in the TCTP, the harder the efforts, the shorter the intervals and the lower the total amount of "work time" during an interval session. During a VO_2max session you might do 16 minutes of total work at VO_2max intensities, whereas you might spend 24 to 36 minutes at lactate threshold intensities during LT workouts.

Originally, the TCTP was designed to deliver race-winning fitness relatively quickly, with the understanding that this peak fitness would be short lived—sort of a "make hay while the sun shines" program. Then we noticed that athletes grew incrementally stronger each time they used the program—provided they took 4 to 6 weeks to recover and focus on endurance-paced rides. Their program-starting field test results were higher the second, third, and fourth time around. And so were their peak power numbers for PowerIntervals. Race results provided the final confirmation of these incremental gains. Now that the program and the book have been around for several more years, we've had the opportunity to see its impact on long-term fitness and performance.

Take Taylor Carrington as an example. His training, lifestyle, and race results in those back-to-back Elite Cyclocross National Championships made him the poster child for the TCTP. But a few years after the first edition of this book was released, Taylor called Jim to let him know he was embarking on an ambitious project at work. If he succeeded, it would be one of those career-making, life-altering, dragon-slaying kind of accomplishments. The cost would be 18 to 24 months of nose-to-the-grindstone work. It would completely disrupt the balance of his life, but he had weighed the costs and benefits and realized this was a relatively short-term cost to take a giant leap forward in his career and prosperity. And with that he hung up his race wheels for two years.

Fast-forward two years, and Taylor's time in purgatory had reached its end. It took 24 months but he closed a monster of a deal. And then he called Rutberg to ask about Masters Cyclocross World Championships. It was late August, and he wanted to race Worlds in January. The biggest unknown was how much detraining had occurred during his time away from structured training and competition.

They reviewed Taylor's activity level over the preceding two years. During the busiest parts of putting the deal together, Taylor rode 1 to 2 times a week. When times were a bit easier, he managed to squeeze in 3 rides a week. And perhaps due to his earlier experiences with the TCTP, or because hard intervals are great stress-relievers, his rides were endurance miles, big climbs, or PowerIntervals. Lots of 1- and 2-minute PowerIntervals.

Remember the string analogy I used earlier? By consistently challenging the top end of your capacity (VO_2max), even for just 10 to 20 minutes a week, you pull up the right (VO_2max) side of the string; in turn, that pulls up on your power at lactate threshold and at more moderate effort levels.

Instead of making incremental gains from cycling through the TCTP 2 to 3 times in a 12-month period, Taylor and other athletes have used the concepts from the TCTP to minimize detraining during prolonged periods away from competition. Contrast this with most people's usual idea of time off from a structured, multi-month training plan, which is to get out on the bike when they can and take it easy because they can't believe their bodies can handle a tough workout.

The science of high-intensity training shows that by sticking with the concepts of the TCTP—or the program itself—when you're severely time-crunched or need to buckle down and focus on something in your career or personal life, you can maintain a large portion of the fitness you've already earned. If you don't have time for the long stuff, make sure to stick with the hard stuff. And when your schedule frees up and you can recommit to some racing goals, you'll find that you haven't lost all that much power.

In Taylor's case, his field test power outputs were only about 10 watts lower than they had been two years earlier. But while his ability to produce power was good, the efforts took more out of him, and it took him longer to recover from intervals and from hard workouts. Rutberg used a modified version of the TCTP with Taylor to ramp him up for Masters Worlds from September into January. Though Taylor's fitness and power responded quickly, his somewhat rusty racing skills yielded a mixture of race results. Nevertheless, he became good in time for his big race and finished 9th in the Men's 35–39 race, behind winner and fellow CTS athlete Scott Frederick. It's not an earth-shattering result, but it's testament to the power of short high-intensity workouts to keep you in the game—or within shouting distance of the game—during prolonged periods away from competition.

WILL HIGH-INTENSITY TRAINING KILL ME?

Last summer I rode the 78-mile Copper Triangle event with my teenage son, Connor. It was his longest ride ever, in mileage, elevation gain, and time on the bike. He did great, and I loved sharing the experience and the day with him. As we both climbed Vail Pass with our hearts pounding away, I thought about the "Cycling to Extremes" article in *VeloNews* magazine and similar articles that have asked the question of whether high-intensity training is dangerous to the hearts of athletes, particularly athletes above the age of 40. It's a subject people ask about frequently, so, after consulting with cardiologists, cardiac surgeons, and electrophysiologists, here are my thoughts on the matter.

If you haven't read the *VeloNews* article, the quick summary goes like this: Some endurance athletes develop atrial fibrillation (AF, an electrical problem in the heart that causes atria to quiver instead of pumping blood properly), myocardial fibrosis (stiffening and thickening of the heart muscle), or tachycardia (an abnormally high heart rate that may feel like your heart is skipping a beat). The question is whether long-term participation in endurance sports increases an athlete's risk for developing these conditions, and the article leans heavily in the direction that it does.

This is obviously a cause for concern for many athletes. I'm 56 years old and I've been training and competing since I was 9. What did I do after reading the article? I went for a bike ride, complete with intervals, and I was far more worried about getting run over by a distracted driver than about potentially damaging my heart.

The physicians I've consulted generally agree with me. On balance, they believe the health benefits of exercise—including strenuous exercise—outweigh the risks of developing electrical or structural problems within the heart by a large margin. That's not to say the risk isn't there, but rather that exercise is only one of many factors that contribute—positively and negatively—to the health of your heart.

But that's not really news. Everyone knows that some exercise is better for you than none, and for the people reading this book, the choice is not between your current training workload and nothing at all. You're not going to hang up your wheels and just sit on the couch. What athletes struggle with is whether the choice is between strenuous exercise and a more leisurely level of activity. Here are a few things to consider.

Cardiac Problems Are Extremely Rare for Time-Crunched Athletes

In the past 16 years, CTS coaches have worked with more than 17,000 athletes, the vast majority of whom fit the profile of a time-crunched athlete. We are neither physicians nor medical researchers, but in that time we know of only a handful of athletes who have developed heart rhythm issues, structural heart issues, or suffered a heart attack or stroke while exercising. For example, throughout our coaching programs, our athletes have the opportunity to put a medical hold on their membership, and when they do so we ask them about their medical condition. Few have cited heart issues as a reason to suspend training. Similarly, when athletes stop working with CTS, we always ask why they are leaving. As part of our quality assurance program we also ask the coaches for information about athletes who cancel. The few athletes who have developed AF were open and eager to tell us, which leads me to believe other athletes would be similarly honest and forthcoming. Yet we are not seeing any increase in the number of athletes reporting arrhythmias or other cardiac problems.

CTS is one of the largest endurance coaching companies in the United States. The vast majority of the athletes we coach are men between the ages of 40 and 65. Some have been training consistently for 30-plus years while others are relatively new to endurance sports. All of them do interval training. If years of cumulative endurance training—including high-intensity training—were leading to a significant increase in arrhythmias in athletes over 40, I would expect we would be one of the first organizations to see it happening. It would be troubling and noticeable if more and more athletes were requesting medical holds or canceling or dying because of cardiac health problems. But we are not seeing that.

You know what we see a lot of? Cancer. At any given time of the year, there are a significant number of athletes on medical holds because of cancer. I know of one athlete who has been on hold for an entire year; he's not canceling because the idea of coming off hold and returning to training provides him with motivation and hope.

Atrial Fibrillation Diagnoses Are Increasing in the Overall Population

The incidence of AF naturally increases with age, and there are an estimated 75 million Baby Boomers (ages 53–71 in 2017) like me who have reached an age when genetics and decades of lifestyle choices start expressing themselves. Things start going wrong, like your heart's electrical system. If there is an increase in the number of AF diagnoses in athletes over the age of 50, perhaps it is because we are representative of a growing population of people over 50. The physicians I consulted also commented that technology has improved their ability to detect arrhythmias earlier, so more people of all ages are finding out they have them. Indeed, a 2015 study by Schnabel et al. of 50-year trends of atrial fibrillation indicates that the increases in incidence and prevalence are at least partly due to increased effort and efficacy of looking for them.

A Lifetime of Factors Contribute to Cardiac Health and Disease Risk

The decisions you made in the past 4 to 6 decades have made you what you are, for better and worse. High-stress careers can be rewarding and lucrative, but being a hard-charging Type-A person means dealing with a lot of stress. Maybe you thrive on it, but your body can still be negatively affected by it. And not all 50-plus athletes have been athletes for their entire lives. Many of you spent decades gorging on cardiac risk factors: excess bodyweight, high cholesterol, high blood pressure, poor eating habits, little to no exercise, high-stress environments, heavy drinking and/or recreational drug use, and smoking. Dropping bad habits and becoming an athlete have done people a ton of good and probably saved some lives, but good habits in the past decade may not completely negate or reverse the damage you did decades ago.

Even before your good and bad habits started building your profile for cardiac risk factors, your genetics dealt you a hand to play. Those cards may predispose you to high cholesterol, or blood clots, or arrhythmias. Could high-intensity exercise help to reveal an underlying problem? The physicians I consulted said yes. But they also said it's likely not just the exertion, but a combination of acute factors like lifestyle stress, fatigue, dehydration, prescription drug interactions, heat stress . . . and exertion. Furthermore, a physician who specialized in electrophysiology pointed out that this could be a good thing. He noted that experiencing an arrhythmia event isn't a sure sign of a life-threatening or long-term problem. A perfectly healthy heart can skip a beat (often the description of what ventricular tachycardia feels like) and return to normal rhythm. Athletes are also more attuned to their bodies and sometimes notice arrhythmia before a sedentary person would, making it more likely to discover an underlying cardiac issue, if there is one, sooner.

Where Do We Go from Here?

The only thing I know for absolute certain is that we're all going to die. The best we can do to prolong our lives is to continue doing things that reduce our risk factors for a wide range of diseases. Exercise, including strenuous exercise, is one of those things. But so is taking a more serious approach to rest and recovery.

The heart is a muscle, and like any muscle it adapts to stress. As an athlete, you have a higher stroke volume (your heart pumps more blood per stroke) and a lower resting heart rate than people in the general population. These are positive adaptations from exercise. As with any other muscle, recovery is key to maximizing positive adaptation and reducing injury risk. As such, it isn't a huge leap to consider that overtraining or under-recovery may negatively impact the heart muscle in similar ways that under-recovery negatively impacts skeletal muscle, joints, connective tissue (ligaments and tendons), and the immune system. It is my belief that structured training that incorporates appropriate amounts of rest and recovery is instrumental in avoiding overtraining or under-recovery.

The large populations of CTS athletes and *Time-Crunched Cyclist* readers train 3 to 5 days per week and have 3 to 6 weeks per year away from training, consisting of either planned or unanticipated time (typically family or work related). CTS coaches worked with more than 17,000 athletes between 2000 and 2016, and we are not seeing an increased incidence of cardiac disease or injury. If there is increased risk for athletes, perhaps it isn't the workload or the intensity of the training that's the problem, but rather the lack of recovery in poorly designed programs.

THE TIME-CRUNCHED PERIODIZATION PLAN

Taylor's and Sterling's experiences with the TCTP demonstrate not only that the program works but also that it calls for a shift in the way endurance training is typically organized. As I mentioned in Chapter 1, the general concept of periodization is to break up the training year into progressively smaller segments to focus the training stressors. Perhaps most important, the technique organizes the scheduling of rest days and weeks to ensure athletes get the right amount of time to adapt to their training.

The periodization plan most often used by athletes in a classic endurance training program starts with a base-building period in the winter and follows with a preparation period that focuses on improving sustainable power at lactate threshold. These workouts prepare the athlete for the high-intensity workouts in the specialization—or competition—period, which leads an athlete to a planned peak of conditioning and competitive readiness.

Depending on the length of the athlete's season, there may be a second period of preparation training, followed by another specialization period and peak, before moving on to a transitional period of lighter, less-structured training. This final period is meant to help the athlete recuperate from the cumulative mental and physical fatigue of a long season.

Just about any cycling training book will include a year-long periodization plan that looks something like what I have just described. It's what most people use, because it works very well for athletes who plan on being strong or competitive from April through October. Time-crunched cyclists should definitely do their best to ride and train year-round, but the TCTP follows a very different periodization plan because of the nature of the workouts you'll be doing and the kind of fitness you'll be developing.

The principal reason a year-long periodization plan is necessary for high-volume trainers is that the volume's contribution to overall workload is so high that it takes a long time to gradually add small increments of intensity. If you try to accelerate the process by quickly ramping up the intensity on a high-volume trainer, you'll soon reach the point where you can't recover and adapt quickly enough to continue making progress. Low-volume training plans can progress faster because the intensity contributes a greater percentage of the total workload, and there's plenty of built-in recovery time. At the same time, the intensity of the program leads to a lot of fatigue, which limits the length of time an athlete can successfully maintain top fitness before needing to back off and recover.

If you think of the classic endurance periodization plan as a dimmer switch where workload and fitness move up and down slowly and gradually, the TCTP is more like an "on/off" switch. When you're "on," it's full on, and you go straight through until you flip the switch to "off." The classic endurance periodization plan has four major periods: foundation (base aerobic training), preparation (aerobic and lactate threshold work), specialization (high-power work and event-specific training), and transition (recuperation and active recovery). The TCTP essentially cuts this down to two hybrid periods: preparation/specialization ("on") and foundation/preparation ("off").

Dear Chris,

I just wanted to take this opportunity to say that I think The Time-Crunched Cyclist *is the new standard. I'm 40 years old and coming back to the sport after a 15-year absence. After 8 months back on the bike and following your training plans, I joined my first fast club ride. I felt and rode like I never missed a beat. I felt good drafting, jumping, and riding at high speeds in a pack of riders at 40–45 km/hr [25–28 mph]. Now I know what I have to do to improve my conditioning and make my way to the front again.*   *—Simon J.*

PREPARATION/SPECIALIZATION (GO TIME)

This period is pretty much defined by the 11 weeks that constitute the TCTP included in this book (see Chapters 6, 7, 8, and 9). You'll notice that the plans start off with a few moderate-intensity interval workouts and then rapidly progress to incorporate more maximum-intensity PowerIntervals. In 3 to 4 weeks you should start seeing dramatic improvements in your power output and performance in group rides or races, and you'll reach your peak performance about 8 weeks into the program. Some athletes, especially less experienced riders, may start to see performance declining about 10 weeks into the program, whereas riders with more than 5 years of experience can typically maintain peak performance through the 11th week.

It's important to incorporate this information into your planning. If you're going to compete in a local criterium series that lasts 8 weeks, start the program 3 to 4 weeks before the first race. You won't be in optimal condition for the first event, but the racing will enhance your training, and your performance will improve all the way through the rest of the series. If you're preparing for a series of events over a 3- to 5-week period, you should start the TCTP 4 to 5 weeks before the first event so you will have made more training progress before you start racing.

Normally, CTS programs follow a pattern that features a recovery week after 3 weeks of training. There are some recovery or regeneration weeks built into the TCTP program as well, but because of the already low training volume we're really only talking about backing off the intensity for 1 or 2 workouts, 4 weeks into the program.

I mentioned previously that some athletes may be able to stretch their fitness for up to an additional month. Cyclists who have raced for many years will have greater success extending the period of time they can maintain their high-performance fitness. For instance, Sterling and Taylor each have 10 to 15 years of miles in their legs and have been able to stay competitive for 14 to 16 weeks after starting the program. Still, their best performances were in the 8- to 12-week period.

FOUNDATION/PREPARATION (MAINTENANCE)

For high-volume trainers, the scientifically proven recipe to prevent detraining is to decrease the volume and retain—or even increase—the intensity. This is the technique most often used to taper athletes before big events and hold on to hard-earned fitness through an end-of-season break or transition period (Mujika et al. 2003). In reality, the technique leverages the same science this program is based on, just for a slightly different purpose. During the TCTP, you're using intensity to increase your workload above what you'd normally be able to achieve, to generate enough stimulus to improve your power at VO_2max and lactate threshold. In contrast, high-volume trainers use a short period of high-intensity, low-volume training to reduce their overall workload while retaining just enough stimulus to keep power at VO_2max and lactate threshold from declining.

Recovery and maintenance are the goals of the periods between the times when you're using the TCTP, but unlike high-volume trainers, aerobic endurance should be your highest priority. When you're done and you flip the switch to "off," you have to back off the intensity. But you can and should maintain your volume. In other words, if you're riding 6 to 8 hours when you're on the program, you should continue riding for 6 to 8 hours a week during the time between build periods. The intensity is what you have to recover from, not the volume. If anything, you should stick to your riding schedule so the time doesn't get siphoned away to other priorities.

Your rides during this period should be less structured but focused on maintaining steady intensities at about 65 to 85 percent of your maximum sustainable power output. This means maintaining a good tempo that's more challenging than an easy cruising pace. You will see a significant decline in your high-end fitness (power at VO_2max and your ability to handle repeated maximal efforts), but that's normal, and those performance markers respond quickly when you return to high-intensity training. By riding at a more challenging tempo, you'll still be getting a reasonable amount of energy from the glycolytic energy system, which will help prevent significant detraining of your aerobic system and power at lactate threshold. Including some intense efforts once a week will further aid in preventing significant detraining, which means that I encourage you to continue going on the local group ride or pushing yourself on the local climb.

Four weeks is the minimum amount of time you must allow between the end of any use of the TCTP and the start of another. Six weeks is better, or you can make the maintenance period as long as you like. At CTS we have had the most success cycling athletes through the program twice in a year.

Depending on an athlete's goals and location, it is sometimes possible to add a third cycle. The TCTP is perfect for having a great spring season and another surge in performance in the late summer or early fall (late fall or early winter for cyclocross racers). To fit in three cycles, you have to start early (February) to be prepared for an early spring season, then prepare again for a midsummer peak, and then prepare again for one in the fall. Although this can work for anyone, it is most often an option for athletes in warm climates because their season can start earlier and end later than the cycling season in northern states.

For specific week-by-week recommendations on the "off" period, see the "Frequently Asked Questions" section at the end of Chapter 5. If you're looking for structure during this period, I've included a 4-week program that you can follow or modify to suit your own needs and training schedule.

4

MEASURING INTENSITY IN THE INFORMATION AGE

ADVANCED TRAINING TECHNOLOGY MAY BE the most important factor working in your favor as a cyclist with a busy schedule. Looking back at my years as a professional cyclist, it saddens me to think about all the energy I wasted. I trained religiously and was advised by many of the sport's top coaches and sports scientists, but training technology hadn't advanced to the point where I could accurately determine how hard I was working. My extreme training volume masked its inefficiency; somewhere in all those hours I managed to ride at the intensities necessary to improve performance, but I also wasted a ton of time at ineffective power outputs or riding when I should have been resting.

Journalists have asked me innumerable times to explain how and why today's pros are so much faster than they were 20 or 30 years ago. There are many factors, including improved road surfaces, lighter and stiffer bikes, slipperier aerodynamics (for riders as well as their equipment), and far superior wheels and bearings. But beyond the mechanical and aerodynamic advancements, today's cyclists have the ability to train with greater precision than any previous generation.

Precision comes from having detailed, real-time performance data you can use to monitor, evaluate, and adjust your training. And by far the best piece of equipment for providing that information is a power meter, which measures the true amount of work you produce as you ride.

Cyclists are fortunate because we have access to more accurate data than any other endurance sport. The most accurate power meters use strain gauges located in the crank or rear wheel to directly measure the mechanical work you're producing (kilojoules) and how rapidly you're producing that work (watts). This information is only now becoming available to runners, but not to swimmers or athletes in any sport played on a field, court, or rink.

Even if you don't own a power meter, as a cyclist you have benefited from the fact that others do. The work coaches have done with power-equipped athletes has broadened our understanding of how the body responds to training and fatigue, and that knowledge has led to positive changes in how workouts are arranged and prescribed. So although I highly recommend investing in a power meter and using it to advance your training, I also know—from experience—that the TCTP works whether you're training with power or heart rate.

TRAINING WITH A POWER METER

Your power meter provides a detailed record of every ride, with heart rate, power output, speed, and cadence information for every effort you put forth. As you'll see in the following sections, that information is crucial during your ride, but it's also very important afterward. One of the most important things you can do with a power meter is download the data from every ride, race, or event to your computer and into software products that can log and analyze the information.

To make sure the data you gather are accurate, it's crucial that you "zero" your power meter before every ride. This simple procedure only takes a few seconds (see the manufacturer's instruction manual for directions), but it means the difference between getting valuable information and recording junk. And more than just ensuring accuracy for individual workouts, setting zero offset is especially important when you're adding data to cumulative training logs. The accuracy of the analysis performed by software programs depends on the accuracy of the data you input.

Tips for Buying and Using a Power Meter

The number of power meters on the market continues to grow, and the features change rapidly as technology improves. For this reason, any list of power meters I include here will be obsolete within months. Instead, let's take a look at the essential aspects you should look for—or be aware of—when it comes to purchasing and using a power meter.

Accuracy is different than consistency. Obviously, you want your power data to be accurate, so manufacturers spend a lot of time telling you their meter is accurate within a certain range—let's say 2 percent. That's great, but it's actually more important that your power meter measures workload consistently from day to day. If it's within 2 percent today, it needs to be within 2 percent tomorrow and next month. If it is measuring 2 percent low today and 5 percent high tomorrow, that's a problem. Consistency is important because you are typically using the same power meter over and over again, so even if it is less accurate (measures 10 watts less than you actually produce, for instance) you will still be able to accurately track and measure your progress as long as its level of precision is consistent over time.

A power meter is only accurate to itself. Your power readings are likely to be different on different power meters, despite the obvious fact that your actual ability to produce power hasn't changed. As quality control and technology improve, these differences are getting smaller, but it is still important to always use the same power meter for workouts and races you want to be able to compare. Now that power meters have come down in price and increased in variety and compatibility, many athletes put them on multiple bikes. This is great, but comparisons of power files from the same athlete using different power meters on different bikes in different conditions can be difficult, especially if the athlete does not consistently zero the meters or take good care of them.

Single-leg versus double-leg measurement. Innovative companies have successfully put strain gauges in a variety of places to measure power. You can get a power meter that measures strain at the crank spider (where the chainrings attach), the chainrings themselves, the rear hub, the pedals, or from within the non-driveside crank arm. Some meters directly measure strain from the entire pedal stroke (spider, chainrings, rear hub). Others can only measure one half of the pedal stroke and essentially double it to calculate your power output. And some pedal-based systems measure power in both pedals and then combine the data to deliver an overall power output. There are pros and cons to each method. The single-leg meters tend to be less expensive, more easily compatible with a wider range of bikes, and more easily swapped from bike to bike. I prefer power meters that measure double-leg data, because then all of your data is the result of direct measurement instead of arithmetic.

Set head unit to record at least once a second. To help extend battery life and manage data storage, some head units allow you to change how frequently they record data from the power meter. More data points yield greater accuracy, so if possible set the recording frequency at one second or faster. For the vast majority of your training sessions and rides, battery life isn't going to be a limiting factor. If you are getting ready to ride the Dirty Kanza 200 or some other ultraendurance event, you could reduce this recording frequency.

Set "zero offset" before each ride. The "zero offset" on your power meter measures the sensor value when there is no torque applied to the strain gauges. This establishes the baseline value so your workload above zero can be measured accurately. It's important because heat, humidity, vibration, and other environmental factors can affect the zero offset of your power meter from ride to ride. Two hundred watts today is not 200 watts tomorrow if the zero offset is wrong. Many power meters can set zero offset automatically, so the important point is to make sure you either have it set to do that or that you do it manually.

Check compatibility before you buy. We have sold a lot of power meters in the past 16 years, and one of the most frustrating experiences for an athlete is ordering a power meter and then realizing it won't work with existing equipment. It's not just whether it will fit onto your existing crank or bottom bracket, or whether the hub has the right spacing for your bike's frame. It's also whether you'll be able to ride the pedals or wheels or other equipment you want to use in different situations. If you want to race different wheels than you train on, a crank- or pedal-based power meter is a better option than a hub-based meter. If you ride multiple bikes, a pedal-based system may be easiest to move between bikes.

Keeping It Simple

There are a thousand ways to slice and dice the massive amount of data athletes generate from their power meters, and some very serious minds have spent enormous amounts of time doing just that. I have a few of these people on my staff, including Dean Golich, who has been one of the leading experts on training with power for more than 20 years. There are athletes who love numbers, too, and many spend their free time analyzing and reanalyzing data from power files. If you're one of them, I recommend the book *Training and Racing with a Power Meter* by Hunter Allen and Andrew Coggan. It is the most complete resource I have seen for anyone who wants to delve into the nitty-gritty details of training with power.

In my view, however, athletes on the Time-Crunched Training Program need to focus on only three main pieces of information. Those pieces are power, kilojoules, and fatigue, and we'll cover them next.

Power

Power, expressed in watts, is derived from the following equation:

Power in Watts = Torque × Angular Velocity

To generate more power, you can push harder on the pedals to generate more torque, or you can pedal faster to create greater angular velocity, or you can do both. Power is a direct measure of the work you are doing right now, and it is unaffected by many of the factors that can distort heart rate data, including dehydration, heat, humidity, anxiety, excitement, and stimulants such as caffeine. These factors can influence your motivation or ability to produce power on the bike, but they don't alter the validity of the numbers you see on the power meter readout.

The two primary uses of power are to determine the demands of the rides, events, and races you want to participate in, and to establish training intensity ranges that you can use to develop the fitness necessary to meet those demands. That is why it is very helpful to race with a power meter and examine power files from centuries, group rides, and other events.

For instance, let's say there's a particular climb on the local group ride where you frequently get dropped. Looking at your power file, you may see that you're able to stay with the group when your power output for the 5-minute effort is 250 watts, but you get dropped when you have to ride at 265 watts on the same climb. To avoid getting dropped there, your training program has to be designed to increase the wattage you're able to maintain for 5 minutes from 250 to 265.

POWER-TO-WEIGHT RATIO

Along with providing athletes with an accurate way of measuring workload, a power meter gives us a good method for comparing the relative climbing strengths of two athletes. Your ability to go uphill quickly depends on the amount of power you can produce and the amount of weight you need to move against gravity. We can quantify this with a power meter by determining your power-to-weight ratio (PWR).

The PWR can be used to compare your abilities as a climber before and after a period of training, or to compare your abilities as a climber against those of a rider who is a different size. For instance, right now you may be able to sustain 250 watts on a local climb, and if you weigh 70 kilograms (154 pounds), your PWR would be 250/70 or 3.57 watts per kilogram. After completing the TCTP, your sustainable power may increase to 275 watts and your weight may decrease to 68 kilograms, bringing your PWR to 275/68 or 4.04 watts per kilogram. Even without climbing-specific workouts, you should reach the summit of the local climb faster with a PWR of 4.04 watts per kilogram than with a PWR of 3.57.

When comparing riders of relatively equal fitness, a taller and heavier rider will tend to have more muscle mass and longer levers with which to generate greater power than a smaller rider. However, the bigger rider also has more mass to carry uphill, so you need more than just the two riders' sustainable power outputs to determine which one has an advantage on a climb.

This is where PWR comes into play. Let's say Big Boy weighs 85 kilograms (187 pounds) and has a sustainable power output of 320 watts, and Little Guy weighs 65 kilograms (143 pounds) and has a sustainable power output of 250 watts. Despite having the strength to sustain 320 watts, Big Boy would reach the summit of the climb behind Little Guy, because his PWR is 3.76 watts per kilogram and Little Guy's is 3.85.   >

A higher PWR also gives a cyclist a tactical advantage, because it gives you a greater ability to accelerate on a steep pitch. You're able to use more power to lift each kilogram of your body weight against gravity, which means that during a hard acceleration on a steep pitch you'll go faster than a rider with a lower PWR.

If you know you have a lower PWR than other riders in the group, your best option is to keep the pace high on the flat roads before the climb and any moderate grades on the climb itself in an effort to make the smaller riders work harder. If your tactic works, you'll effectively reduce the other riders' PWRs by tiring them out and reducing the power outputs they're able to sustain on the steep sections.

If you're the little climber with a high PWR, you want to conserve energy before the climb and hit the big guys hard as soon as you come to a really steep pitch. You'll force them to make a choice: dig deep to stay with you, or let you go and hope you'll tire so they can gradually catch you.

It's important to realize that PWR is entirely dependent on time. You can't just say a rider has a PWR of 4.0 watts per kilogram. That value has to have a time associated with it, like 4.0 watts per kilogram for 20 minutes. The shorter the climb, the higher your PWR will be.

For instance, I've often said that I consider 6.8 watts per kilogram for 30 minutes to be a performance marker that a rider needs to accomplish to be considered a contender for overall victory at the Tour de France. That doesn't mean that a Tour contender can ride a 45-minute climb during the Tour at 6.8 watts per kilogram. Beyond the fact that the climb is longer than the 30-minute test, climbs in the Tour are contested after many days of racing and sometimes after more than 4 hours of hard riding earlier in the stage. That's why top riders average PWRs in the 4 to 5 watts per kilogram range at the Tour, even though they can hit the 6.8 watts per kilogram threshold during a pre-Tour test.

An athlete's weight and stature can make a big difference in time trials and the cycling portion of a triathlon, not only because these characteristics impact PWR but because they also affect the relationship between aerodynamics and power production. No matter how aerodynamic you make a bicycle, the human on top of it is the biggest impediment to going faster. But as athletes get bigger, the hole they have to punch in the air doesn't grow proportionally with their height and weight. As a result, tall athletes tend to have an advantage over shorter ones when riding in an aerodynamic position; they generate more power because of longer levers and more muscle mass, but the hole they have to punch in the air isn't that much larger than that of a much shorter rider.

When smaller riders excel in time trials, it is often because they have tremendous power relative to their muscle mass and their small stature enables them to minimize the height differential between saddle and aero bars. By essentially hiding behind their hands and tucking their heads to fill the gap between their upper arms in order to smooth the airflow around their bodies, some small riders can rival their taller peers.

On courses with significant climbs, smaller athletes can level the playing field by using their superior PWR to gain time on the hills. Instead of using a steady effort level (which is often the preferred plan on low rolling hills or flat courses), you may benefit from surging up and over the top of climbs, and then get into your best aerodynamic position to maximize speed and minimize power output during the descents and flat portions of the course.

On descents and flat ground, bigger riders can use their power advantage to go faster, but that extra speed costs them a lot of energy. When you go faster uphill, you can take significant amounts of time away from them, and the energy cost of gaining that time is lower than trying to out-ride them on flat ground. Over a 40-km course of rolling hills, the rider with a higher PWR will eventually ride away from a bigger rider who has more power and more weight to drag along.

Many athletes have less specific goals for improving their power output; they just want to be able to go faster and ride longer. For these athletes, and even for athletes who are trying to meet specific demands, increasing sustainable power at lactate threshold and increasing power at VO_2max are the best ways to improve cycling performance. In addition, it's important not only to focus on achieving higher wattages at these levels but also to work on increasing the amount of time you can sustain those intensities.

In order to increase the power you can produce for efforts ranging from a few seconds to several hours, you need to establish training ranges that challenge your body and lead to the adaptations you seek. I cover this subject in more detail later in this chapter.

Kilojoules

I don't have to tell you that pedaling a bicycle is work, but the number of kilojoules you produce during a ride provides an accurate accounting of exactly how much work you do during each ride. A kilojoule is a unit of mechanical energy, or work produced, and 4.184 kilojoules is equal to 1 kilocalorie. You expend kilocalories to produce kilojoules, but the human body is not a perfectly efficient machine, so only a portion of the kilocalories you expend do the mechanical work of turning your pedals. In fact, a cyclist's efficiency is about 20 to 25 percent, meaning that about 75 to 80 percent of the energy you expend is lost, mostly as heat, which is why strenuous exercise is such a sweaty affair.

If every calorie you expended was used for producing kilojoules, you would have to multiply your kilojoule count by 4 to come up with the number of kilocalories you burned during your workout (X kilojoules $\times$ 4.184 = Y kilocalories). However, because of the 25 percent efficiency of the system, it takes about 4 kilocalories to produce 1 kilojoule of mechanical work. That brings the ratio of energy expended to work produced back to about 1:1. In other words, when you return from a ride or race, you can generally consider the number of kilojoules displayed on your power meter to be equal to the number of kilocalories you burned during your time on the bike. There is actually some error in this number, in that your efficiency may have been between 20 and 25 percent, but the error is typically so small that it's not worth worrying about.

Kilojoules can be a more accurate way of prescribing the desired workload for a ride than either time or mileage. Basing workout duration on distance is convenient but notoriously bad in terms of determining the actual work done during the ride. From downtown Colorado Springs, for instance, I can complete 30-mile rides that are either entirely flat or extremely hilly. When I return home I've completed 30 miles, but the workload and training effect of the flat ride would be completely different than those of the hilly ride.

Similarly, basing workouts on time has some of the same problems. A 2-hour ride on a hilly route and a windy day could be far more challenging than a 2-hour ride on flat terrain on a windless day. Based on time, you'd cover more distance on the 2-hour flat ride (let's say 40 miles), but the workload could still be lower than covering 30 miles on the hilly ride on a windy day. And if I rode really hard on the flat ride but easy on the hilly ride, the flat ride could actually end up being harder than the hilly one.

With so many variables and so little objective data (even heart rate is relatively easily influenced by outside factors), it can be difficult to accurately determine the true workload of your rides. With a power meter, however, you can make an apples-to-apples comparison of one ride with another. A 1,500-kilojoule ride is a 1,500-kilojoule ride, whether it took you 90 minutes or 2 hours to complete, and whether it was uphill into a headwind or ripping along on flat roads with a tailwind.

It's important to note, however, that while kilojoules provide raw information about the endurance component of your training, this information must be considered in conjunction with time and intensity. That is, you need to think about how you produced those kilojoules to evaluate the ride's impact on your fitness, performance, and fatigue.

Races and events are among the most useful places to gather kilojoule data. If you're doing 45-minute criteriums and you race with a power meter, you can see how many kilojoules of energy you produced during your event. Let's say you return from a local race and your power meter says you produced 800 kilojoules. That's the total energy demand of your event, which means you can use that information to guide your training. For instance, to develop the endurance for your events, you may want some of your rides to be at least 800-kilojoule sessions. But your training rides aren't as intense as your races, so it may take you 60 to 75 minutes to reach 800 kilojoules in training, compared to 45 minutes during a race.

For century riders and athletes preparing for cycling tours, it's difficult to match the energy expenditure of your goal event in training. During a 6-hour century, you might produce 3,000 to 4,000 kilojoules, and during even the hardest training sessions it's difficult for any athlete to achieve more than 1,200 kilojoules in an hour. As a matter of perspective, a 170-pound cyclist is likely to produce 800 to 1,000 kilojoules during the 75- to 90-minute interval sessions featured in the TCTP. Ideally, you would complete a few challenging 3- to 4-hour rides that pushed your energy production to about 3,000 kilojoules, but you can be adequately prepared for your long days without these rides if necessary.

There's an inverse relationship between power output and exercise duration, meaning that your average power output—and hence the kilojoules produced per hour—will decline as the length of rides increases. Most cyclists realize this without ever being told; it's called pacing. When you leave your house for a 90-minute ride, you know you can afford to ride more aggressively than when you roll out for a 5-hour ride. If you didn't know this and attempted to ride aggressively right from the start of a century, you'd ride at a high power output and energy expenditure for the first 2 hours and end up crawling home at a very low output in the last hour. Almost every novice cyclist makes this mistake at least once. It's like a rite of passage that helps us learn how to pace ourselves.

The inverse relationship between power output and exercise duration also means that relatively short training sessions can prepare you for longer events. As you build a bigger aerobic engine, you're gaining the fitness necessary to produce more kilojoules per hour through primarily aerobic metabolism. Let's say that right now 600 kilojoules an hour is an endurance pace you can comfortably sustain for 3 hours. As I discussed in Chapter 2, riding at 600 kilojoules an hour for an additional hour isn't going to do you much good in terms of increasing your mitochondrial density, a key marker of increased oxidative capacity in skeletal muscle. However, because shorter, higher-intensity interval workouts can increase mitochondrial density and give you the tools to burn more fat and carbohydrate through aerobic channels, these workouts can increase the number of kilojoules you can produce aerobically each hour. This increased fitness can be used two ways: You can use it to ride at a higher power output that may get you up to 700 kilojoules an hour, or you can ride at 600 kilojoules an hour for more hours because you're relying more on fat and carbohydrate through aerobic metabolism and deriving less energy from the glycolytic system.

Fatigue

Fatigue gets a bad rap, but it is not always a bad thing; it's actually one of the most important components of an effective training program. It is always created in the process of overloading a physical system, which makes it an integral part of the stimulus your body is responding to as you adapt and grow stronger. And like any other part of training, fatigue has to be managed properly so it can enhance your performance rather than destroy it. A power meter can be a very effective tool for helping you manage fatigue, not only during individual workouts but also within entire periods of training.

Power is a direct measure of the work you're doing right now, so it provides an accurate way to tell if you're too tired to continue with effective intervals. As you fatigue, you'll see a decline in the power output you're able to sustain for interval efforts as well as endurance-pace riding. But there's a difference between knowing that you're getting tired and making the right decisions about what to do about it. This is covered in more detail in the section "Knowing When to Say When" in Chapter 5; for now it's important to realize that there are times when you will want to push through the fatigue and complete your intervals but also times when skipping those intervals will be the better choice.

One of the most important things cycling coaches learned once we started training athletes with power was that there were times when athletes were less fatigued than we originally believed. Before power meters were widely used, we used heart rate and perceived exertion to judge an athlete's level of fatigue and then adjusted training accordingly. The day after a lactate threshold or VO_2max interval session, we noticed that an athlete's exercise heart rate was often suppressed (lower heart rate values at similar paces) and ratings of perceived exertion were often elevated (efforts at similar paces felt harder). This suggested that the athlete was fatigued and needed more recovery before performing another effective interval workout.

In fact, heart rate and perceived exertion were lying. Once riders started using power meters, we saw that despite the suppressed heart rates and elevated ratings of perceived exertion, athletes were often able to complete interval workouts on back-to-back days at matching—and sometimes even higher—power outputs. Yes, there was fatigue present, as illustrated by heart rate and perceived exertion, but the power meter provides context for that fatigue. In the days before power meters, we knew fatigue was present but couldn't tell how much.

When a power meter reveals that an athlete can sustain efforts at outputs equal to those of the day before, despite a suppressed exercise heart rate and an elevated rating of perceived exertion, that means there's fatigue, but not enough to warrant a full recovery day. On the other hand, if during the second consecutive day of intervals an athlete's power output is more than 10 to 15 percent lower than on the previous day, exercise heart rate is suppressed more than 10 percent, and perceived exertion is elevated, this indicates the athlete's level of fatigue is high enough that a rest day is a better option than another training session.

Power meters have led to an increase in the use of 2-day training blocks, and they are featured prominently in the training programs in this book. The benefit of block training is that you generate a strong training stimulus by completing the second day of interval training in a somewhat fatigued state. Put simply, you're reinforcing the training stimulus from the first day and giving your body a more urgent request for adaptation.

TRAINING WITH HEART RATE

After the preceding discussions of the benefits of training with power, it should come as little surprise when I tell you that heart rate training is not as effective as using a power meter. However, power meters are still quite expensive ($500 to $5,000), and it's unrealistic to expect all cyclists to invest in them.

In terms of effectiveness, the difference between training with power and with heart rate is a matter of degree. The fact that training with power is more effective doesn't mean that training with heart rate is not effective at all. My coaches and I have been working with heart rate for more than 20 years, and our athletes have won and continue to win races and achieve personal goals using heart rate alone.

Research backs me up. Scientists (Robinson et al. 2010) at the University of Florida divided 20 men and women into two groups: one assigned to train with power meters, and one with heart rate monitors. At the end of 5 weeks of 90-minute sessions of once-a-week, high-intensity lactate threshold intervals, both groups saw roughly the same improvement in power. So if all you can afford is a heart rate monitor, don't sweat it. You're still using a powerful tool, and you won't be short-changing your training.

In fact, the nature of the TCTP actually makes it better suited to heart rate training than many other programs. There are two main types of workouts in the program: lactate threshold intervals and VO_2max intervals. As you'll see in the description of the CTS Field Test, it's relatively easy to establish accurate heart rate and power training intensities for intervals that improve your sustainable power at lactate threshold.

In terms of VO_2max intervals, heart rate has never been a good way to evaluate these efforts anyway. They're very short (1 to 4 minutes), and because your heart rate is an observation of your body's response to effort, it lags too far behind these efforts to provide useful information. Most likely your heart rate will steadily increase throughout the interval even though your power output may stay relatively constant, or decline.

Whether you're using a power meter or a heart rate monitor, VO_2max intervals are governed by a relatively unscientific prescription: You go as hard as you can. Power meters provide more accurate information about exactly how hard you went, but at the end of the day, these intervals can be just as effective whether you have that detailed information or not.

One of the greatest disadvantages of using heart rate alone to gauge training intensity is "cardiac drift." Because up to 75 percent of the energy produced in muscles is lost as heat, your body has to work to dissipate that heat to keep your core temperature from rising out of control. As you exercise—and especially as you ride at higher intensities—your body uses your skin as your car uses its radiator. Heart rate increases, not only to deliver oxygen to working muscles but also to direct blood to the skin so it can donate fluid for sweat. The sweat then evaporates, which carries much of this excess heat away from the body. Much of the fluid that appears as sweat on your skin was most recently part of your bloodstream. As you lose blood plasma volume to produce sweat, your heart has to pump even faster to continue delivering the same amount of oxygen to working muscles. As a result, your heart rate will increase slightly as exercise duration increases, even if you maintain the same level of effort.

The impact of cardiac drift will be lower if you're better at staying hydrated; you're replacing the fluid lost by sweating and helping to maintain a higher overall blood volume. However, no matter how diligent you are about consuming fluids, some level of cardiac drift is unavoidable during intense endurance exercise.

You can see the impact of cardiac drift in Figure 4.1. In this power file from a lactate threshold interval workout, the athlete performs three intervals at roughly the same power output, but his or her heart rate gets progressively higher for each effort. When athletes train with heart rate alone, they are instructed to maintain the same heart rate range for each interval. Ideally this would result in efforts of equal intensity, but as a result of cardiac drift, this often means that the first interval is actually completed at a higher power output than the subsequent ones. To the athletes, heart rate and perceived exertion seem right on target, but they don't realize that power output is actually falling, and as a result, the workout loses some of its potential effectiveness.

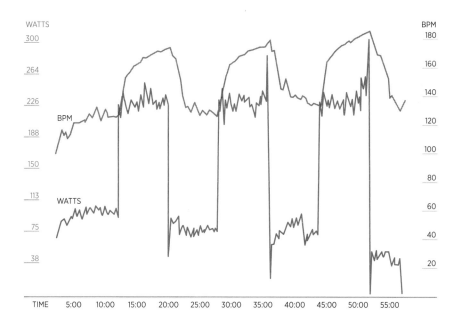

Cardiac Drift

You can see how the rider's heart rate (BPM) increases from the first hard effort to the third. This is a clear example of cardiac drift, where workload remains relatively stable but heart rate increases by an average of 10 beats from the first to the final interval. (Note: cadence and speed traces have been removed from all power files for clarity.)

The next logical assumption is that athletes training with heart rate should adjust their heart rate ranges during interval workouts to compensate for cardiac drift. In other words, some athletes ask if they should ride their first interval at 160 to 165 beats per minute, the second one at 163 to 166, and the last one at 166 to 169. The problem with this idea is that without a power meter you can't accurately determine the extent to which an athlete's performance is being affected by cardiac drift. Raising your heart rate ranges during a series of intervals could either under- or overcompensate for cardiac drift. The best option for heart rate trainers is to focus on staying hydrated and controlling core temperature (to minimize cardiac drift) and stick to the prescribed heart rate ranges for all intervals in a given workout.

Again, the fact that the workouts in the TCTP are short works to the advantage of athletes training with heart rate. Cardiac drift is more pronounced during workouts longer than 2 hours, so the relatively short nature of the workouts in this program helps to minimize its detrimental impact on actual interval intensities.

RATING OF PERCEIVED EXERTION (RPE): THE NO-TECH WAY TO MEASURE INTENSITY

Even as technology has delivered remarkably accurate data about an athlete's true workload, a seemingly archaic measure of intensity refuses to disappear. Rating of perceived exertion, or RPE, is the ultimate in simplicity, nothing more than a scale of how hard you feel you are exercising. Not one single piece of data is collected, and you don't need any special equipment. All you need is the scale.

In the physiology lab, my coaches and I use the Borg Scale, which ranges from 6 to 20 (6 being no exertion at all and 20 being a maximum effort). Why 6 to 20? Well, Borg's research has shown that there's a high correlation between the number an athlete chooses during exercise, multiplied by 10, and his or her actual heart rate at that time. In other words, if you're on an ergometer during an LT test and tell me that you feel like you're at 16, there is a pretty good chance your heart rate is around 160 beats per minute. This isn't absolutely true of all athletes, but you'd be surprised how accurate the 6 to 20 scale tends to be.

Outside the lab, however, I haven't found the Borg Scale to be as helpful for athletes. Most athletes find it easier to relate to a simpler 1 to 10 scale (1 being no exertion at all and 10 being a maximum effort). Using this scale, an endurance or "cruising" pace would be 4 to 5, a challenging aerobic tempo would be 6, LT work occurs at about 7 to 8, climbing and time trial efforts are a solid 8 (sometimes 9), and VO_2 intervals and all-out sprints are the only efforts that reach 10. Just as the Borg Scale multiplies the perceived exertion number by 10 to correlate with heart rate, the number chosen on the 1-to-10 scale, multiplied by 10, seems to correlate closely to the percentage of VO_2max that an athlete is currently maintaining.

With power meters providing an accurate and direct measure of workload, some athletes are tempted to relegate RPE to the trash bin of sports science history, but power meters have actually made RPE more important than ever. Although it's true that 200 watts today is the same workload as 200 watts tomorrow, RPE provides valuable context for your power files. When you're fresh, 200 watts may feel like a moderate spin, but when you're fatigued you may feel like you're working harder than normal for those same 200 watts (sluggish, heavy legs, pedaling through peanut butter, and similar terms may come to mind). RPE is a great early warning device for revealing fatigue; your body is telling you it can still do the job but that even though the work being done is the same, the effort to complete it is greater.

RPE can also indicate progress, even without a change in your power outputs. For example, at the beginning of the season, a 20-minute climb at 250 watts average power may feel strenuous enough to rate a 7 or even an 8. Later in the season, when your fitness has improved, riding at 250 watts up the same climb may take less out of you and feel more like a 6. An RPE of 7 to 8 on the climb may end up being 275 watts at the height of the season.

I have included RPE values with each workout in this book, and I encourage you to record your RPE during each effort in the CTS Field Test. Not only is perceived exertion important for providing context for power and heart rate files, but it also helps you learn to accurately evaluate your intensity level in the absence of all other technologies. Part of becoming a skilled cyclist is learning to use technology effectively while also reducing your dependence on it.

USING STRAVA FOR DATA ANALYSIS

The funny thing about training data is that athletes now generate a ton of it, but not many athletes either download it from their devices or upload it directly to web- or app-based analysis tools. Even those who do gather the data rarely do more than glance at their latest ride and go on with their day. The data you're generating are immensely valuable, but only if you can put it to good use.

A wide range of personality types are drawn to endurance sports, and some people love to geek out over analyzing their data files. Others only want to see some highlights. And there are some who are more than happy to have a coach do the analysis for them. Regardless of which type you currently fall into, I recommend recording all of the data you generate and uploading it to an online analysis tool. If at some point you decide to work with a professional coach, that historical data will be very valuable for your coach to review.

The two most widely used analysis tools are TrainingPeaks and Strava. If you are looking to deep-dive into your training data, you will likely prefer TrainingPeaks. For athletes who want a more user-friendly interface and want to focus on the essentials, Strava is a great choice.

While Strava is best known for its social tools, including segments, leaderboards, clubs, and the ability to "follow" other riders and provide kudos, you can also use it to analyze your performance, track your progress, and monitor the interplay between training stress and recovery. These tools may not be quite as robust as TrainingPeaks, but they are far more accessible to the average time-crunched athlete and provide the essential information you need.

Key Strava Analysis Tools

There are a variety of analysis tools within Strava, and they will be most helpful when you train with a power meter and upload all of your data from each training session. If you plan to do a substantial amount of your training indoors, I recommend purchasing a smart trainer like the KICKR or KICKR SNAP from Wahoo Fitness. With a smart trainer and an interactive training platform like Zwift, you can generate and upload training data files to Strava from both outdoor and indoor rides. Once your data is on Strava, there are analysis tools available for athletes with free accounts and even more tools available for athletes with Strava Premium accounts.

Personal Leaderboard. While it is interesting to see where you stack up on the overall leaderboards for local segments, that ranking only tells you where you fall within a population that ranges from pros to newbies. The overall leaderboards can also contain a lot of errors, as when an athlete's cycling computer is still recording data when the bike is on the roof of a car.

A far more relevant use of leaderboards is to select a segment from your ride and filter the leaderboard by "My Results." To view all of your results, click "View Full Leaderboard." This provides you with a visual representation of how your times have changed on a specific segment over time. Initially this will be a text list of your times. Once you have accumulated enough data over that segment, you will see a graph that plots each segment time on the y-axis. As you get stronger, you will see the general trendline get faster. Remember, though, that segments are recorded whether you were trying to go fast or not. As a result, you will not see steady improvement in segment times each time you ride them.

In the short term, the times will be all over the place. This will be particularly true of segments that you consistently ride during interval rides, endurance rides, and recovery rides. Your speed will reflect the purpose of the workout, and because those three categories of rides have very different purposes, your personal leaderboard for those segments will look more like a scattershot. Even so, over the course of a few months, even with these heavily used segments, you should see a general trend toward faster times.

Another key advantage to the personal leaderboards is the ability to compare your segment times with your competitors. If there are segments defined for a race course, like specific climbs or descents, or even the entire lap, you can navigate to this segment and click "Compare." On the Compare screen you can filter the results by "Today," for instance, to see how your speed compared to everyone else in that event. This helps coaches and athletes see where athletes lost time or made up time, which helps identify strengths and weaknesses. For instance, you may notice that you were consistently one of the fastest riders on the climbs but lost time on descents. Using the Effort Comparison tool (described later), you can gain further insights to see where within the segment you gained or lost time to other athletes. This is a level of analysis that is not possible with TrainingPeaks, which only allows you to compare your own efforts.

Analysis Tab. When you upload a ride to Strava and view it online, you will initially see the Overview. To analyze the whole ride or specific segments, click on the "Analysis" tab. Below the map displayed on the next page you will see an elevation profile, and below that you will find your power, speed, and cadence data displayed for the entire ride. By selecting portions of the ride on the elevation profile you can zoom in on the data for that section; the most important thing you're looking for is your average power for that section of the ride. You can select defined segments or larger sections of the ride, such as a series of climbs or the second hour of the ride.

On longer rides, one of the things you are likely to notice is that power output gradually declines. This will be especially true for rides over 3 hours. You may also notice that your average power for climbs later in the ride will tend to be lower than your power for climbs earlier in the ride. Although this makes sense, it is also something many athletes overlook when planning their rides. Remember that to develop fitness it is important to perform your highest-quality work when you are freshest. If you have an interval session planned, this means doing your intervals early in your ride, right after you warm up. If you wait until later in the ride to do ClimbingRepeats or PowerIntervals, you may not achieve the power outputs you are aiming for.

As you make progress with the TCTP program, you should notice you are able to maintain a more consistent power output throughout a 2- to 4-hour ride and see less of a drop-off in the final hour (you should see this same trend as you cycle through the TCTP a few times). The consistency will depend greatly on how you pace your ride. If you start out harder than you should, you will see a more significant drop-off in power output in the final hour regardless of improved fitness.

Watching how your power output trends throughout a ride can also help you evaluate the success of your hydration and nutrition strategy. When you overheat, get dehydrated, or run low on fuel, your power output will drop more significantly as your ride progresses. Many riders use the same training routes over and over, so it can be useful to compare the overall trend of your power data from a cool day to a very hot one. Although there are a variety of factors that could lead to changes between two rides, monitoring your data over time may help you identify problems with nutrition or hydration, and similarly confirm improvements in how you eat and drink if you are making the right changes.

Effort Comparison. Many athletes use the same segment over and over again for intervals. Instead of using time to delineate ClimbingRepeats, for instance, some athletes modify the workout slightly to use landmarks on a climb that approximates the desired interval time. If you climb that same segment four times in a workout, and multiple times over a period of weeks, you can use the Effort Comparison tool in Strava to see how your speed changes from one effort to another.

You need to have a Strava Premium account to use the tool. First, select a segment from a recent ride. When you open the details for that instance, click on "Compare." On the next screen you have the opportunity to compare your current performance to your personal record (PR) on that segment. You can also choose up to five records to compare. I recommend using this tool for longer segments (5+ minutes) and use your PR as the baseline record. If your PR was set a long time ago in very different conditions (a strong tailwind and you weighed 10 pounds less), then a better baseline effort would be one that is more indicative of the performance you are aiming to get to in the next few months.

The Effort Comparison tool can give you insight on pacing for longer segments. If you use your PR as the baseline effort, the distance between baseline and the line representing your current effort or selected rides will increase as you get slower or faster than PR pace at that point in the segment. The best use of this tool is to see where you suddenly slow compared to your PR time.

As your fitness improves, the lines on the Effort Comparison graph will get closer as your segment times become more consistent. For longer segments, however, you will likely notice a point at which the slower instances start to get progressively slower; the lines representing these efforts will get farther from the baseline effort. If you are making progress with your fitness you will notice that it takes longer and longer to reach this point of divergence, meaning you are gaining the fitness to stay at or near PR pace longer. When you add more efforts to the comparison you should see not only that it takes longer to reach the point of divergence but that the extent of slowing from PR pace also diminishes.

This description assumes you have a previous PR you are working to get back to and eventually exceed. If you are making steady progress and setting new PRs, you should still use the comparison tool with your PR as the baseline effort. But instead of looking for the places where a lack of fitness is causing you to slow down, you can use the tool to see where your newfound fitness gave you the power to move ahead of previous efforts.

The Effort Comparison tool can also be good for pacing, as it will show you what happens when you push the pace in one area of a long segment versus saving that energy for another area. For instance, if there is a quarter-mile steep pitch in the middle of a 10-minute segment, you could charge that pitch and go 20 seconds faster, but will expending that energy mean you have to slow down substantially after the pitch lessens? With the Effort Comparison tool, you can try both strategies and see whether gaining those 20 seconds costs you a minute later on, or whether the effort is worth the cost because you can recover quickly afterward.

The weakness of the Effort Comparison tool is that it is based on speed and not power, so it is susceptible to variations from wind, temperature, hydration status, and so on. As a result, it's important to consider the context of the efforts you're comparing and try to compare efforts that were performed in reasonably similar conditions.

The Effort Comparison tool can give you great insights by enabling you to compare your efforts to your competitors'. Obviously this only applies to competitors who upload data to Strava, but when they do you can see where you were faster and slower than other riders on a given segment. This can provide valuable information for your training when you see patterns emerge. For example, while comparing data you may find that you are consistently losing time after the 5-minute mark of a longer climb. Or you might see that you are faster than the competition on the climbs but losing time on technical descents, which means that more skill and technique work is necessary. Remember, races are not won by the biggest aerobic engine but by the smartest and most skillful riders.

The Effort Comparison tool is another significant point of difference between TrainingPeaks and Strava. Even comparing your own efforts is far more labor-intensive in TrainingPeaks than Strava, and the ability to compare your efforts to others' is currently not an option in TrainingPeaks at all.

Power Curve. The Power Curve is another feature of a Strava Premium account. To access this feature, go to the "Training" tab on the top menu and select "Power Curve." The screen you will see shows your Power Curve for the preceding 6 weeks and gives you the opportunity to compare it against another time frame. You can also view the Power Curve for any individual ride by opening up that activity and selecting "Power Curve" from the left side menu.

The concept of the Power Curve is to slice your data and graph your peak power outputs at a range of times. The general trend of this data will be from highest power values for the shortest periods to lowest power values for longer time frames. This makes logical sense, as it is pretty obvious that you'll do the best 5 minutes of your ride at a higher power output than your best 20 minutes.

The shape of the curve matters, too. As your training improves various aspects of your fitness, you will see that improvement reflected in your Power Curve. For instance, as your power at VO_2max increases, the height of the curve in the 0–5 minute area will rise. This should subsequently lead to an increase, albeit a smaller one, in the height of the curve in the 10–30 minute range. The more you focus your training on power at lactate threshold, the more the middle portion of the curve may flatten out. As your improved fitness enables you to maintain LT power longer, you will see less decline as the efforts get longer.

Over time, your Power Curve can also help you identify areas of your physiology that are more adaptable than others. Sometimes athletes think of this along the lines of their strengths and weaknesses. VO_2max is somewhat trainable, and power at lactate threshold is perhaps the most trainable part of an endurance athlete's physiology. But different athletes respond to training based on their unique physiology, so some riders may find their power at VO_2max responds quickly and significantly with focused training. Another athlete might do the same training and not see as much of an increase in the peak power in the 1–5 minute range. Similarly, focused training might dramatically increase one athlete's peak power outputs in the 10–20 minute range, but that same athlete might have more trouble raising VO_2max power outputs, even with a similar level of training focus.

Fitness and Freshness. One of the most useful and valuable analysis tools available in Strava Premium accounts is the Fitness and Freshness feature. The purpose of the tool is to aggregate data on training load and fatigue over time in order to provide a snapshot of your current form. "Form" can be thought of as your readiness to perform. If your form is good, you are ready to perform at a high level. In order to have good form, you need to have good fitness and not be burdened by a lot of fatigue. Regardless of how much fitness you have, if your fatigue values are too elevated you won't be able to access the fitness you have, and hence your actual readiness to perform will be low.

The Fitness and Freshness tool uses an impulse-response model to determine the impact individual rides will have on your fitness. This model assigns a "Training Load" (if you're using power) and/or "Suffer Score" (if you're using heart rate) to each ride you record. These scores are based on the distribution of efforts during the ride compared to your maximum sustainable power and/or heart rate. Strava utilizes functional threshold power (FTP), which is calculated from your best 20-minute power. Your FTP number calculated by Strava will be slightly different than your result from the CTS Field Test, as I'll explain later in this chapter. The more time you spend at high power outputs during a ride, the higher the Training Load will be. Training Load will also be high from long rides, even though the distribution of power outputs will favor lower, sub-threshold values.

The dose-response model, originally described by Dr. Eric Bannister, essentially says that following a dose of training stress, fitness will increase and then gradually decrease. Additional doses of training will improve the response, meaning there's an additive effect of repeated doses of training stress on fitness. For best results, though, the doses of training stress have to be appropriately sized and spaced apart. What we see with athletes who only train on weekends is that the time between the application of training stress is too long. The fitness stimulus from the previous weekend has declined too much for the coming weekend's training to significantly build on it.

The dose-response model can be applied to fatigue in a similar fashion. The big difference between using this model to look at fitness and fatigue is that Training Load affects fitness more slowly and fatigue more quickly. In other words, today's hard ride increases fitness a little but spikes fatigue more greatly. Fatigue accumulates faster than fitness builds. But with rest, fatigue disappears faster than fitness declines. This difference in how fitness and fatigue respond to recovery is crucial to developing your form—your ability to perform at a high level.

Form is the difference between fitness and fatigue (Fitness – Fatigue = Form). Therefore, when fitness is high and you are well rested, form is very good. But to get there you have to accumulate enough training load to increase your fitness. This drives up your fatigue, and because fatigue rises faster than fitness, your form during hard training periods will be in negative numbers. The key is to keep your form from getting too negative, which indicates you tilted the balance too far toward being more fatigued than you can adequately recover from and continue with productive training.

If your form goes below –30 during a period of purposeful training, it indicates you may need more recovery between training sessions or a reduction in the workload of your training sessions. On the other end of the spectrum, once you have been resting or lightly active for several days or more, you don't want your form value to get above about 10 to 15 before returning to training. If you are peaking for a big event, getting form values closer to 20–25 is good, but more than that isn't necessarily better because your training load is now so low—and has been so low for so long—that you will start losing fitness.

For users of TrainingPeaks software, Strava's Fitness and Freshness tool will sound very familiar. The model is essentially the same as TrainingPeaks' Training Stress Balance (TSB), which subtracts fatigue (defined as Chronic

Training Load, or CTL) from fitness (defined as Acute Training Load, or ATL) to calculate TSB.

ESTABLISHING EFFECTIVE TRAINING INTENSITY RANGES: THE CTS FIELD TEST

Performance testing is a crucial part of training, because an accurate test provides a snapshot of your current level of fitness and allows athletes and coaches to determine whether progress has been made. As you grow stronger, testing provides a means for adjusting training intensities so you can continue to challenge yourself.

There are two primary categories of performance testing: lab and field. In the lab we put you on an ergometer and run you through a series of steps at ever-increasing power outputs. At the same time, you're breathing into a tube so we can analyze the composition of your inspired and expired air, and we're pricking your finger to measure the amount of lactate present in your blood. At the end of a combined lactate threshold/VO_2max test, the information is analyzed, and we can provide you with an accurate determination of your power output at lactate threshold, power at VO_2max, and blood lactate levels at both points.

In the field, we can determine the power output and/or heart rate you can sustain for an effort of a given duration. Although that probably sounds like a paltry amount of information compared to a lab test, the fact is that there's a strong correlation between the accuracy of lab and field tests. Having tested thousands of athletes using both methods, I generally prefer field testing, because it is easier to fit into an athlete's schedule, it's cheaper and more accessible to more athletes, and it provides data that are just as useful for achieving all the aforementioned goals for performance testing.

In addition, because the field test is often completed in real-world conditions out on the road, it provides athletes with greater context for their performance. They experience all the sensations (speed, wind, road feel, etc.) of riding an all-out effort, which can help them better judge their efforts during rides and races when they may not be able to see information from a power meter or heart rate monitor.

There are numerous methods for field testing involving efforts of varying durations. The CTS Field Test consists of two 8-minute, all-out time trials separated by 10 minutes of easy spinning recovery. If you have read my previous books, you'll notice this is different from the original recommendation of two 3-mile time trials. The difference is mostly one of semantics: Instead of gauging improvement by completing 3 miles faster, I have changed the test so you can gauge improvement by covering more distance in 8 minutes. This updated recommendation also translates better to indoor trainers, where distance isn't typically measured at all. It also reflects the increased use of power meters, because training with power relies heavily on information about your sustainable output for a given period of time rather than on distance.

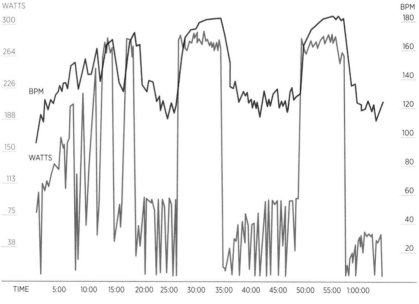

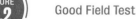

FIGURE 4.2

Good Field Test

The test depicted shows a proper warm-up with some high-intensity efforts before two steady field test efforts. Power is consistent in the first 8 minutes. The second 8 minutes also show a relatively even effort until the final drop in power, indicating that the athlete has reached fatigue. This is a good indicator that the field test was run properly and that the athlete gave a full effort.

In a study published in the *Journal of Strength and Conditioning Research* (Klika et al. 2007), the CTS Field Test was shown to be an effective method for establishing training intensities. Fifty-six participants performed both a lactate threshold test in a lab and the CTS Field Test on an indoor trainer before a CTS-designed, 8-week, power-based indoor training program. At the end of 8 weeks, participants performed both tests again and, on average, experienced a 12.9 percent increase in power at lactate threshold. There was a statistically significant correlation between their improvement in the lab and their improvement as measured by the CTS Field Test. The study concluded that the CTS Field Test is "a valid measure of fitness and changes in fitness, and provided data for the establishment of training ranges." Figures 4.2, 4.3, and 4.4 show examples of results from the CTS Field Test.

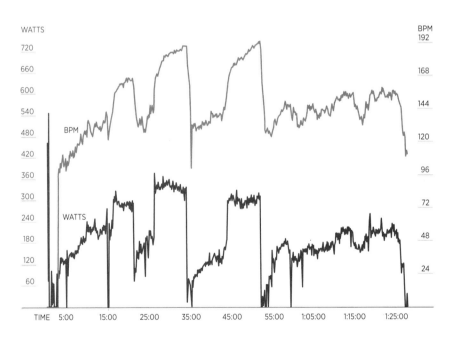

Inexperienced Field Test

FIGURE 4.3

In contrast to the steady effort in Figure 4.2, this graph shows a strong first field test followed by a significant drop in power (watts) for the second test. This indicates that the rider, while strong, lacks endurance and the ability to hold high power for repeatable efforts. This is not a "bad" field test; in fact, it reveals a tremendous amount about the athlete's specific need to develop the aerobic energy system.

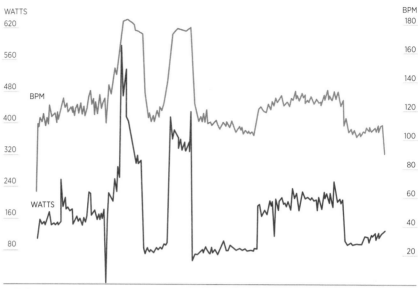

 FIGURE 4.4

Bad Field Test

You can see from the sharp spike in power at the start of the field test and the rapid decline that this athlete did not pace himself well for the entire 8-minute effort. He went out too hard, had to slow down, and then pushed again at the end of the effort (indicated by the sharp upward slope of the wattage data). To achieve a better field test result, you want to use the first 45–60 seconds of each effort to gradually get up to speed.

Why 8 Minutes?

Some athletes and coaches ask me about the rationale behind the two 8-minute efforts that make up the CTS Field Test. My field test is unique in its brevity; it's not a 60-minute or even a 20-minute time trial because I've found that I don't need to put athletes through such an effort to gather the necessary data. It's not that a 60- or 20-minute time trial effort won't work; in fact, those tests work quite well. However, my coaches and I work with a very broad spectrum of athletes, and a field test of two 8-minute efforts can be performed well by novices as well as by experienced masters competitors and even pros.

I prefer two 8-minute efforts over one longer effort because I believe there's valuable information to be gained from observing your ability to recover from and repeat a hard effort. With a 10-minute recovery period between efforts, an athlete with a well-developed aerobic engine will be able to complete the second effort with an average power output within 5 percent of the first effort. If your average power from your second effort is more than 10 percent lower than your first effort, that doesn't change your training prescription, but it gives you one more marker by which you can evaluate progress the next time you complete the test. For example, if the average power outputs for your two field test efforts become more equal, it indicates that your training has improved your ability to recover between efforts. The first effort took less out of you, and you were able to recover from the effort more quickly, leading to the ability to perform a second effort at an equal power output after just 10 minutes of easy spinning recovery.

Sometimes an athlete has a higher average power on the second effort of the CTS Field Test, and this can often be attributed to one of two factors: He or she was cautious on the first effort and held back, or he/she didn't warm up well enough before the field test (the first effort, then, was in essence the end of the athlete's warm-up). In either case, training ranges are established from the higher of the athlete's two average power outputs or heart rates, so the fact that the CTS Field Test consists of two efforts allows us to establish accurate training ranges despite a poor performance on one part of the test.

In a test that consists of one longer effort, either the learning curve of the test or a poor warm-up is more likely to result in training intensities that are lower than they should be. In the long run, this isn't all that harmful to an athlete's training, because training intensities will most likely be corrected by subsequent tests, and most athletes make performance gains even if their training intensities are a little lower than they could be. Nevertheless, through testing thousands of athletes with the CTS Field Test, I have found that it provides greater accuracy the first time around as well as in subsequent tests.

WHAT ABOUT VO$_2$MAX TESTING?

An athlete's VO$_2$max is defined as the maximum amount of oxygen the body can take in and use per minute, and it's often expressed relative to body weight. During their professional careers, some elite cyclists have recorded VO$_2$max values of more than 80 milliliters per kilogram per minute (ml/kg/min.). The average sedentary human has a VO$_2$max of about 40, and a well-trained cyclist will often have values from 55 to 65 ml/kg/min.

Genetics play a pivotal role in determining your VO$_2$max, but it also responds to training. You can increase your absolute VO$_2$max, the power you can produce at VO$_2$max, and how long you can sustain efforts at this maximal intensity. However, on a percentage basis, lactate threshold responds to training better than VO$_2$max does. An untrained athlete could conceivably double his or her power at lactate threshold but would not be able to raise a starting VO$_2$max of 40 ml/kg/min. all the way to 80 unless he or she was born with the genetics to have a VO$_2$max of 80 ml/kg/min. In other words, you can improve your power at threshold to a greater extent than you can your power at VO$_2$max. On the other hand, a relatively small improvement in power at VO$_2$max—and the amount of time you can sustain that power—can have a significant impact on performance at lower intensities.

A scenario we often aim for in training is to improve both power at VO$_2$max and power at lactate threshold, with the overall goal of getting an athlete's LT power to be a higher percentage of his or her VO$_2$max power. For example, when CTS Premier coach Nick White was coaching triathlete Craig Alexander in preparation for the 2008 Ironman World Championships, he found that Craig's LT power was only 77 percent of his power at VO$_2$max. Through training, Craig's power at VO$_2$max increased, but perhaps more important, his power at threshold increased to about 85 percent of his VO$_2$max power. That meant he was able to use a greater percentage of his aerobic capacity for sustained efforts. In Kona he stayed near the leaders in the swim, rode conservatively on the bike to save energy, and came from minutes behind during the marathon to win his first Ironman World Championship.

Interestingly, ultramarathon runners typically have the opposite problem, in that their lactate threshold is sometimes 95–97 percent of their VO_2max. Based on the paragraph above, this would seem like an ideal situation, but CTS coach Jason Koop, who works with many top ultramarathon runners and is author of *Training Essentials for Ultrarunning*, recognized that in the ultrarunning community the problem was that not enough attention had been paid to maximizing VO_2max. Elite ultrarunners could sustain paces so close to their maximum aerobic capacity because they weren't training to improve maximum capacity! By incorporating VO_2max intervals into ultramarathon training plans (which seemed crazy since paces for 100-mile running races generally reflect low-to-moderate-intensity running), he essentially raised the performance ceiling for ultrarunners, which then provided room to raise their lactate threshold running paces.

Because VO_2max intervals are a major part of the TCTP (CTS PowerIntervals are VO_2max intervals), many athletes want to know whether they should have a VO_2max test done. There's certainly no harm in getting a VO_2max test, especially because it can often be tacked onto the end of a lactate threshold test. However, if you can't get your VO_2max tested, don't worry about it. The reason that LT testing or field testing is so important is that we need to establish an accurate training range for efforts that are somewhere between moderately challenging and very strenuous. Accuracy counts because riding too easy won't provide the necessary stimulus, and riding too hard means you'll fatigue before you accumulate enough interval time. With VO_2max intervals, the intensity is as hard as you can go, which simplifies matters greatly because it means the intervals can be just as effective whether you've had a VO_2max test or not.

The CTS Field Test Versus Other Performance Tests

The other major question my coaches and I are asked about field testing is whether the power or heart rate we use to establish training ranges is equal to an athlete's power or heart rate at lactate threshold. The answer is no, but the results from the CTS Field Test correlate predictably with results from laboratory testing, so a conversion factor can be applied to your numbers to establish accurate training ranges.

One of the reasons some coaches prefer longer field test efforts is that longer tests result in average power numbers that are closer to actual lab-tested lactate threshold power outputs. The reason for this is that you can maintain an effort well above your lactate threshold for a short period of time, but because LT pretty much defines the upper limit of your sustainable power output, if you ride long enough you'll settle into a pace that's very close to—and most likely below—your lactate threshold power output.

This is another situation in which sports science doesn't necessarily work to an athlete's benefit. Yes, a 60-minute time trial could provide a relatively accurate estimation of your lactate threshold power output, but only if you can stay motivated to ride all-out for a full hour. If you can't—and there's no shame in that; most novices and amateur racers struggle with such a long, intense effort—your numbers are going to be low, and you'll establish training intensities that are lower than they should be. Even if you could stay motivated enough to complete a great 60-minute time trial, it would be difficult to integrate that into your training program on a regular basis because it's such a demanding workout in and of itself.

After thousands of tests, my coaches and I have found that the CTS Field Test generates average power outputs that are about 10 percent above an athlete's lab-tested lactate threshold power output. In the calculations that I present for establishing your own training intensity ranges, this 10 percent is already factored into the equations in the tables. In other words, you'll take your actual power output or heart rate from the field test and plug it directly into the equation.

We have been using the CTS Field Test and the corresponding training intensity calculations for many years, and the accuracy of this method was proven in the Klika et al. study (2007), which was conducted in Aspen, Colorado. The study found that participants' maximum sustainable power outputs, as measured by the CTS Field Test on an indoor trainer, were 7.5 percent higher than their lab-tested power at lactate threshold. However, it is important to remember that the study was conducted at an elevation of 9,000 feet, where not only is power at lactate threshold lower than at sea level, but the ability to sustain efforts above threshold is even more limited. Therefore, I have continued to use the 10 percent conversion factor for calculating training intensity ranges from CTS Field Test data.

One popular field test, published in *Training and Racing with a Power Meter* by Hunter Allen and Andrew Coggan, is a 20-minute time trial. This test is a good one; it's short enough that many athletes can complete a high-quality effort. Allen and Coggan also use a conversion factor to account for the difference between an athlete's field test power and his or her predicted lactate threshold power. In their system, athletes record their average power output from a 20-minute time trial, multiply this number by 0.95, and then apply a series of percentages to the resulting power output to establish power training intensities. They multiply by 0.95 initially because an athlete's 20-minute power output will be about 5 percent higher than that same athlete's power output in a 60-minute effort—which is also about equal to an athlete's lab-tested lactate threshold power output. Essentially, if you consider a 60-minute test to be roughly equal to power at lactate threshold, then a 20-minute test will give you a power output 5 percent higher than that, and the CTS Field Test will give you a power output another 5 percent above that.

The CTS Field Test

The CTS Field Test establishes the baseline for your training, so you should complete the test before you begin the TCTP. If you decide to use the program more than once in a season, you should perform a new field test each time before starting the program again.

When you view the workouts and training programs, you'll notice that the CTS Field Test is not included as a workout at the very beginning of the schedule. That's because it is a separate process that precedes the programs, and I want you to complete it a few days before you begin any of the training programs.

Make sure you're well rested before taking the test. Don't perform the test the day after a major race or hard century ride because you won't be able to determine how fatigue affects your results. When performing the CTS Field Test, collect the following data:

- Average heart rate for each effort
- Max heart rate for each effort
- Average power for each effort
- Average cadence for each effort
- Weather conditions (warm vs. cold, windy vs. calm, etc.)
- Course conditions (indoors vs. outdoors, flat vs. hilly, point-to-point vs. out-and-back, etc.)
- Rating of perceived exertion (RPE) for each effort (how hard you felt you were working on a scale of 1 to 10)

The field test itself consists of two 8-minute efforts, but it's important to be properly fueled and warmed up before beginning the first time trial. Refer to the pre-workout nutrition tips in Chapter 11 for more information on optimal pre-workout meals and snacks. When you get on the bike, you'll need time to complete the warm-up, the field test, and a good cool-down, so budget a total of an hour for the entire field test workout.

FIELD TEST WARM-UP

Start with 10 minutes of easy to moderate-intensity riding and then complete the following warm-up routine (details on FastPedal and PowerInterval workouts can be found in Chapter 5):

1 minute FastPedal (in a light gear, bring your cadence up as high as you can without bouncing in the saddle)

1 minute easy spinning recovery

2 minutes FastPedal

1 minute easy spinning recovery

1 minute PowerInterval (maximum-intensity interval at 90 to 95 rpm; bring the intensity up gradually over the first 30 seconds and hold that effort level through the end of the interval)

2 minutes easy spinning recovery

1 minute PowerInterval

4 minutes easy spinning recovery

Begin CTS Field Test

STEP 1
Find a Suitable Course

The CTS Field Test can be completed on an indoor trainer, which offers the ultimate in controlling conditions, but I have found that many athletes achieve higher power outputs with outdoor tests. I believe this isn't due to any inherent problem with indoor trainers but rather that the sensations of speed and wind outdoors help motivate some athletes to perform better tests outside. The difference tends to be minor, however, so there is no need for a conversion factor between a field test completed indoors and one completed outdoors.

If you're completing the test outside on the road, try to find a relatively flat course or one that is a consistent climb of no more than about a 5 to 6 percent grade. A course that contains rolling hills or a significant descent is not going to produce a good test. Likewise, a test performed on a steep climb is problematic because you end up in a situation where you're just doing whatever you need to in order to keep the pedals turning over; the terrain dictates your effort more than you do. Above all, find a course that's safe and allows you to complete the 8-minute efforts without having to stop for stop signs, traffic lights, and school buses.

For the sake of being able to compare one effort with the other, and one test with another, complete the test in weather conditions that are reasonably common for your area (not on a particularly hot or cold or windy day). You should also use the recovery time between efforts to return to your original starting point so you can complete the second effort over the same section of road.

STEP 2
Begin Effort No. 1

Begin the effort from a standing start. Your gear selection should allow a fast, stable start, not so small that you spin the gear out before you are able to sit down, and not so large you can barely get it moving.

As you gain speed, but before you spin out your starting gear, shift up one gear and accelerate until you have reached a cadence of 90 to 100 rpm. Shift again and bring your cadence back up to 90 to 100, then sit and select the gear you're going to use to maintain a high power output at 90 to 100 rpm. Resist the urge to start too fast; you should reach your top speed about 45 to 60 seconds after you start, not before.

STEP 3
Find Your Pace and Gear

Keep accelerating and shifting until you reach a speed you feel you can barely maintain for the length of the effort. Focus entirely on completing this effort at the highest power output you possibly can. Avoid the temptation to mash big gears; your leg muscles will fatigue quickly, and your power output will drop precipitously before the end of the effort.

Try to maintain a cadence above 90 rpm on flat ground or an indoor trainer, and above 85 rpm if you're completing the test on a climb. The effort will be challenging from this point on, but do your best to keep breathing deeply. If you're hyperventilating (panting uncontrollably) during the first half of the effort, you started too fast.

STEP 4
Stay on It

Every pedal stroke counts, so it's important to force the pace all the way through the end of the effort. Again, don't think about the second effort; just live for the one you're doing now. When you get to the final minute of the time trial, really open the throttle. As I repeatedly remind athletes during the indoor trainer classes at Carmichael Training Systems, you can do anything for 1 minute. Don't let up at 7:30 or even 7:55. Push all the way through to 8:00.

STEP 5
Recover and Prepare for Effort No. 2

When you reach the end of Effort No. 1, you should be drained. But don't stop pedaling. Shift into an easy gear and keep turning the pedals over. Active recovery spinning helps your body circulate oxygenated blood to your tired muscles and flush away waste products.

In the first minute of this recovery period, you may feel there's no way you can possibly repeat the effort you just completed, but you can if you spend these 10 minutes wisely. Take a drink of water, sit up with your hands on the tops of the bars, and relax as you spin. If you're completing the test outdoors, return to the same starting point you used for the first effort. If it takes you a little more than 10 minutes to get back there, that's OK. It's more important for the efforts to be completed over the same stretch of road than for the recovery time to be exactly 10 minutes.

STEP 6
Complete Effort No. 2

Just as you did at the beginning of Effort No. 1, slow until you're nearly standing still and use your gears and cadence to accelerate to your top speed over the first 45 to 60 seconds of the effort. If you're using a power meter, avoid the temptation to pace your effort based on the average power output from your first effort. There's a good chance your second effort will result in a higher power output, but the only way you'll know that is if you give it everything you have.

STEP 7
Cool Down; Record Your Data

Once you finish Effort No. 2, you're done with the CTS Field Test. All that's left is to cool down with some easy spinning for 15 to 30 minutes (or however long it takes to get home). When you get off the bike, make sure to consume carbohydrates and fluids per the post-workout recommendations in Chapter 11, and record your CTS Field Test data in a training log or software program. You can also use Table 4.3 to record your data.

CALCULATING TRAINING INTENSITIES FOR CTS WORKOUTS

In the spirit of keeping things simple, I use a relatively small number of training intensity ranges (see Table 4.1). The whole idea of intensity ranges is to focus your efforts on specific regions of the energy system continuum. As I mentioned in Chapter 2, you're always using all your energy systems, but the percentage of energy coming from each system changes as you move from lower to higher intensities. One of the key principles of interval training is that by spending focused time at specific points along this curve, you can stimulate greater training adaptations than by riding at self-selected speeds.

To calculate your individual training intensities for the CTS workouts (Part II), you need to know either the highest of the two average power outputs or the highest of the two average heart rates from your CTS Field Test. If you have both pieces of information, calculate both power and heart rate training intensities, but use power to gauge your interval efforts whenever possible.

Instructions for Calculating CTS Training Intensities

1. Find the higher of the two average power outputs and/or the higher of the two average heart rates from your CTS Field Test.

TABLE 4.1

Establishing Training Intensities

WORKOUT NAME	PRIMARY TRAINING GOAL	% OF CTS FIELD TEST POWER	% OF CTS FIELD TEST HEART RATE
EnduranceMiles	Basic aerobic development	45–73	50–91
Tempo	Improved aerobic endurance	80–85	88–90
SteadyState	Increased power at lactate threshold	86–90	92–94
ClimbingRepeat	Increased power at lactate threshold	95–100	95–97
PowerInterval	Increased power at VO_2max	Max effort (101 at absolute minimum)	100–max

2. Multiply the power output and/or heart rate by the percentages listed in Table 4.1 to establish the upper and lower limits of your training ranges.

Training Intensities for Joe Athlete

Let's say Joe Athlete completed the CTS Field Test and recorded average power outputs of 300 watts and 296 watts. During the same efforts, his average heart rates were 172 and 175, respectively. He would use the 300 watts and the 175 heart rate for calculating his training intensities, even though they came from different efforts during the CTS Field Test.

The lower limit of Joe Athlete's SteadyState intensity ranges would come out to $300 \times 0.86 = 258$ watts. The upper limit of his SteadyState intensity range would come out to $300 \times 0.90 = 270$ watts. So Joe Athlete should complete SteadyState intervals at a power output between 258 and 270 watts. Table 4.2 shows Joe Athlete's intensity ranges.

Intensity Ranges for Joe Athlete

TABLE 4.2

WORKOUT NAME	PRIMARY TRAINING GOAL	% OF CTS FIELD TEST POWER	CTS POWER INTENSITY RANGE (WATTS)	% OF CTS FIELD TEST HEART RATE	CTS HEART RATE INTENSITY (BPM)
Endurance Miles	Basic aerobic development	45–73	135–219	50–91	88–159
Tempo	Improved aerobic endurance	80–85	240–255	88–90	154–158
Steady State	Increased power at lactate threshold	86–90	258–270	92–94	161–165
Climbing Repeat	Increased power at lactate threshold	95–100	285–300	95–97	166–170
Power Interval	Increased power at VO$_2$max	Max effort (101 at absolute minimum)	300+	100–max	175–max

YOUR CTS TRAINING INTENSITIES

After completing the CTS Field Test, use Table 4.3 to record your intensity outputs and calculate your CTS training intensities. You should also record your data in a training log or software program, whichever you use.

Recording Your CTS Intensities

WORKOUT NAME	PRIMARY TRAINING GOAL	% OF CTS FIELD TEST POWER	CTS POWER INTENSITY RANGE (WATTS)	% OF CTS FIELD TEST HEART RATE	CTS HEART RATE INTENSITY (BPM)
Endurance Miles	Basic aerobic development	45–73		50–91	
Tempo	Improved aerobic endurance	80–85		88–90	
Steady State	Increased power at lactate threshold	86–90		92–94	
Climbing Repeat	Increased power at lactate threshold	95–100		95–97	
Power Interval	Increased power at VO_2max	Max effort (101 at absolute minimum)		100–max	

PART II

Training Programs

When I originally designed the Time-Crunched Training Program, I focused it on short competitions and century rides. The short competition category included criteriums, cross-country mountain bike races, cyclocross races, and amateur road races. These races last anywhere from 45 minutes to about 2 hours; even road races are typically less than 3 hours for everyone other than elite amateurs. The century training programs were designed for events lasting 5 to 7 hours, but with different—and generally lower—power demands compared to the competitor programs.

In the years since the first edition of this book was published, however, athletes have shown over and over again that the time-crunched training concepts can be successfully applied to events far beyond short competitions and moderate-intensity century rides. As a result, I have expanded the number of training plans available in this book and categorized them by the duration of the events you're preparing for.

In Chapter 6 you will find the training programs for short competitions lasting up to 3 hours: crits, road races, cyclocross races. Training programs for middle-distance events lasting 5–7 hours are detailed in Chapter 7. The time-crunched ultradistance training plan, which includes gravel rides and events, can be found in Chapter 8. And if your commute to and from work is a major component of your time on the bike, consider the Commuter Training Plan in Chapter 9.

5

TIME-CRUNCHED CYCLIST WORKOUTS

IN THE COMING CHAPTERS YOU'LL FIND complete training programs for events lasting everywhere from 45 minutes to 12 hours, and all of those programs are built from the workouts in this chapter. We can use the same building blocks to create the structure needed to prepare you for this wide range of events because each workout is designed to address the principles and components of training discussed in Part I.

After spending the vast majority of my life either training as an elite athlete or coaching athletes, I can tell you that while it is trendy to come up with complicated workouts and intricate systems for prescribing training intensity, the truth of the matter is that there's nothing complicated about effective workouts. Sometimes the process of scheduling workouts, balancing work and recovery, and juggling an athlete's personal schedule can get very complex, but the individual workouts used to apply physiological stress aren't complicated.

Another truth about effective workouts is that they are rarely sexy. For instance, two of the most effective cycling workouts are Tempo and SteadyState. Tempo is a moderate-intensity aerobic interval that lasts 20–60 minutes. You just pedal steadily in a somewhat heavy gear (to keep you cadence relatively low) at a power output a little above your cruising pace and well below your lactate threshold. I can try to make it exciting by throwing in little accelerations or making you breathe out of one nostril at a time, but the only thing that really matters is that you accumulate a lot of time at this specific intensity.

SteadyState is the other cornerstone workout for cyclists that is at once extremely effective and extraordinarily ordinary. SteadyStates are 6- to 20-minute intervals near your lactate threshold power output, separated by easy spinning recovery periods half the duration of the intervals. Workouts that target lactate threshold intensity are featured in every endurance coach's arsenal, and people have tried all manner of manipulating workout components in an attempt to create something unique and special. I've been there and done that, and my coaches and I always come back to the simplest, least complicated, easiest to communicate, and easiest to execute versions of workouts.

Training isn't that complicated, and it shouldn't take an advanced degree or a spreadsheet to understand what you need to do on the bike. Furthermore, simplicity is exactly what time-crunched athletes need. These workouts get the job done. If they seem too simple, remember that they were designed for simplicity. You have enough complication in your life; it shouldn't take mental calculus to correctly execute a workout. Remember Ed Burke's advice: Keep it simple. If you follow the instructions for each workout faithfully, you will gain power, endurance, form, and fitness.

CTS WORKOUTS

The selected workouts included here are featured in the training programs that appear throughout this book. Not every workout is used in every training program. Power and heart rate training intensities are included for every workout and are based on your CTS Field Test (see Chapter 4). Rating of perceived exertion (RPE) is also included for each workout, using the 1-to-10 scale described in Chapter 4.

FASTPEDAL (FP)

Training Intensities for FastPedal
RPE: 7
HR: NA
Power: NA

This workout should be performed on a relatively flat section of road. The gearing should be light, with low pedal resistance. Begin slowly working up your pedal speed, starting out with around 15 to 16 pedal revolutions per 10-second count. This equates to a cadence of 90 to 96 rpm. While staying in the saddle, increase your pedal speed, keeping your hips smooth, with no rocking. Concentrate on pulling through the bottom of the pedal stroke and pushing over the top. After 1 minute of FP you should be maintaining 18 to 20 pedal revolutions per 10-second count, or a cadence of 108 to 120 rpm for the entire time prescribed for the workout. Your heart rate (HR) will climb while doing this workout, but don't use it to judge your training intensity. It is important that you try to ride the entire length of the FP workout with as few interruptions as possible, because it should consist of consecutive riding at the prescribed training intensity.

ENDURANCEMILES (EM)

Training Intensities for EnduranceMiles

RPE: 5

HR: 50–91% of highest CTS Field Test average

Power: 45–73% of highest CTS Field Test average

This is your moderate-paced endurance intensity. The point is to stay at an intensity below lactate threshold for the vast majority of any time you're riding at EM pace. The heart rate and power ranges for this intensity are very wide to allow for varying conditions. It is OK for your power to dip on descents or in tailwinds, just as it is expected that your power will increase when you climb small hills. One mistake some riders make is to stay at the high end of their EM range for their entire ride. As you'll see from the intensity ranges for Tempo workouts, the upper end of EM overlaps with Tempo. If you constantly ride in your Tempo range instead of using that as a distinct interval intensity, you may not have the power to complete high-quality intervals when the time comes. You're better off keeping your power and/or heart rate in the middle portion of your EM range and allowing it to fluctuate up and down from there as the terrain and wind dictate. Use your gearing as you hit the hills to remain in the saddle as you climb. Expect to keep your pedal speed up into the 85 to 95 rpm range.

NOTE ON COMBINATIONS

When a combination workout calls for "60 min. EM with 3 × 8 min. SS," that 60 minutes is your total ride time; your warm-up, SteadyState Intervals, recovery periods between intervals, and cool-down are all to be included within that 60 minutes.

TEMPO (T)

Training Intensities for Tempo

RPE: 6

HR: 88–90% of highest CTS Field Test average

Power: 80–85% of highest CTS Field Test average

Tempo is an excellent workout for developing aerobic power and endurance. The intensity is well below lactate threshold, but it's hard enough that you are generating a significant amount of lactate and forcing your body to buffer and process it. The intervals are long (15 minutes minimum, and they can be as long as 2 hours for pros), and your gearing should be relatively large so that your cadence comes down to about 70 to 75 rpm. This combination helps increase pedal resistance and strengthens leg muscles. Also, try to stay in the saddle when you hit hills during your T workouts. It is important that you try to ride the entire length of the T workout with as few interruptions as possible—T workouts should consist of consecutive riding at the prescribed intensity to achieve maximum benefit. This workout is not used in the TCTP but is featured in the supplemental Endurance Block training in Chapter 14.

STEADYSTATE (SS)

SS

Training Intensities for SteadyState

RPE: 7

HR: 92–94% of highest CTS Field Test average

Power: 86–90% of highest CTS Field Test average

These intervals are great for increasing a cyclist's maximum sustainable power because the intensity is below lactate threshold but close to it. As you accumulate time at this intensity, you are forcing your body to deal with a lot of lactate for a relatively prolonged period of time. SS intervals are best performed on flat roads or small rolling hills. If you end up doing them on a sustained climb, you should really bump the intensity up to ClimbingRepeat range, which reflects the grade's added contribution to your effort. Do your best to complete these intervals without interruptions from stoplights and so on, and maintain a cadence of 85 to 95 rpm. Maintaining the training zone intensity is the most important factor, not pedal cadence. SS intervals are meant to be slightly below your individual time trial pace, so don't make the mistake of riding at time trial pace during them. Recovery time between SS intervals is typically about half the length of the interval itself.

WHY ARE THERE GAPS IN THE INTENSITY RANGES?

One of the questions we get from athletes relates to the gap between the power intensity ranges for SteadyState and ClimbingRepeats. The power range for SS is 86–90 percent of the CTS Field Test, and the range for ClimbingRepeats is 95–100 percent of field test power. What about the 90–95 percent area? Or the 73–80 percent gap between the top of the EnduranceMiles power range and the bottom of the Tempo range?

While it would be more convenient for the power intensity ranges to butt up against each other, they are separated and purposely narrow because of

CLIMBINGREPEATS (CR)

Training Intensities for ClimbingRepeats

RPE: 8

HR: 95–97% of highest CTS Field Test average

Power: 95–100% of highest CTS Field Test average

This workout should be performed on a road with a long steady climb. The training intensity is designed to be similar to that of a SS interval but reflect the additional workload necessary to ride uphill. The intensity is just below your lactate threshold power and/or heart rate, and it is critical that you maintain this intensity for the length of the CR. Pedal cadence for CR intervals while climbing should be 70 to 85 rpm. Maintaining the training intensity is the most important factor, not pedal cadence. It is very important to avoid interruptions while doing these intervals. Recovery time between intervals is typically about half the length of the interval itself. This interval is not used as a stand-alone training intensity in the TCTP, but it is used as a component of the OverUnder intervals.

human nature. By giving you a smaller target to aim for—a 5 percent range instead of a 10 percent range—you are more likely to actually achieve the power I want you to achieve. If I asked you to shoot an arrow at the broad side of a barn, you wouldn't focus very much on the quality of your effort. Good or bad, you'll hit a big target. But if I ask you to shoot an arrow at a 5-foot square on the side of that same barn, you're going to pay more attention to your shot. You might still miss a bit, but you'll be closer than if I gave you a bigger target to begin with. That's why I keep the training intensity ranges for CTS workouts smaller. I know you might wander a bit above or below the range, but you'll be closer to the target intensity because a smaller range focuses your attention.

POWERINTERVALS (PI)

PI

Training Intensities for PowerIntervals

RPE: 10

HR: 100% max

Power: 101% of highest CTS Field Test average

PowerIntervals are perhaps the most important workouts in the entire TCTP. These short efforts are the way you're going to apply the concepts of high-intensity training to your program to make big aerobic gains in a small amount of time. These intervals are maximal efforts and can be performed on any terrain except sustained descents. Your gearing should be moderate so you can maintain a relatively high pedal cadence (100 rpm or higher is best). Two types of PI are used in this program: SteadyEffort and Peak-and-Fade.

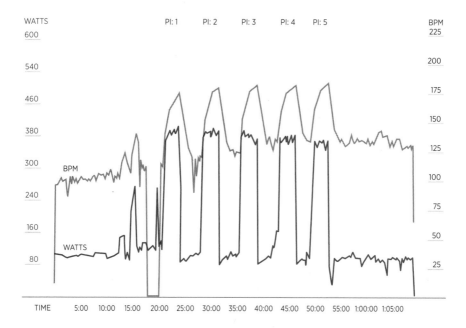

SteadyEffort PowerInterval

This athlete completed five relatively consistent power intervals. Notice the wattage data from each interval forms a mostly stable horizontal line, while heart rate lags behind and continues to rise throughout. This is a good example of why training with power is so useful in providing a picture of actual workload.

SteadyEffort PowerIntervals (SEPI)

Try to reach and maintain as high a power output as possible for the duration of these intervals. Ideally, these efforts should look like flat plateaus when you view your power files (see Figure 5.1). Take the first 30 to 45 seconds to gradually bring your power up and then hold on for the rest of the interval. The point here is to accumulate as much time as possible at a relatively constant and extremely high output. These are the PIs featured in the earlier weeks of the TCTP.

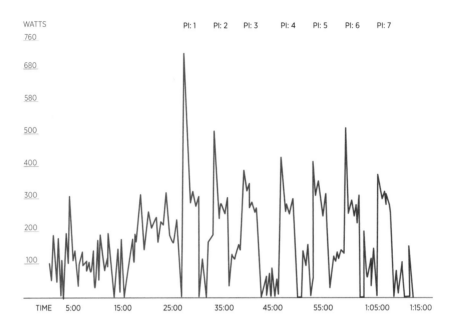

FIGURE 5.2 Peak-and-Fade PowerInterval

During a Peak-and-Fade PowerInterval, you should accelerate hard at the beginning of the interval and continue working as hard as you can throughout. Your power files will show a sharp spike in power followed by a rapid decline. Your goal is to minimize the decline and develop the ability to surge again at the end. (Note: heart rate removed for clarity.)

Peak-and-Fade PowerIntervals (PFPI)

These intervals start with a big acceleration rather than a gradual increase in intensity. Go all-out right from the beginning and keep your power output as high as possible as the interval progresses (see Figure 5.2). Because of the hard acceleration, your power output will fall after the first 40 to 60 seconds. That's expected and perfectly normal; just keep pushing. Keep a high cadence (above 90 rpm) for the entire interval. Don't let fatigue lead you to start mashing gears in the second half of the effort. PIs generate a great deal of lactate and are reserved for the later weeks of the TCTP.

The rest periods between PIs are purposely too short to provide complete recovery, and completing subsequent intervals in a partially recovered state is a key part of what makes these efforts effective. Typically, recovery times are equal to the interval work time, which is sometimes referred to as a 1:1 work-to-recovery ratio.

OVERUNDER (OU) INTERVALS

OU

Training Intensities for OverUnders

RPE: 9

HR: 92–94% (Under) of highest CTS Field Test average, alternating
with 95–97% (Over)

Power: 86–90% (Under) of highest CTS Field Test average, alternating
with 95–100% (Over)

OverUnder intervals are a more advanced form of SS intervals. The "Under" intensity is your SS range, and the "Over" intensity is your CR range. By alternating between these two intensity levels during a sustained interval, you develop the "agility" to handle changes in pace during hard sustained efforts (see Figure 5.3). More specifically, the harder surges within the interval generate more lactate in your muscles, and then you force your body to process this lactate while you're still riding at a relatively high intensity.

This workout can be performed on a flat road, on rolling hills, or on a sustained climb that's relatively gradual (3 to 6 percent grade). It is difficult to accomplish this workout on a steep climb, because the pitch often makes it difficult to control your effort level. Your gearing should be moderate, and pedal cadence should be high (90 rpm or higher) if you're riding on flat ground or small rollers. Pedal cadence should be above 85 rpm if you're completing the intervals on a gradual climb.

To complete the interval, bring your intensity up to your SS range during the first 45 to 60 seconds. Maintain this heart rate intensity for the prescribed Under time and then increase your intensity to your Over intensity for the prescribed time. At the end of this Over time, return to your Under intensity range and continue riding at this level of effort until it's once again time to return to your Over intensity. Continue alternating this way until the end of the interval.

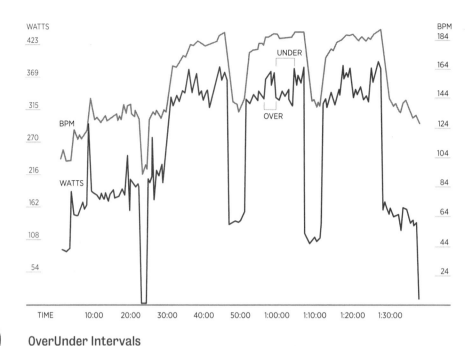

FIGURE
5.3

OverUnder Intervals

In this particular power file the athlete performed three OverUnder intervals, alternating between "Under" and "Over" twice per interval. Note the high-higher-high-higher pattern in each. This athlete also did a great job riding easy during recovery periods.

OverUnder intervals always end with a period at Over intensity. Recovery periods between intervals are typically about half the length of the work interval. (A more advanced version of this interval would alternate between SS and PI intensities instead of SS and CR intensities.)

Note: *In the training programs, the parameters of the OU intervals are written as 3 × 12 OU (2U, 1O), 5 minutes RBI. This should be read as follows: Three intervals of 12 minutes. During the 12-minute intervals, the first 2 minutes should be at your Under intensity (2U). After 2 minutes, accelerate to your Over intensity for 1 minute (1O), before returning to your Under intensity for another 2 minutes. Continue alternating in this manner—in this example you'd complete 4 cycles of Under and Over—until the end of the interval. Spin easy for 5 minutes and start the next interval.*

THRESHOLDLADDERS (TL)

Training Intensities for ThresholdLadders

See Table 4.1, Establishing Training Intensities, to calculate your training intensities for the PI, CR, and SS workouts that make up the ThresholdLadders.

ThresholdLadders mimic the accelerations and sustained power requirements used in breakaways, the start of races, and anytime you need to accelerate hard and then gradually settle into a sustainable pace. They begin with a 1- to 2-minute all-out PowerInterval, followed immediately by 3 to 4 minutes at ClimbingRepeat intensity (95–100 percent of threshold power), and end with 5 to 6 minutes at SteadyState power (86–90 percent of power at threshold).

I won't lie: These suckers hurt. But so does racing, where success is the ability to separate yourself from the peloton and then continue hammering away until you open up a significant gap on the rest of the field. ThresholdLadders generate tremendous amounts of lactate in the first segment of the interval, but then there's no recovery period.

You go directly to ClimbingRepeat intensity, which is still at or even above your lactate threshold intensity. Your body has to learn how to continue producing power while coping with elevated levels of lactate, and that's what stimulates it to produce more mitochondria to process the lactate faster. This adaptation boosts your power at threshold as well as your ability to attack time after time after time.

KNOWING WHEN TO SAY WHEN

As an athlete, listening to your body is one of the most important things you can do to enhance the effectiveness of your training. Even with a perfectly structured training schedule, many factors will influence your ability to complete every workout exactly as it's written. Perhaps you didn't sleep well last night and you're not quite as recovered as you should be from your previous workout. Or maybe a meeting ran long, and you didn't get a chance to eat a good lunch before your afternoon workout.

All athletes experience a workout or a period of time when their bodies are sending them signals that the workload is too high. If you recognize these signals and adjust your workouts accordingly, it's easy to stay on track. On the other hand, if you ignore the signals and blindly plow forward, you could do yourself more harm than good. There are two times when you really have to know when to say when: during an interval session and between workouts.

When to Stop an Interval Session

Interval workouts are only effective when you can maintain an intensity level high enough to address the goal of the session. A good example is a PI workout. To be effective, these intervals have to be maximum-intensity, high-power efforts. Ideally, the recovery periods between intervals give you the ability to complete all the efforts at consistent power outputs. However, because they are so strenuous, you're going to fatigue, and you'll be fighting harder to reach that high power output during the final set. The big question is, as your power outputs start dropping, how do you tell if you should continue with the next interval or shut down and go home?

I've seen a few methods that attempt to quantify the drop in power output over a series of intervals to provide a clear point at which further intervals are not recommended. One of the better ones is provided by Hunter Allen and Andrew Coggan in *Training and Racing with a Power Meter*. They recommend using the third interval of a VO_2max-interval workout as your benchmark and stopping if your power output in subsequent intervals drops to more than 15 percent below that level. I think that method works best when you're doing one long string of VO_2max intervals, which I prescribe for some advanced athletes, but for most athletes I prefer to break VO_2max intervals (PowerIntervals in the programs in this book) into smaller sets. In the TCTP, for example, most PI sessions consist of three sets of three PIs with a 1:1 work/recovery ratio during the set and 5 to 8 minutes of easy spinning recovery between sets. Breaking the session into sets typically allows athletes to accumulate more total work at high power outputs.

Breaking PI workouts into sets, however, makes it more difficult to provide a clear-cut stopping point based on fatigue. For example, it's possible that the third interval of your second set could be 15 percent or more below your power output from the intervals in your first set. But with 5 to 8 minutes of easy spinning recovery before you begin the third set, you may recover enough to match or even exceed your performance earlier in the workout.

Rather than automatically cutting your workout short if your power outputs are starting to fade, I recommend first adding some time to the recovery period between intervals. This means that if your power output from one PI to the next falls by 15 percent or more, add 1 minute to the recovery period immediately following that effort. If the next interval is no better than the one before it—despite the extra recovery time—then you're done for the day. Don't add more than 1 additional minute of easy spinning between efforts, and don't change the recovery periods between sets. If the added recovery time allows you to get through the end of the workout—or even just a few intervals closer to the end—that's great. Completing the work will help you perform your next PI workout without having to add recovery time.

Even if you don't spend the time or mental effort to figure out if your last interval was equal to or X percent lower than the one before it, PIs are pretty much self-limiting. If you're doing them correctly, meaning that each interval is an all-out effort, then your power output isn't likely to decline gradually and

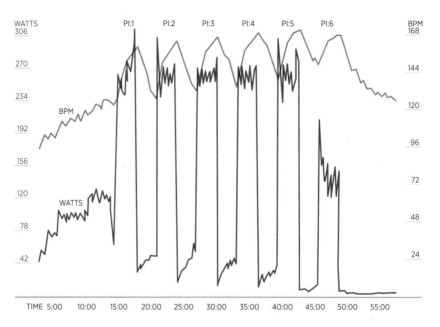

FIGURE 5.4 Reaching Overload

This rider started with 5 strong PowerInterval (PI) efforts but quickly ended on the sixth interval when average power dropped by over 100 watts. It was clear to the athlete that the workout was over. He had reached overload and wisely chose to skip interval number 7.

imperceptibly (see Figure 5.4). Your power won't be just a little lower than before—it will tank. Your legs will feel like bricks, your pedal mechanics will become very ugly, and you'll feel like you're pedaling through wet concrete while breathing through a straw.

When your body tells you it's done, you're done for the day. Grunting your way through one more interval won't make you more of a man or woman, and listening to your body now is going to prevent you from doing more damage to muscles that are already in need of recovery and replenishment.

When it comes to SS and OU intervals, which target improvements in power at lactate threshold, it's not uncommon for athletes to struggle in the final 2 to 3 minutes of an individual interval. After all, these efforts are 8 to 12 minutes long, and they are not that far below the workload from your CTS Field Test (see Chapter 4). However, struggling in the final 2 to 3 minutes of an SS or OU interval is not cause to skip the next effort. More than likely, following several minutes of easy spinning recovery, you'll be able to repeat or exceed your performance in the previous effort.

You'll know it's time to stop if you can't reach the prescribed training intensity within the first 60 seconds of an interval, or if the perceived effort to stay at that power output makes the interval feel like an all-out, do-or-die time trial. SteadyState intervals should feel like 7 on a 1-to-10 scale of perceived exertion, with CRs at 8 and OUs at 8 or 9. Only PIs should feel like 10, and if you're not going anywhere, on top of feeling like your eyes are going to pop out of your head, then you're done for the day.

Hi Chris and Team,

Your program has proven to be very successful for me. I knocked 12 minutes off last year's time in a 100-km participation ride, finishing in 2:44 [22.7 mph]. I found the program to be very hard, and I missed some sessions (although I tried not to miss the PI sessions) due to being tired or family commitments. No one said it would be easy though. I was using a heart rate monitor for my training as I did not have access to a power meter, and although not as responsive, I still gained a great deal from your program. My fitness, speed, and staying power have improved. I will be using the program again. —Jeff J.

When to Skip an Interval Workout

I can't tell you the number of times I've rolled away from the CTS office in Colorado Springs completely convinced I was too tired to have a good workout, only to return 90 minutes later after hitting every single power output I was shooting for during my intervals. Fatigue can be a tricky thing to judge, especially when you're training on a low-volume, high-intensity program. The interval workouts generate a lot of fatigue even though the work times only range between about 18 and 27 minutes for any individual session. At the same time, there are only 4 workouts scheduled per week, leaving 3 complete rest days. For many athletes, this is enough recovery to have consistently strong performances during their workouts. Nonetheless, the intensity in this program may be enough—especially coupled with your busy work and family schedule—to make you too tired to complete a workout here or there. The trick is understanding whether you need a kick in the butt to get you out the door or an extra day of rest so you can get back to kicking butt on the bike.

Since you have so little time each week to ride anyway, your decision shouldn't be whether or not to ride, but rather whether or not you should complete the scheduled interval workout. You should get on your bike regardless, if for no other reason than to ensure that your already limited training time isn't siphoned away any further. Similarly, although I understand the need to occasionally move workouts around in the schedule due to business trips or family obligations, I'm not a big fan of rescheduling interval workouts that are skipped due to fatigue. If you're too tired to complete a workout on Tuesday and you move it to Wednesday, it's likely you'll then be too tired to have a good workout again when you try to get back on schedule during Thursday's workout. I'd rather see you skip the interval session completely and get back on track with a series of great efforts during the next scheduled workout.

But let's get back to deciding whether to complete the day's scheduled interval session. If you're feeling tired when you get on your bike, it's a good idea to start with a focused warm-up and see if that kick-starts your motivation and energy systems. After 5 to 10 minutes of moderate-paced riding, complete the following:

- 1 minute FastPedal
- 1 minute easy recovery
- 1 minute FastPedal
- 1 minute easy recovery
- 1 minute SteadyEffort PowerInterval

By this point you should be about 15 minutes into your ride, and you have completed a few efforts. That should give you enough real information to evaluate whether you're ready to have a high-quality interval session. If you felt like you were really dragging in the SteadyEffort PI, or your power output for the effort was considerably lower than normal for a 1-minute effort, I recommend skipping the scheduled interval session and instead completing a moderate-paced endurance ride. If you were merely struggling with motivation to get out the door, your body will respond positively to these short efforts, and they will effectively "blow the crap out of the carburetor" (a reference that may be completely lost on athletes too young to remember when cars had carburetors instead of fuel injection; for them let's just say you need to clear out the system to fire on all cylinders). But if your body doesn't come around after these short "openers," you're most likely too fatigued to have a high-quality interval session today.

ADJUSTING THE PROGRAMS FOR YOUR PERSONAL SCHEDULE

When my coaches and I work directly with an athlete, it's rare that we can go more than 2 weeks without needing to adjust that athlete's training based on a schedule conflict. It's simply a reflection of the complexity of modern life. When you have a full-time career and a family your schedule changes, and you have to be flexible with your training. After all, when push comes to shove, family and career will come before training.

Because we won't be in your living room with you as you try to adjust the training programs in this book to fit your schedule, I have developed the following guidelines to help you.

Two-Day Interval Blocks Only

If you have to rearrange the workouts within a week, it's OK to put two interval workouts back-to-back on consecutive days, but after the second day it's imperative that you take a rest day. A 3-day block would create a workload that is too high, and it's likely that you'll be too fatigued to perform a high-quality interval workout on the third day. Ideally, you should take 2 days of recovery after a

2-day interval block, but if you need to ride Wednesday, Thursday, Saturday, and Sunday, you'll most likely be fine. Be careful to monitor your training the following week, however, and if you struggle in your next workout, you should back off and convert that day to an EM ride rather than an interval workout.

Hardest Intervals First

If you rearrange your schedule to group your workouts into 2-day blocks, always complete the hardest interval workout on the first day of the block. You'll be freshest on this day, so you'll have the power to complete a high-quality training session. For example, if the two workouts in question are a PI session and an OU session, complete the PIs on the first day and the OUs on the second day. The following list of workouts is arranged in order from highest intensity/workload to lowest:

Highest

PowerIntervals

OverUnders

SteadyState

Tempo

EnduranceMiles

Easy Spinning/Recovery Ride

Lowest

No Makeup Days

If you unexpectedly have to skip a workout, I recommend simply moving on rather than trying to reschedule it. Although you have limited training time and must make every workout count, missing a training session now and then is not going to derail your progress. Constantly rearranging your riding schedule is more likely to cause problems with both your training progress and your work/family/training balance.

Intervals Take Priority

If you have to cut a ride short, strip it down to the essentials. Complete a short warm-up, complete the interval set, and complete a short cool-down. This may be necessary if you have to cut a 2-hour weekend ride to an hour or a weekday ride to 45 minutes. The intervals are the primary source of training stimulus in these programs, so your primary goal should be to complete as much time as possible at the prescribed interval intensities.

FREQUENTLY ASKED QUESTIONS

In the course of working with our athletes on the TCTP over the years, we've fielded quite a few questions about it, in part because it is so different from the programs they had used previously. Here are answers to the most common questions we've received.

Why 11 weeks?

The TCTP is structured a little differently from most event-based training programs. Many programs are designed with one specific goal event in mind, such as a particular century or criterium. In contrast, the athletes who led the development of these workouts sought to perform at their best for a series of races or a period lasting several weeks. As a result, the TCTP is designed to deliver peak performance at about week 8, and then provides training necessary for maintaining this level of fitness for another 3 weeks. For racers who are competing in a local criterium series, you should start racing at about week 6, and your best performances are likely to occur during the weekend at the end of week 8 or 9. Depending largely on your fitness level at the beginning of the program, you may find you can maintain race-winning performance levels all the way through week 11, but it's not unusual for racing performances to start declining at week 10.

The TCTP does not include a longer buildup (say, 12 to 16 weeks to peak performance instead of 8) because we have found that it's difficult for athletes to maintain the focus necessary to complete such a high-intensity training program for 3 to 4 months. These workouts also generate a great deal of fatigue, and extending them to 12 to 16 weeks often leads to a cumulative workload that is higher than most athletes can handle.

 Can I complete a Century program and move right into a Competitor program?

No. You can certainly upgrade from using a Century program to completing a Competitor program, but you still need to separate the programs with a 4- to 6-week recovery/maintenance period (see the last question in this section and Table 5.1 for my suggestions on creating a structured recovery period). Even though these are low-volume programs, the high-intensity interval sessions generate a great deal of fatigue, and you need to allow time for recovery before you will be able to benefit from another period of intense training; the same goes for any of the workouts and programs in this book. A recovery/maintenance period is necessary after using any one of the programs.

Keep in mind, however, that the periods between being on the TCTP don't have to be weeks of easy spinning. You can—in fact I encourage you to—go on group rides, long rides, training crits, and even epic mountain bike rides. Your fitness isn't going to disappear overnight. It's just important that you back off from doing two or three structured, high-intensity interval workouts per week for a while.

 Can I go straight from an Endurance Training Block to the TCTP?

At the very least, you should allow 1 recovery week between the end of an Endurance Training Block (Chapter 14) and the start of the TCTP. If you were to finish an Endurance Block on Sunday and start your high-intensity training program on Tuesday, you'd be coming into the program with a lot of fatigue, and it would be difficult to adequately recover between training sessions in the following weeks.

 Should I do my interval workouts in the morning, afternoon, or evening?

 In more than 40 years as an athlete and a coach, I've yet to see any compelling evidence that one time of day is any better than another for training. However, there's no doubt that individual athletes are better off choosing times that are the least disruptive to their families and professional schedules.

If early mornings work for you because you can get up and be done with your training before helping to get the kids fed and off to school, then mornings are your best training time. If you hate mornings but you're a night owl and you have the energy to train after the kids go to bed, then evenings are your best training time. And if you have the opportunity to train in the middle of your workday. . . well, I'd take it.

Personally, I'd rather go into the office early and ride at lunchtime, because it gives me something to look forward to during the morning, and I often return from my midday rides fired up and ready for a productive afternoon. The most important thing is to find a workout time that fits into your daily schedule and enhances what you're able to accomplish during the rest of the day. If your workout time is disruptive, you're more likely to find reasons to skip workouts.

How can I tell if I should end the program before week 11?

Some athletes will be able to maintain their high-performance fitness longer than others, and some may find that their performance starts to diminish as early as the beginning of week 9. The point at which you're no longer able to adequately recover from the intensity of the workouts in the TCTP will largely depend on your fitness level at the beginning of the program and the amount of prior cycling experience you have before starting it. From week 9 to week 11, the weekly workouts do not progress. The workload remains constant because you are working to maintain the fitness you gained in the first 8 weeks. Ideally your power outputs are going to stay the same for identical workouts in weeks 9, 10, and 11. If your power outputs are a bit low one day, that's not cause for alarm. If they get progressively worse as the week goes on, even if it's in week 10, it's time to start your recovery period.

 Do I need to repeat the CTS Field Test each time I start the TCTP?

Yes. Whether you're using the training workouts in this book or you're on a year-round coaching program, your fitness will fluctuate over the course of a year. As a result, your maximum sustainable power output will rise and fall, and it's important to repeat the CTS Field Test at regular intervals to make sure your training intensities are appropriate for your current fitness level. Most often, when cyclists use the TCTP twice in one season (in the spring and again in the late summer, for example), their field test power outputs are higher the second time. As a result, their training intensities are higher, and they make greater progress.

Over the winter, riders' power outputs tend to fall more than during a recovery/maintenance period that covers a portion of the summer. (This is because you're more likely to continue riding more hours during the summer, even if you're between periods of structured training.) As a result, field test results in the spring are often equal to or sometimes lower than field test results from the previous summer/fall. This is why a good winter training program is important; it's difficult to make progress from year to year if your fitness goes backward for 3 months over the winter.

How can I incorporate indoor cycling videos if I'm doing the Time-Crunched workouts on an indoor trainer?

Many cyclists have a library of training DVDs or video downloads and ask about substituting video workouts for workouts in the program when they have to use an indoor trainer. This is understandable because in addition to the workouts, the videos (whether they're ones CTS has produced or someone else's) provide music and encouragement, which makes indoor trainer time more pleasant and often more productive.

Anyway, the short answer to the question is yes, you can substitute training videos if you're going to be training indoors. However, I think it's best to limit such substitutions to one workout per week, and it's important to choose videos that feature workouts that address the same—or at least similar—goals as the training session that was originally prescribed. For example, if you have a PI workout scheduled, look for a training video that features short maximum-intensity intervals, even if the exact number of sets and interval durations are a little different. CTS-produced videos that fit this description are *Speed Intervals*, *Tour of California Workouts*, *Max Power*, *Race Power*, *Climbing Speed*, *Race Simulation*, *Criterium*, and *Cycling for Power*. Similar workouts from other companies will often refer to being race-specific, high-intensity, or just plain hard.

If you have SS or OU intervals scheduled and you're looking for a training video to use, find one that focuses on intervals that increase maximum sustainable power or power at lactate threshold. These will likely be longer sustainable efforts of 6 to 15 minutes, but the key is that the intervals are subthreshold or in or around your SS intensity level. CTS-produced videos that fit this description are *Epic Climbing*, *Time Trial*, *Climbing*, *Climbing II*, and *Threshold Power*, and titles from other companies will often refer to being applicable to time trials or power at lactate threshold.

Can I use the TCTP even if I don't have any specific racing or touring goals?

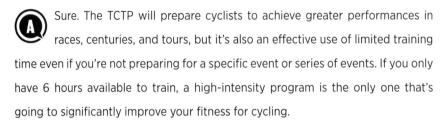 Sure. The TCTP will prepare cyclists to achieve greater performances in races, centuries, and tours, but it's also an effective use of limited training time even if you're not preparing for a specific event or series of events. If you only have 6 hours available to train, a high-intensity program is the only one that's going to significantly improve your fitness for cycling.

We have athletes who have used the Century programs two or even three times in a year simply to increase the average speed they can maintain on their weekend rides. As I've said all along, the purpose of training is to give you the opportunity to get greater enjoyment from your rides. For some riders that simply means being able to ride faster rather than slower when they get a chance to go for a substantial ride on the weekends, and you can absolutely use this program to accomplish that goal.

 How do I adjust the training schedule if I'm racing on a Saturday or a Sunday?

As you may have noticed, several of the training plans in this book have interval workouts scheduled for Saturdays and endurance or group rides on Sundays. Generally speaking, you can replace the Saturday interval workout with a bike race and continue the rest of the program as is. The intensity and variability of the race will do everything the workout would have, and more. However, if you're going to be racing on Saturday, you might want to go out for 30 to 40 minutes of easy spinning on Friday, and throw in three to five 1-minute PowerIntervals just to stay sharp and primed for Saturday.

If you're going to be racing on Sunday, you'll want to lighten up the Saturday workout from what's laid out in the training plan. It's rare for an athlete to see a diminished race performance the day after a 60- to 90-minute endurance ride with three to five 1-minute PowerIntervals and two 3-minute OverUnders (2U, 1O). Keep recovery equal to the interval times for both types of intervals. In the first 6 weeks of any of the training programs, I wouldn't recommend racing twice in one weekend. After that, if you have the opportunity to race Saturday and Sunday, go for it!

 What's the best plan to follow in the 4 to 6 weeks between two TCTP periods?

Although I don't generally believe you need to incorporate too much structure into this 4- to 6-week "off" period, I've been asked to be more specific about the recommendations for it. So here's a breakdown; note that the outline and terms here will make more sense once you have followed the training program at least once.

First week. The week after completing the program should be a recovery week. That means no riding Monday through Wednesday. Start again on Thursday with a light spin for 45 to 60 minutes. Over the weekend, bring the volume back up to normal but don't add structured workouts until the following week.

Second week. Starting the second week, continue riding Tuesday/Thursday/Saturday/Sunday if you can, or more if you're currently riding more frequently. It's important to retain your training time, lest it be siphoned away to other tasks. In other words, the volume of your weekly training won't go down, but the intensity must decrease. During the first 2 weeks that you're back riding (after the recovery week), your rides should be primarily at EnduranceMiles intensity, with 20 minutes spent near the top of your EM heart rate or power range during a 60- to 90-minute ride, and 30 minutes during a ride 2 hours or more.

Third and fourth weeks. Incorporate some efforts at or even above lactate threshold, but there's no need for structure. This would be a good time to jump into

TABLE
5.1

Maintenance Program

WEEK	MONDAY	TUESDAY	WEDNESDAY	THURSDAY
1	Rest day	Rest day	Rest day	45–60 min. easy spinning
2	Rest day	60–90 min. EM	Rest day	75–90 min. EM with 15 min. at upper end of EM power or HR range
3	Rest day	60–90 min. EM	Rest day	75–90 min. EM with 20 min. at upper end of EM power or HR range
4	Rest day	60–90 min. EM with 10–20 min. at SS intensity	Rest day	60–90 min. EM with 6–8 PI-type efforts

EM: EnduranceMiles; **PI:** PowerIntervals; **SS:** SteadyState.

local group rides, and go out and hit the gas on a few climbs. Once you get back into the program there will be a lot of structure and a ton of intervals, so take advantage of this time to avoid following a plan. I've found that athletes are more likely to be able to focus on high-quality interval sessions during the program if they've been good about reducing the structure of their rides for a while before they start. Otherwise, the constant focus on intervals and structured training just wears them down.

Fifth and sixth weeks: As I mention in Chapter 3 (see the section on "Foundation/ Preparation (Maintenance)"), you don't absolutely have to take 6 weeks off, but you should if you can. During these weeks, continue riding as in weeks 3 and 4. Enjoy your rides, avoid too much planning, and keep your volume up while maintaining EnduranceMiles intensity.

I've also prepared a 4-week program (Table 5.1) that you can use as a guide or starting point.

FRIDAY	SATURDAY	SUNDAY
Rest day	Group ride or 90–120 min. EM	90–120 min. EM in hilly terrain
Rest day	Group ride or 90–120 min. EM with 15–20 min. at upper end of EM power or HR range	90–120 min. EM in hilly terrain
Rest day	Group ride or 120–150 min. EM with 30–40 min at upper end of EM power or HR range	90–120 min. EM in hilly terrain
Rest day	Group ride or 120–150 min. EM with 30–40 min. at upper end of EM power or HR range	120–150 min. EM or group ride

6

CRITERIUM, ROAD RACE, AND CYCLOCROSS TRAINING PROGRAMS

THE COMPETITOR PROGRAMS IN THIS CHAPTER focus not only on building greater aerobic fitness but also on preparing you for the repeated high-power efforts of racing. You need to be able to accelerate and to handle rapid changes in pace. You need the power for all-out efforts and also the ability to recover from those efforts while still riding at a high speed. As a result, these programs focus more on maximum-intensity PowerIntervals (PIs) that build power for all-out efforts and help your body learn to process and tolerate more lactate. (See Chapter 5 for the workout description for PowerIntervals and all the other workouts mentioned here.)

There are New Competitor and Experienced Competitor programs in this chapter. The differences between them are subtle but reflect the fact that more experienced riders are generally able to handle a higher workload because they have more years and miles in their legs. If you're an experienced cyclist who has been riding for 5, 10, 15 years or more, you'll be happy to know that even if you're currently not riding very much, the training adaptations from all those years of riding haven't completely disappeared. Your current fitness may be quite low compared to what it once was, but riders who have several years of training behind them are able to handle greater workloads when they initially return to more structured training, and they adapt more quickly and regain a greater percentage of their former fitness.

However, it's important to realize that each of the programs starts with lactate threshold intervals right out of the gate. If you have been riding two to four times a week, participating in group rides or training races, and consider yourself in decent riding condition, you should be able to jump right in and start one of the TCTPs immediately. But if you have been off the bike for a while or have been only riding occasionally, and you can't remember the last time you rode hard enough to go above lactate threshold, you need to spend a week or two just going on 60- to 90-minute rides that include 20, 30, or 40 minutes of time at Tempo (T) intensity to get back up to speed before jumping into one of the programs in this book.

More detailed descriptions of each program, and the riders they're best suited to, follow.

NEW COMPETITOR PROGRAM

If you've been riding fewer than 5 years and want to prepare for criteriums, cross-country or short-track mountain bike races, cyclocross races, or road races up to about 60 miles in length, this is the program you should choose. The weekly workload in the New Competitor program (see Table 6.1) is most appropriate for cyclists who have fewer years of miles in their legs, meaning it's lower than the Experienced Competitor program. The progression also spends more time on lactate threshold workouts before moving on to PIs. Some riders, especially those who have been riding 3 to 4 years, may be able to handle the workload of the Experienced Competitor program, but I encourage you to use the New Competitor program at least once before you decide to complete the harder one. Due to the intensity featured in these programs, it's wise to be conservative with your choice. This is similar to the program CTS coach Jim Rutberg used with John Fallon (read about John in Chapter 16).

EXPERIENCED COMPETITOR PROGRAM

This is the program that riders like Sterling Swaim (see Chapter 1) and Taylor Carrington (see Chapter 3) used because they were experienced racers whose accumulated years of training meant they could handle a high initial workload. Experienced riders also adapt quickly, so the progression in this program is more rapid than in the New Competitor program. If you've been riding and/or racing for 5 years or more, this program is for you (see Table 6.2). That being said, if your current fitness is particularly low because you've done very little training (one or two rides a week) or haven't been training at all in the past 6 months, you may be better off working through the New Competitor program once before moving on to this program (following a 4- to 6-week recovery/ maintenance period, of course). If you have any doubt about whether you should use the New or the Experienced Competitor program—perhaps you've been riding for 10 years but you've barely trained or raced in the past 2 years— it's wise to start with the New Competitor program.

CYCLOCROSS PROGRAM

If you live in a region with an active cyclocross scene, consider yourself lucky. You've got a built-in reason for staying on your bike deep into the year and enjoying the rush of competition without burning yourself out. Since 'cross races are short—30 to 45 minutes on average for the majority of amateur events—they provide a great training stimulus that hits your high-end energy systems, and you can be surprisingly competitive with only a few hours of training each week.

The Cyclocross program has its roots in the Competitor plans; the biggest difference is that you will ramp up more quickly to the point where

TABLE 6.1

New Competitor

WEEK	MONDAY	TUESDAY	WEDNESDAY
1	45–60 min. EM	60–90 min. EM with 3 × 8 min. SS (5 min. RBI)	Rest day
2	Rest day	75–90 min. EM with 3 × 10 min. SS (6 min. RBI)	Rest day
3	Rest day	60–90 min. EM with 2 × [3 × 3 min. SEPI (3 min. RBI)] (8 min. RBS)	Rest day
4	Rest day	Rest day or 45 min. easy spinning	Rest day
5	Rest day	60–90 min. EM with 2 × [3 × 3 min. SEPI (3 min. RBI)] (6 min. RBS)	60–90 min. EM with 2 × [3 × 3 min. SEPI (3 min. RBI)] (8 min. RBS)
6	Rest day	60–90 min. EM with 5 × 3 min. SEPI (3 min. RBI)	60–90 min. EM + 3 × [3 × 2 min. PFPI (2 min. RBI)] (8 min. RBS)
7	Rest day	60–90 min. EM with 3 × [3 × 2 min. PFPI (2 min. RBI)] (6 min. RBS)	Rest day
8	Rest day	60 min. EM with 4 × 3 min. FP (3 min. RBI)	Rest day
9–11	Rest day	60–90 min. EM with 6 × 2 min. SEPI (2 min. RBI)	Rest day

RBI: Rest between intervals; **RBS:** Rest between sets; **Week 8:** End of progression, really good weekend to race; **Weeks 9–11:** Holding on to the fitness; **EM:** EnduranceMiles; **FP:** FastPedal; **OU:** OverUnders; **SS:** SteadyState; **PFPI:** Peak-and-Fade PowerIntervals; **SEPI:** SteadyEffort PowerIntervals.

THURSDAY	FRIDAY	SATURDAY	SUNDAY
60–90 min. EM with 3 × 8 min. SS (5 min. RBI)	Rest day	Group ride or 90–120 min. EM	90–120 min. EM (hilly terrain)
75–90 min. EM with 3 × 10 min. SS (6 min. RBI)	Rest day	Group ride or 90–120 min. EM	90–120 min. EM or group ride
75–90 min. EM with 3 × 9 min. OU (2U, 1O) (6 min. RBI)	Rest day	90–120 min. EM with 3 × 9 min. OU (2U, 1O) (5 min. RBI)	90–150 min. EM
60–90 min. EM + 2 × [3 × 3 min. SEPI (3 min. RBI)] (8 min. RBS)	Rest day	90–120 min. EM with 2 × [3 × 3 min. SEPI (2 min. RBI)] (6 min. RBS)	120–150 min. EM or group ride
Rest day	Rest day	90–120 min. EM with 3 × 10 min. OU (3U, 2O) (6 min. RBI)	90–150 min. EM or group ride
Rest day	Rest day	90–150 min. EM with 3 × 12 min. OU (2U, 2O) (8 min. RBI)	90–150 min. EM or group ride
60–90 min. EM with 3 × [3 × 2 min. PFPI (2 min. RBI)] (6 min. RBS)	Rest day	90–150 min. EM with 3 × 12 min. OU (2U, 1O) (8 min. RBI)	90–150 min. EM or group ride
60–90 min. EM with 4 × 2 min. PFPI (1 min. RBI); rest 8 min.; 4 × 3 min. OU (2U, 1O) (3 min. RBI)	Rest day	90–150 min. EM or group ride	90–150 min. EM or group ride
60–90 min. EM with 4 × 2 min. PFPI (1 min. RBI); rest 8 min.; 4 × 3 min. OU (2U, 1O) (3 min. RBI)	Rest day	90–150 min. EM with 3 × 12 min. OU (2U, 2O) (8 min. RBI)	90–150 min. EM or group ride

TABLE
6.2

Experienced Competitor

WEEK	MONDAY	TUESDAY	WEDNESDAY
1	45–60 min. EM	60–90 min. EM with 3 × 10 min. SS (5 min. RBI)	Rest day
2	Rest day	75–90 min. EM with 3 × 12 min. SS (6 min. RBI)	Rest day
3	Rest day	60–90 min. EM with 2 × [3 × 3 min. SEPI (3 min. RBI)] (8 min. RBS)	Rest day
4	Rest day	Rest day or 45 min. easy spinning	Rest day
5	Rest day	60–90 min. EM with 2 × [3 × 3 min. SEPI (2 min. RBI)] (6 min. RBS)	60–90 min. EM with 2 × [3 × 3 min. SEPI (2 min. RBI)] (6 min. RBS)
6	Rest day	60–90 min. EM with 6 × 3 min. SEPI (3 min. RBI)	60–90 min. EM with 3 × [3 × 2 min. PFPI (1 min. RBI)] (6 min. RBS)
7	Rest day	60–90 min. EM with 3 × [3 × 2 min. PFPI (2 min. RBI)] (6 min. RBS)	Rest day
8	Rest day	60 min. EM with 4 × 3 min. FP (3 min. RBI)	Rest day
9–11	Rest day	60–90 min. EM with 6 × 2 min. SEPI (2 min. RBI)	Rest day

RBI: Rest between intervals; **RBS:** Rest between sets; **Week 8:** End of progression, really good weekend to race; **Weeks 9–11:** Holding on to the fitness; **EM:** EnduranceMiles; **FP:** FastPedal; **OU:** OverUnders; **SS:** SteadyState; **PFPI:** Peak-and-Fade PowerIntervals; **SEPI:** SteadyEffort PowerIntervals.

THURSDAY	FRIDAY	SATURDAY	SUNDAY
60–90 min. EM with 3 × 10 min. SS (5 min. RBI)	Rest day	90 min. EM with 3 × 10 min. SS (5 min. RBI) or 90–120 min. group ride	90–120 min. EM
75–90 min. EM with 4 × 6 min. OU (2U, 1O) (5 min. RBI)	Rest day	90–120 min. EM with 4 × 6 min. OU (2U, 1O) (5 min. RBI)	90–120 min. EM
60–90 min. EM with 2 × [3 × 3 min. SEPI (3 min. RBI)] (8 min. RBS)	Rest day	90–120 min. EM with 3 × 9 min. OU (2U, 1O) (6 min. RBI)	90–150 min. EM or group ride
60–90 min. EM with 2 × [3 × 3 min. SEPI (3 min RBI)] (8 min. RBS)	Rest day	90 min. EM with 2 × [3 × 3 min. SEPI (2 min. RBI)] (6 min. RBS)	120–150 min. EM or group ride
Rest day	Rest day	90–120 min. EM with 3 × 10 min. OU (3U, 2O) (6 min. RBI)	90–150 min. EM or group ride
Rest day	Rest day	90–150 min. EM with 3 × 12 min. OU (2U, 2O) (8 min. RBI)	90–150 min. EM or group ride
60–90 min. EM with 3 × [3 × 2 min. PFPI (2 min. RBI)] (6 min. RBS)	Rest day	90–120 min. EM with 1 × [6 × 3 min. SEPI (3 min. RBI)]	90–150 min. EM or group ride
60–90 min. EM with 4 × 2 min. PFPI (1 min. RBI); rest 8 min.; 4 × 3 min. OU (2U, 1O) (3 min. RBI)	Rest day	90–150 min. EM or group ride	90–150 min. EM or group ride
60–90 min. EM with 4 × 2 min. PFPI (1 min. RBI); rest 8 min.; 4 × 3 min. OU (2U, 1O) (3 min. RBI)	Rest day	90–150 min. EM with 3 × 12 min. OU (2U, 2O) (8 min. RBI)	90–150 min. EM or group ride

PowerIntervals (PI) become the mainstay of your training. You will also do more of them in a given workout, often in 1 long set instead of split among 2 to 3 sets. Here's why:

Leveraging summer fitness: If you were on the TCTP in the summer, you'll have that fitness to build on. If you were on another program or just riding when you could, you're still likely to be more fit in the fall than you were coming out of last winter.

Preparing for flat-out racing: Cyclocross is raced all-out from the starting gun to the finish line. There are no breaks, no times where you can settle in for a few laps or miles and catch your breath. The races are a lot of fun and take a lot of focus, and to prepare your body for that kind of stress you'll need to spend time pushing your body to VO_2max.

Increase the time you can sustain VO_2max power: Raising power at VO_2max is one goal, but another goal is increasing the amount of time you can spend at VO_2max. In this case, that's what the specificity in this program delivers.

During my first season of 'cross, I couldn't break the top 30. After training with the Time-Crunched Cyclist Program, I placed second overall in the series—and the leader was only one point ahead of me! This year, I've even decided to try road racing. Thanks for the book. It's changed how I do everything on my bike, as well as teaching me about nutrition and the science of how my body functions. Thanks! —Justin B.

Supplemental Workouts for the Cyclocross Training Plan

On specific training days, you'll ride your 'cross bike to complete PowerIntervals with a dismount and run at the end or doing practice laps on a makeshift 'cross course you've mapped out. The key word I want you to remember here is "practice." These days are to build skills first, fitness second.

PowerIntervals with Run-ups

PIs with Run-ups have to be done on your 'cross bike. First, find a stretch of pavement, grass, or dirt (something relatively solid, not sand) leading to a small steep hill (grass or dirt is fine) or a staircase. Start your PI on the bike, following the SteadyEffort PowerIntervals format (SEPI), and head toward the hill or staircase. Time your approach so that it does not take longer than 45 seconds to reach the hill/stairs. When you reach the bottom, dismount and shoulder the bike, and then run up the hill/stairs as fast as you can. At the top, remount the bike and take a couple pedal strokes to finish the PI. Take a minute to spin back down to the start and repeat. These are very hard, but effective at making you quicker on your feet when it comes to race-day run-ups.

Skills Practice

On skills practice days, map out or create your own cyclocross loop in a neighborhood park that takes you 3 to 5 minutes to complete. Use sandy playgrounds, hills, staircases, little bits of singletrack, logs, homemade barriers—whatever you can find—to construct a reasonable course. Except for the last 10 minutes, complete your laps at a moderate pace that allows you to focus on technique. Use this time to work on being smooth through a section of barriers, on practicing a variety of inside and outside lines through corners, and so on. During the last 10 minutes or last two laps, go all out, hitting the course at race pace. This way you'll test the skills practiced earlier in the workout and see how they work at full speed. Skills practice days often include EnduranceMiles (EM) in addition to the practice. The idea is to spend 30 to 45 minutes on your cyclocross bike practicing your skills (mounts, dismounts, run-ups, sand, turning at high speed on wet grass, off-camber turns, and so on) and then going for a 60- to 90-minute road ride on either that bike or your road bike.

TABLE 6.3

Cyclocross

WEEK	MONDAY	TUESDAY	WEDNESDAY
1	Rest day	60–90 min. EM with 3 × 8 min. SS (4 min. RBI)	Rest day
2	Rest day	60–90 min. EM with 3 × 9 min. TL 1/3/5 (5 min. RBI)	Rest day
3	Rest day	60–90 min. EM with 3 × 9 min. TL 1/3/5 (5 min. RBI)	Rest day
4	Rest day	Rest day, or 30 min. easy 'cross practice	Rest day
5	Rest day	60–90 min. EM with 8 × 2 min. PI (2 min. RBI)	60–90 min. EM with 15 × 1 min. PI (1 min. RBI)
6	Rest day	60–90 min. EM with 5 × 2 min. PI (2 min. RBI), then 8 min. easy, then 5 × 1 min. PI with Run-up (1 min. RBI)	60–90 min. EM with 15 × 1 min. PI (1 min. RBI)
7	Rest day	Rest day, or 30 min. easy 'cross practice	Rest day
8	Rest day	60–90 min. EM on 'cross bike with 10 × 1 min. PI (1 min. RBI)	Rest day
9–11	Rest day	60–90 min. EM with 8 × 1 min. PI (1 min. RBI); Run-up optional	Rest day

RBI: Rest between intervals; **Run-up:** During last 15 sec. of PI dismount, run up a hill or stairs, remount to complete PI; **CR:** ClimbingRepeats; **EM:** EnduranceMiles; **FP:** FastPedal; **OU:** OverUnders; **PI:** PowerIntervals; **SS:** SteadyState; **TL 1/3/5:** ThresholdLadders = 1 min. PI, 3 min. CR, 5 min. SS; **TL 2/4/6:** ThresholdLadders = 2 min. PI, 4 min. CR, 6 min. SS.

THURSDAY	FRIDAY	SATURDAY	SUNDAY
60–90 min. EM with 3×8 min. SS (4 min. RBI)	Rest day	Group ride or 90–120 min. EM	90–120 min. EM over hilly terrain
75–90 min. EM with 3×10 min. SS (5 min. RBI)	Rest day	30–45 min. 'cross practice PLUS group ride or 90–120 min. EM	90–120 min. EM, or group ride
60–90 min. EM with 3×9 min. TL 1/3/5 (5 min. RBI)	Rest day	90 min. EM with 3×12 min. SS (5 min. RBI)	30–45 min. 'cross practice PLUS group ride or 90–120 min. EM
60–90 min. EM with 3×2 min. PI (2 min. RBI)	Rest day	Race or 30–45 min. 'cross practice PLUS 60–90 min. EM with 8×2 min. PI (2 min. RBI)	120–150 min. EM, or group ride
Rest day	Rest day	Race or 30–45 min. 'cross practice PLUS 90 min. EM with 3×12 min. OU (1 min. O, 1 min. U), 6 min. RBI	90–150 min. EM, or group ride
Rest day	Rest day	Race or 30–45 min. 'cross practice PLUS 90–120 min. EM with 3×12 min. TL 2/4/6 (6 min. RBI)	90–120 min. EM, or group ride
60–90 min. EM with 5×2 min. PI (2 min. RBI), then 8 min. easy, then 5×1 min. PI with Run-up (1 min. RBI)	Rest day	Race or 30–45 min. 'cross practice PLUS 90–120 min. EM with 3×12 min. TL 2/4/6 (6 min. RBI)	120–150 min. EM, or group ride
60–90 min. EM with 5×1 min. PI (1 min. RBI), then 8 min. easy, then 3×6 min. OU (1 min. O, 1 min. U), 3 min. RBI	Rest day	Race	120–150 min. EM with 3×12 min. OU (1 min. O, 1 min. U), 6 min. RBI
60–90 min. EM with 5×1 min. PI (1 min. RBI), then 8 min. easy, then 3×6 min. OU (1 min. O, 1 min. U), 3 min. RBI	Rest day	Race	90–120 min. EM with 2×12 min. TL 2/4/6 (6 min. RBI)

Additional Tips

Start racing early: You have the green light to start racing as early as week 4 in this program. You won't be in prime shape by then, but you need the experience of tackling the barriers, run-ups, sand pits, and weather in a competitive environment.

Race often: Cyclocross season is short and only comes around once a year. There's not much point in doing cyclocross-specific training and then skipping a bunch of the available races. Plus, the experience you pick up will serve you well once you reach peak competition fitness during weeks 9 through 11.

Train on your 'cross bike as much as you can: If you're training with power, swap your power meter onto your 'cross bike. You can also put road wheels on it and train on the road.

Use clinics to improve skills: Find some local 'cross clinics and group cyclocross practices to gain hands-on skills instruction. Another good reference for cyclocross skills is Simon Burney's book *Cyclocross Training and Technique.*

7

CENTURY AND GRAN FONDO TRAINING PLANS

THE TRAINING PLANS IN THIS CHAPTER are designed to prepare you for a middle-distance event like a century or a Gran Fondo. It is interesting that these events now need to be categorized as middle-distance. A generation ago, a century (100 miles) was the benchmark for long-distance cycling. Sure, ultradistance events like brevets and double-centuries and cross-state or cross-country races have been around for a long time, but for the vast majority of cyclists a century represented the longest ride they were aiming to complete. With the emergence of Gran Fondos, gravel races, and endurance mountain bike events, many cyclists are pushing beyond the 100-mile mark, or at least beyond the 5–7 hour time frame that typically characterizes a 100-mile road ride.

I love the 5–7 hour duration for centuries and Gran Fondos. For time-crunched athletes, I think this category of events represents a significant and different challenge compared to the shorter competitions. In criteriums, cross-country mountain bike races, and road and cyclocross races, the biggest challenges for the time-crunched athlete are developing acceleration power, high-end speed, and the ability to repeat hard efforts over and over again. The distance and the duration of the events are rarely issues; it's the physical demand required in that short period of time that's the problem. In middle-distance events like centuries and Gran Fondos, though, the acute physical demands tend to be lower, although the distance, duration, and cumulative amount of elevation change take a toll instead.

People often ask what's different between a century and Gran Fondo. A Gran Fondo sits between a traditional road race and a noncompetitive century ride. Unlike traditional road races, Gran Fondos are mass start events. As in a century ride, everyone from beginners to pros starts at the same time. In contrast, road races are strictly divided into categories and you must race within your category at your given time. A Gran Fondo is run like an open race, in that finishing times and standings are recorded and there are typically age-group rankings, but you can cooperate with anyone out on the road. The lead group on the road might contain pros and age-groupers from their 20s to 50s. And beyond the overall finishing times and standings, you can often compete for rankings on timed segments like particular climbs. Riders who aren't in the front group are still eligible for these prizes and rankings because they are simply based on your recorded time from start to finish of that segment.

To make matters more confusing, the term *Gran Fondo* is—at least in the United States—being applied very liberally to events ranging from 40 miles to 130 miles, and including anywhere from a few hundred feet of climbing to more than 10,000 feet of elevation gain. For the sake of this book, however, let's set the minimum for a Gran Fondo at 100 miles and 7,000 feet of climbing. Why? Because in addition to incorporating components of competition, an event with 7,000 or more feet of climbing in a timed 100-mile ride is a step up from a noncompetitive century in terms of physical challenge.

There are three training plans in this chapter: New Century, Experienced Century/New Gran Fondo, and Competitive Gran Fondo. Compared with the short competition programs in the previous chapter, these programs include fewer maximum-intensity intervals and focus more on building power at lactate threshold. The primary goal of these programs is to increase the pace you can comfortably sustain for your long rides, meaning you'll be doing more SteadyState (SS) and OverUnder (OU) workouts and fewer PowerIntervals (PI). The OU workouts are especially important because they will help you handle the changes in pace and power demands that come with riding in pace lines and over undulating terrain.

NEW CENTURY PROGRAM

The New Century program (see Table 7.1) is the easiest program in this book and is therefore the best choice for a novice cyclist or a rider who is returning to the sport after several years off the bike. Even though it's the easiest of the programs, it is still quite challenging. The ideal candidate for the New Century program is a cyclist who has been riding recreationally for a few years, has perhaps completed a century or two, and is looking for improved fitness and higher average speeds on long rides.

Hi Chris,

I have followed the Experienced Century program this year in preparation for the Étape du Tour, Act 2 [a 130-mile ride through the mountains of central France]. I found the plan really helpful, as it is the first formal approach I have used—up to now it had only been best endeavors. I followed the program pretty close. I generally did all midweek sessions on an indoor trainer and got out into the real world on weekends. I also commute a massive 3 miles to work and back each day, although there's a nice hill on the way home. I'm pleased to say I achieved a successful result at L'Étape. —Dan R.

EXPERIENCED CENTURY/NEW GRAN FONDO PROGRAM

Of all the programs in this book, I have a hunch this one will be used most often. There are a lot of new and experienced racers out there, but there are many more of you who have been cyclists for several years and either have no interest in racing or are quite happy being former bike racers. This is the program that will give you the ability to complete your favorite long rides at

TABLE 7.1

New Century

WEEK	MONDAY	TUESDAY	WEDNESDAY
1	45–60 min. EM	60–90 min. EM with 4 × 6 min. SS (5 min. RBI)	Rest day
2	Rest day	60–90 min. EM with 3 × 8 min. SS (4 min. RBI)	Rest day
3	Rest day	Rest day	75–90 min. EM with 3 × 10 min. SS (5 min. RBI)
4	Rest day	Rest day	Rest day or 45 min. easy spinning
5	Rest day	60–90 min. EM with 3 × 9 min. OU (2U, 1O) (6 min. RBI)	Rest day
6	Rest day	60–90 min. EM with 3 × 9 min. OU (2U, 1O) (6 min. RBI)	60–90 min. EM with 3 × 10 min. SS (5 min. RBI)
7	Rest day	90 min. EM with 3 × 12 min. OU (2U, 2O) (8 min. RBI)	60–90 min. EM with 3 × 12 min. SS (6 min. RBI)
8	Rest day	45 min. easy ride with 4 × 3 min. FP (3 min. RBI)	Rest day
9–11	Rest day	60–90 min. EM with 3 × 10 min. SS (5 min. RBI)	Rest day

RBI: Rest between intervals; **RBS:** Rest between sets; **Week 8:** End of progression, really good weekend to race; **Weeks 9–11:** Holding on to the fitness; **EM:** EnduranceMiles; **FP:** FastPedal; **OU:** OverUnders; **SS:** SteadyState; **SEPI:** SteadyEffort PowerIntervals.

THURSDAY	FRIDAY	SATURDAY	SUNDAY
60–90 min. EM with 4 × 6 min. SS (5 min. RBI)	Rest day	90–120 min. EM	90–120 min. EM
60–90 min. EM with 3 × 8 min. SS (4 min. RBI)	Rest day	90–120 min. EM or group ride	90–120 min. EM
60–90 min. EM with 3 × 8 min. SS (4 min. RBI)	Rest day	90 min. EM with 2 × [3 × 2 min. SEPI (3 min. RBI)] (8 min. RBS)	90–120 min. EM or group ride
60–90 min. EM with 3 × 8 min. OU (3U, 1O) (6 min. RBI)	Rest day	120–150 min. EM	120–150 min. EM or group ride
90 min. EM with 2 × [4 × 2 min. SEPI (3 min. RBI)] (8 min. RBS)	Rest day	90 min. EM with 6 × 3 min. FP (3 min. RBI)	120–150 min. EM or group ride
Rest day	Rest day	90 min. EM with 2 × [4 × 2 min. SEPI (2 min. RBI)] (8 min. RBS)	120–150 min. EM or group ride
Rest day	Rest day	120 min. EM with 2 × [4 × 2 min. SEPI (2 min. RBI)] (8 min. RBS)	150 min. EM or group ride
60–90 min. EM with 4 × 2 min. SEPI (2 min. RBI); rest 8 min.; 4 × 3 min. OU (2U, 1O) (3 min. RBI)	Rest day	150–180 min. EM or group ride	90–150 min. EM or group ride
60–90 min. EM with 4 × 2 min. SEPI (2 min. RBI); rest 8 min.; 4 × 3 min. OU (2U, 1O) (3 min. RBI)	Rest day	90–150 min. EM or group ride	90–150 min. EM or group ride

higher average power outputs, bump up your average speed for your next century, and finish strong in the front half of a Gran Fondo peloton. If you are preparing for a multiday tour, such as a Tour de France camp, this is also the program I'd recommend.

The workouts in this program are designed to increase your sustainable power output. Note that even though the Experienced Century/New Gran Fondo program includes a healthy dose of PIs, they are being applied here in an effort to give your lactate threshold training a boost rather than create the high-end power to handle repeated maximal efforts. For that, you need the structure of the Competitor programs in Chapter 6.

COMPETITIVE GRAN FONDO PROGRAM

It's not the first 3,000 feet of climbing that's going to get you; it's the last 3,000 feet. This training program is a step up from the Experienced Century program because it incorporates more back-to-back training days and a greater focus on climbing. Consecutive training days are important for time-crunched cyclists preparing for longer or harder single-day events because it is as close as you can come to replicating the cumulative kilojoule workload of the event in training. If a 5-hour Gran Fondo will require 3,300 kilojoules but you don't have the time to accumulate that workload in training (which would take more than 6 hours by yourself at a lower average power output), the best thing you can do is to accumulate those kilojoules over consecutive days. In order to achieve this in the training program, you will see back-to-back interval days during the week as well as back-to-back longer endurance rides on the weekends.

Compared to the New Gran Fondo plan, this one will incorporate more total weekly hours, which may push the limits for some time-crunched athletes. There will also be more time-at-intensity, meaning more intervals or longer intervals within workouts of similar durations. I recommend this training program for athletes who want to finish in the first third of Gran Fondo peloton or who have been competing in shorter races (criteriums, road races) within the past year.

Tips for Having a Great Gran Fondo

Be rested. This is a one-day event, so go in fresh and be ready to completely drain the tank. In the days leading up to the event, have confidence in your training and avoid the temptation to squeeze in "one last interval session."

Start fast. Staying with a fast group is important. You can always drift back through groups later on, but if you're too conservative early on you'll be surrounded by riders who can't help you move up into stronger, faster groups.

Keep your head up. Gran Fondos aren't distinctly categorized like your local criterium; the rider in front of you may have power but little technical skill and even less pack savvy. Don't follow wheels unthinkingly.

Start with plenty of food. If you're trying to finish fast, minimize time in aid stations by carrying more food in your pockets from the start. It doesn't weigh much and means that at some aid stations you can just fill bottles and go.

Be patient. As I alluded to before, being a hero on the early climbs burns matches you're going to need for later. No matter what you do, you will get slower as the day goes by and your sustainable climbing power will decline; but if you charge up the early climbs, you'll crawl up the final ones. Be patient in the early climbs, even if it feels like you're going slower than you could. You'll be rewarded with good climbing legs in the finale. How does this relate to the advice above to start fast? It comes down to balancing your efforts. There's a difference between doing everything you can to conserve energy as you stay with a fast group and going to the front of that fast group to show everyone how strong you are.

TABLE 7.2

Experienced Century/New Gran Fondo

WEEK	MONDAY	TUESDAY	WEDNESDAY
1	45–60 min. EM	60–90 min. EM with 3 × 8 min. SS (5 min. RBI)	Rest day
2	Rest day	60–90 min. EM with 3 × 10 min. SS (5 min. RBI)	Rest day
3	Rest day	Rest day	75–90 min. EM with 3 × 12 min. SS (6 min. RBI)
4	Rest day	Rest day	Rest day or 45 min. easy spinning
5	Rest day	60–90 min. EM with 3 × 9 min. OU (2U, 1O) (6 min. RBI)	60–90 min. EM with 3 × 10 min. SS (5 min. RBI)
6	Rest day	60–90 min. EM with 3 × 12 min. OU (2U, 1O) (6 min. RBI)	60–90 min. EM with 3 × 9 min. OU (2U, 1O) (6 min. RBI)
7	Rest day	90 min. EM with 3 × 12 min. OU (2U, 2O) (6 min. RBI)	Rest day
8	Rest day	60 min. EM with 4 × 3 min. FP (3 min. RBI)	Rest day
9–11	Rest day	60–90 min. EM with 3 × 12 min. OU (2U, 2O) (8 min. RBI)	Rest day

RBI: Rest between intervals; **RBS:** Rest between sets; **Week 8:** End of progression, really good weekend to race; **Weeks 9–11:** Holding on to the fitness; **EM:** EnduranceMiles; **FP:** FastPedal; **OU:** OverUnders; **SS:** SteadyState; **PFPI:** Peak-and-Fade PowerIntervals; **SEPI:** SteadyEffort PowerIntervals.

THURSDAY	FRIDAY	SATURDAY	SUNDAY
60–90 min. EM with 3 × 8 min. SS (5 min. RBI)	Rest day	90–120 min. EM	90–120 min. EM
60–90 min. EM with 3 × 10 min. SS (5 min. RBI)	Rest day	90 min. EM with 2 × [3 × 2 min. SEPI (3 min. RBI)] (8 min. RBS)	90–120 min. EM
60–90 min. EM with 3 × 10 min. SS (5 min. RBI)	Rest day	90 min. EM with 2 × [4 × 2 min. SEPI (3 min. RBI)] (8 min. RBS)	90–120 min. EM or group ride
75–90 min. EM with 3 × 12 min. SS (6 min. RBI)	Rest day	120 min. EM with 3 × 9 min. OU (2U, 1O) (6 min. RBI)	120–150 min. EM or group ride
Rest day	Rest day	90 min. EM with 2 × [4 × 2 min. SEPI (2 min. RBI)] (8 min. RBS)	120–150 min. EM or group ride
Rest day	Rest day	90 min. EM with 2 × [4 × 2 min. SEPI (2 min. RBI)] (8 min. RBS)	120–150 min. EM or group ride
90 min. EM with 3 × 12 min. OU (2U, 2O) (6 min. RBI)	Rest day	120 min. EM with 2 × [4 × 2 min. SEPI (2 min. RBI)] (8 min. RBS)	150 min. EM or group ride
60–90 min. EM with 4 × 2 min. PFPI (2 min. RBI); rest 8 min.; 4 × 3 min. OU (2U, 1O) (3 min. RBI)	Rest day	120–180 min. EM or group ride	90–150 min. EM or group ride
60–90 min. EM with 4 × 2 min. PFPI (2 min. RBI); rest 8 min.; 4 × 3 min. OU (2U, 1O) (3 min. RBI)	Rest day	90–150 min. EM or group ride	90–150 min. EM or group ride

TABLE 7.3

Competitive Gran Fondo

WEEK	MONDAY	TUESDAY	WEDNESDAY
1	Rest day	60–90 min. EM with 4 × 8 min. SS (5 min. RBI)	Rest day
2	Rest day	60–90 min. EM with 2 sets of 3 × 2 min. SEPI (3 min. RBI, 8 min. RBS)	Rest day
3	Rest day	Rest day	60–90 min. EM with 2 sets of 4 × 2 min. SEPI (3 min. RBI, 8 min. RBS)
4	Rest day	Rest day	Rest day or 45 min. easy spinning
5	Rest day	60–90 min. EM with 8 × 2 min. SEPI (2 min. RBI)	90 min. EM with 3 × 15 min. SS (8 min. RBI)
6	Rest day	90 min. EM with 3 × 12 min. OU (2U, 1O) (6 min. RBI)	90 min. EM with 3 × 12 min. OU (2U, 1O) (6 min. RBI)
7	Rest day	90 min. EM with 10 × 2 min. SEPI (2 min. RBI)	90 min. EM with 10 × 2 min. SEPI (2 min. RBI)
8	Rest day	60–90 min. EM with 10 × 1 min. PFPI (1 min. RBI), 8 min. rest then 4 × 3 min. OU (2U, 1O) (3 min. RBI)	Rest day
9–11	Rest day	60–90 min. EM with 10 × 2 min. SEPI (2 min. RBI)	60–90 min. EM with 3 × 12 min. OU (1U, 1O) 6 min. RBI)

RBI: Rest between intervals; **RBS:** Rest between sets; **Week 8:** End of progression, really good weekend to race; **Weeks 9–11:** Holding on to the fitness; **EM:** EnduranceMiles; **FP:** FastPedal; **OU:** OverUnders; **PFPI:** Peak-and-Fade PowerIntervals; **SS:** SteadyState; **SEPI:** SteadyEffort PowerIntervals.

THURSDAY	FRIDAY	SATURDAY	SUNDAY
60–90 min. EM with 3 × 10 min. SS (5 min. RBI)	Rest day	120 min. EM	120 min. EM
60–90 min. EM with 3 × 12 min. SS (6 min. RBI)	Rest day	120 min. EM with 3 × 12 min. SS (6 min. RBI)	120 min. EM
60–90 min. EM with 3 × 12 min. SS (6 min. RBI)	Rest day	120 min. EM with 3 × 12 min. SS (6 min. RBI)	120 min. EM or group ride
90 min. EM with 3 × 9 min. OU (2U, 1O) (6 min. RBI)	Rest day	150 min. EM with 3 × 12 min. SS (6 min. RBI)	120 min. EM or group ride
Rest day	Rest day	120 min. EM with 3 × 9 min. OU (2U, 1O) (6 min. RBI)	120–150 min. EM or group ride
Rest day	Rest day	120 min. EM with 10 × 2 min. SEPI (2 min. RBI)	120–150 min. EM or group ride
Rest day	Rest day	180 min. EM with 3 × 12 min. OU (1U, 1O) (6 min. RBI)	150 min. EM or group ride
60 min. EM with 6 × 1 min. PFPI (1 min. RBI)	Rest day	Gran Fondo! If event is on Sunday, then 60 min. EM with 6 × 1 min. FastPedal (1 min. RBI)	Gran Fondo! If event was on Saturday, today is optional.
Rest day	Rest day	120–150 min. EM or group ride	120–150 min. EM or group ride

8

GRAVEL RACING AND ULTRAENDURANCE MTB TRAINING PLAN

I REALLY WASN'T SURE ABOUT GRAVEL RACING until I was out in the middle of nowhere in the Flint Hills of Kansas, 175 miles into the Dirty Kanza 200. It was early in the evening, with the late-day June sun low in the western sky. Golden hour, the photographers call it, and now I see why. What struck me was the quiet. It took 175 miles, but I had reached a point where the only man-made structure I could see on the vast grassland was the gravel road I was on, and I couldn't see another human ahead or behind me. It was wonderful to be alone on a bicycle in a beautiful landscape of flowing grass.

Having ridden with and talked to a lot of athletes who have completed gravel races and/or ultraendurance mountain bike events, the quiet is one of the common threads that draws people to these events. It may take 8 hours or more to get there, but you reach a point where you are finally alone, and in today's ever-busier world being totally alone is rare.

The other common draw to ultraendurance events is the very real likelihood of failure. In shorter events you may fail to stay in the lead group or you may get dropped from the peloton, but it is rare that you will reach the point of giving up. People get pulled from criteriums because they get dropped, but they rarely sit up and quit of their own volition. In contrast, almost everyone contemplates quitting during a rough patch in an ultraendurance event.

For the highly motivated career professional, the notion of failure is territory you may not have experienced in a long time. You have succeeded in nearly every avenue of life. You have conquered the challenge of building a successful career. You are an expert in your field. You haven't failed, in a substantial way, in years. Yet here you are, many hours into an endurance event, wrestling with the decision of whether to continue or accept personal defeat. Quitting is easy; continuing is hard. For many athletes, the underlying reason to enter ultraendurance events is to reconnect with the visceral challenge of facing and overcoming a true decision between success and failure.

There are many reasons why athletes are increasingly drawn to gravel and ultraendurance mountain bike events, and isolation and the chance of failure are only two. For some athletes, these events are the next logical step after participating and competing in shorter events that no longer offer a substantial challenge. Others are being drawn away from training and competing on pavement because gravel roads and mountain bike trails present a lower risk of being hit by a car. Whatever is drawing you to ultraendurance events, the inescapable fact is that you can't dramatically increase the time you have available for training. This leads to the inevitable question of whether the principles and concepts of time-crunched training can be successfully applied to events lasting 8 to 24 hours.

The short answer is yes. We have successfully used low-volume, high-intensity training principles to prepare athletes for success in ultraendurance events, from the Leadville 100 to Dirty Kanza 200, and the Breck Epic to La Ruta des los Conquistadores.

The training program in this chapter fills the need for an efficient training plan that can be folded into a hectic workweek, splits the all-day weekend ride into two more manageable chunks, and yet still prepares you for the wide range of challenges presented by ultraendurance races.

Be aware that this is not an off-the-couch program that takes you from a life of no exercise to the finish line at Leadville. Before commencing this plan, you should have cycled through either the TCTP Competitor program or Century program and ridden through a 4-week recovery-and-maintenance block (see Table 5.1). The people who achieve the best results with this plan are those who are already experienced cyclists and can leverage some of the long-term aerobic fitness they've accumulated over the years. This program was designed for those looking to tackle a new challenge—one that keeps them riding and enjoying the sport throughout the year. The program can be used equally well to prepare for a long gravel event, an ultraendurance road event, or an ultraendurance mountain bike race. It is designed more to create the fitness necessary for a 100-plus mile event than it is tailored specifically for the technical skills of road, gravel, or mountain biking.

THE ULTRAENDURANCE PROGRAM

There's a massive difference in the physical demands of being able to stay competitive in hour-long criterium races on the weekend versus racing up and down 10,000 vertical feet over the course of 9 to 10 hours. Unlike the weekend racers, competitive ultraendurance racers are usually logging at least 10 hours a week on the bike. Many riders are more in the 16-to-20-hours-a-week category. So keep in mind that like the Century plans, this plan isn't likely to produce race-winning fitness for ultraendurance events; there's simply not enough time on the bike prescribed here for a rider to dominate an 8-plus-hour race. Of course, if you prove me wrong, be sure to let me know.

To match your expectations to the reality of the program in this chapter, I'm confident that a reasonably experienced mountain biker who follows the plan closely has a good shot at finishing the Leadville 100 in around 10 hours. Is a sub–9-hour finish possible? It's been done, but it's a stretch for the program, and the CTS athletes who have accomplished that feat came into the program very fit. Those results assume that you have good weather, no equipment failure, no crashes, and a smart nutrition-and-hydration strategy on race day.

The biggest departure from the other plans in this book is that the Ultraendurance plan (see Table 8.1) requires significantly more weekly training hours. That, of course, leads to the question, How can it still be called a Time-Crunched Training Program? In essence, the program relies on the same science and utilizes most of the same weekday training structure. That's the part that targets metabolic improvements: an increase in your ability to produce energy from carbohydrate and fat, and an increase in your ability to deliver oxygen to working muscles and process lactate before it starts building up. But then there are the unique challenges associated with long days in the saddle, and there's no other way to prepare for those than with long days in the saddle. The Ultraendurance plan requires no fewer than 7 hours a week throughout its 12-week schedule and maxes out at 13.5 to 14.5 hours of training during week 10. However, the weekday workouts can be completed in as little as 90 minutes.

Back-to-Back Training

The bulk of this plan's training time is devoted to back-to-back multihour rides on the weekends. These aren't overly intense or structured rides; they're what I call "ass-in-the-saddle" rides where you prepare your body for the rigors of 10 hours of riding. By splitting up, say, the 8 total hours of weekend rides in week 8, you're logging a huge chunk of saddle time within 24 hours. When you get on the bike on Sunday, you'll be fatigued, your back and joints will be a bit stiff, and your sit bones (the ischial tuberosities) may be a bit tender. Riding through the soreness and fatigue is an important part of preparing yourself for the final third of long endurance races.

Midweek rides are short—less than 90 minutes—but still intense, and placed on back-to-back days. I planned them on consecutive days to increase the cumulative workload and better replicate the training stimulus from a long ride. On these longer rides, I'd have a rider completing several 20-minute SteadyState (SS) intervals, longer ThresholdLadders (TL), or more OverUnder (OU) sets (see Chapter 5 for details on these workouts). When there isn't time to put all that work into one interval session, you can achieve a very similar overload with back-to-back interval days.

Because back-to-back training days serve as the foundation of the Ultraendurance plan, Monday and Friday rest days are even more critical. You need them to recover from the training block and give your body time to adapt so you go into the weekend or week feeling fresh and fitter. Don't skip these rest days. Don't use them to make up a workout. If you can't ride on a given day, especially during the middle of the week, skip it and move on. Just try to keep the skipped workouts to a minimum.

If you have time to get in the optional 45- to 60-minute EnduranceMiles (EM) ride in the middle of the week, great. But remember, the intensity for an EM ride ranges from 45 to 75 percent of your threshold power and 50 to 91 percent of your threshold heart rate. Do your body a favor and keep your power and heart rate at the lower end of the EM range for these rides. All I want you to do here is get more time in the saddle and add more miles to your legs.

Climbing Rides

Half of the Saturday rides in the plan call for climbing. This doesn't mean you have to do climbing repeats up the same trail or dirt road for 4 hours. Aim to spend 40 to 60 percent of your overall ride time (not distance!) going uphill. That means at least 90 minutes of climbing in a 4-hour ride or up to 3 hours of climbing in a 5-hour ride.

I understand that it's easy for me to find routes that will accomplish those goals in my hometown of Colorado Springs, while in some areas of the country it's not realistic at all. If rolling hills are what you have, then use them well. And if you live in a truly flat region, you'll have to make do riding into the wind or somewhat over-geared.

TABLE 8.1

Ultraendurance

WEEK	MONDAY	TUESDAY	WEDNESDAY	
1	Rest day	60–90 min. EM with 3 × 8 min. SS (5 min. RBI)	60–90 min. EM with 3 × 8 min. SS (5 min. RBI)	
2	Rest day	60–90 min. EM with 3 × 10 min. SS (5 min. RBI)	60–90 min. EM with 3 × 10 min. SS (5 min. RBI)	
3	Rest day	45 min. recovery miles	75–90 min. EM with 3 × 12 min. SS (6 min. RBI)	
4	Rest day	Rest day	Optional: 45-60 min. EM ride	
5	Rest day	60–90 min. EM with 3 × 12 min. OU (2U, 1O) (6 min. RBI)	60–90 min. EM with 3 × 12 min. OU (2U, 1O) (6 min. RBI)	
6	Rest day	60–90 min. EM with 3 × 12 min. OU (1U, 1O) (6 min. RBI)	60–90 min. EM with 3 × 12 min. OU (1U, 1O) (6 min. RBI)	
7	Rest day	60–90 min. EM with 3 × 12 min. OU (1U, 1O) (6 min. RBI)	90 min. EM with 3 × 12 min. SS (6 min. RBI)	
8	Rest day	60 min. easy spinning recovery ride	Rest day	
9	Rest day	60–90 min. EM with 3 × 9 min. ThresholdLadder (1,3,5) (5 min. RBI)	60–90 min. EM with 3 × 9 min. ThresholdLadder (1,3,5) (5 min. RBI)	
10	Rest day	60–90 min. EM with 4 × 9 min. ThresholdLadder (1,3,5) (5 min. RBI)	60–90 min. EM with 4 × 9 min. ThresholdLadder (1,3,5) (5 min. RBI)	
11	Rest day	Rest day	60–90 min. EM with 8 × 2 min. PI (2 min. RBI)	
12	Rest day	60–90 min. EM with 4 × 2 min. PI (2 min. RBI)	60 min. easy spinning recovery ride	

RBI: Rest between intervals; **RBS:** Rest between sets; **EM:** EnduranceMiles; **FP:** FastPedal; **OU:** OverUnders; **SS:** SteadyState; **SEPI:** SteadyEffort PowerIntervals.

THURSDAY	FRIDAY	SATURDAY	SUNDAY
Optional: 45–60 min. EM ride	Rest day	120–150 min. EM	120–150 min. EM
Optional: 45–60 min. EM ride	Rest day	150 min. EM	150 min. EM
60–90 min. EM with 3×10 min. SS (5 min. RBI)	Rest day	180 min. EM	150 min. EM or group ride
75–90 min. EM with 3×12 min. SS (6 min. RBI)	Rest day	150 min. EM with 3×12 min. OU (2U, 1O) (6 min. RBI)	150 min. EM or group ride
Optional: 45 min. recovery miles ride	Rest day	180 min. EM with 4×15 min. SS (8 min. RBI)	180 min. EM or group ride
45–60 min. EM ride	Rest day	4 hrs. road or MTB EM with climbing	120–150 min. EM or group ride
60–90 min. EM with 3×10 min. SS (5 min. RBI)	Rest day	4 hrs. road or MTB EM with climbing	180 min. EM or group ride
60–90 min. EM with 1×9 min. ThresholdLadder (1,3,5)	Rest day	5 hrs. road or MTB EM with climbing	3 hrs. road or MTB EM any terrain
Optional: 45–60 min. ride	Rest day	5 hrs. road or MTB EM with climbing	4 hrs. road or MTB EM any terrain
90 min. EM with 3×12 min. SS (6 min. RBI)	Rest day	6 hrs. MTB EM with climbing	4 hours road or MTB EM with climbing
60–90 min. EM with 4×2 min. PI (2 min. RBI), 8 min. rest then 4×3 min. OU (2U, 1O) (3 min. RBI)	Rest day	3 hrs. MTB EM with climbing	2 hrs. road or MTB EM any terrain
60 min. EM with 5×1 min. PI (1 min. RBI)	30 min. easy spinning, with 3–5 accelerations to loosen up	Race!	Rest day

Week 10

Week 10 is the most demanding week in the program—in this entire book, for that matter. It calls for around 14 hours of saddle time dominated by a 6-hour ride on Saturday and a 4-hour ride on Sunday. In addition to the physiological challenges of this weekend block, the stretch of time on your bike—and the long weekend blocks before it—will uncover any issues you have with your gear and with your nutrition-and-hydration strategy.

For example, you may discover that your stomach doesn't tolerate sweet gels or sports drinks after 5 hours of riding. If that's the case, you'll need to ensure you have salty or bland food options available for the last half of the race. During my multiple races at the Leadville 100, La Ruta, Trans Andes, and other epic events, I've consumed every energy bar and gel flavor; chomped through baked potatoes covered in salt, breakfast burritos, and other foods; and downed Cokes because the variety helped settle my stomach, provided me with something I was craving, or kept me interested in eating.

Although it is important to keep eating during long training rides and long races, you have to adjust your consumption based on your energy expenditure. During a hard 2-hour road race, you could burn 850 calories per hour or more, but during a 10-hour mountain bike race your burn rate falls sharply because of your pacing. You're going slower, spending more time at aerobic intensities and less time at intensities at or above lactate threshold. So instead of 850 calories per hour, you may be at 500 to 600 per hour. And you're still only going to want to replenish 20 to 30 percent of those calories (probably closer to 30 percent) by eating and drinking on the bike.

The biggest thing to remember is that you can come back from a calorie crisis in minutes, but it can take several times as long to recover from a hydration crisis. Calories get to their destination quickly, so if you get behind with eating, you can make a pretty rapid recovery if you catch the problem in time. But it takes a lot longer for fluids to replenish the areas they were pulled from as you become more and more dehydrated or overheated.

With regard to gear, pay attention to the fit of your shoes, gloves, bike shorts, and helmet. Things you don't even notice on a 2-hour ride are annoying at 5 hours, painful at 7 hours, and excruciating at 9. If your apparel or gear is causing discomfort during the long weekend blocks starting on week 8, find solutions to those problems as quickly as possible. You want to have time to get used to new equipment before the race.

Pay attention to your bike fit and setup as well. An aggressive position that works great for short track and cross-country races might lead to back, neck, and hand pain during a 10-hour race. You may also want to seek suspension tuning and tire pressure advice from riders experienced with the particular course you'll be racing. The right setup can dramatically improve your levels of comfort and control, which in turn help you go faster!

ROAD RIDING TO A BETTER MOUNTAIN BIKE RACE

You're going to want to do the bulk of your training on your road bike unless you're fortunate enough to have a mountain range out your back door that's riddled with singletrack or forest roads featuring long, sustained climbs that take well over an hour to ride. And if your road bike has a power meter but your mountain bike does not, then you'll definitely want to use it instead of your mountain bike for the midweek interval workouts. There are a few reasons for this:

Time. It's much faster to roll out of your driveway and start your warm-up at the end of the block on your road bike than ride or drive to a trailhead to get on your mountain bike. You can also knock out a workout on an indoor trainer in the predawn hours if necessary.

Terrain. Even with great off-road options, it's rare to find a trail that allows you to climb all-out for at least 12 minutes. Switchbacks, technical sections, or short downhills can throw off your momentum and wreak havoc with the work you need to do. On the road, you can still reach the intensities outlined in the program even if it's pancake flat.

Weather. When I was a kid I loved to ride in the mud (who didn't?), but now I know riding muddy trails leads to more erosion, means I have to spend a lot of time cleaning my bike, and increases the wear and tear on my bike's drivetrain. I don't have time for the cleanup and I can't make my training dependent on trail conditions and weather conditions, so when time is short I often find I can train more consistently by focusing my interval workouts on my road bike.

Comparisons of data from road bike and mountain bike power meters also provide valuable insight into the pros and cons of dividing time between the mountain and road bikes. We have several elite-level mountain bike racers training and racing with mountain-bike power meters, and one interesting finding is that overall workload and pedaling time (total ride time minus the time when cadence equals zero) are very often lower on the mountain bike compared to the road bike for rides of equal duration. In other words, there's a lot more coasting in mountain biking.

On the other hand, the high-power spikes during mountain bike rides are more frequent and reach higher power outputs. It's not uncommon to see 800- to 1,000-watt spikes in the power meter file, and the distribution of points in a cadence/force scatter plot is more spread out for a mountain bike ride.

This means that even if workload is constant between a road ride and a mountain bike ride, the workload was accumulated across a wider range of power outputs and cadence ranges on the mountain bike. There are more high-power, low-cadence efforts (accelerating out of a sharp switchback) and instantaneous power spikes (popping the front wheel over a log).

From a training specificity standpoint, mountain bikers have to ride their mountain bikes. But from an energy system standpoint, you can maintain consistent efforts at the appropriate power levels more easily on the road bike or cyclocross/gravel bike. The crossover point sometimes occurs on forest service roads, if you live in a place where they are prevalent. Living in Colorado Springs, Brevard (NC), Santa Ynez (CA), and Tucson, my coaches are fortunate to have dirt road climbs that provide the opportunity to maintain road-bike-like consistency for anywhere from 25 minutes to 3 hours. There are other parts of the country, though, where mountain biking is pretty much restricted to laps in a park, and it can be difficult to achieve consistent training efforts in that terrain. If that's the case, I recommend focusing your longer SteadyState, ClimbingRepeat, and ThresholdLadder workouts on the road bike. You can do PowerIntervals on the mountain bike, and you can modify the OverUnders to be less structured and more like runners' Fartlek intervals on your local trail system.

Until week 10, you have the option of doing one of the weekend rides on your road bike. From week 10 to race day, all your Saturday/Sunday rides should be done on your mountain bike. This gets your butt, back, hands, shoulders, and neck used to your mountain bike's fit.

If you are preparing for an ultraendurance gravel event, your road bike and gravel bike will be relatively similar in terms of riding position. The closer you get to your event, however, the more hours you should spend on the gravel/cyclocross bike. Even if you don't have access to a lot of dirt to train on, put road wheels/tires on the gravel/cyclocross bike so you become accustomed to the position and handling characteristics of that bike.

USING THE ULTRAENDURANCE PLAN FOR MULTIDAY EVENTS

I developed this plan with a focus on one-day ultraendurance races, but it also works for those of you looking to get the most out of a multiday cycling vacation or a mountain bike stage race like the La Ruta. The volume of back-to-back miles over the weekend closely matches—and in many cases exceeds—the amount of daily saddle time most people face on a cycling vacation.

You can also use it to plan your own epic adventure. In a follow-up to Jim Rutberg and Grant Davis's 2-day, 200-mile weekend in northern New Mexico mentioned in Chapter 15, the two of them set out in September of the following year with Grant's brother-in-law Jeff Klem on a 3-day jaunt along the San Juan Skyway, a 235-mile loop connecting the southwestern Colorado mountain towns of Durango, Ouray, and Telluride. The route rolls through some of Colorado's best scenery, crosses four spectacular 10,000-foot high passes, snakes through tight canyons, and includes a fast downhill that goes on for an unbelievable 50 miles. The area's known as the "Switzerland of the Rockies" for good reason.

To prep for the ride, Grant had used a hybrid modification of the New Competitor TCTP plan with his thrice-weekly bike commute while Jim used the first inklings of the training ideas and workouts outlined in this chapter to get ready for the Leadville 100 race. Jim got through Leadville just fine, took a week off to recover, and then turned his sights to this trip.

During their ride through the San Juans, Grant was pleasantly surprised that his roughly 6 to 8 hours of riding a week had given him just enough fitness to see him through the tour. Jim rode strong over all three days and thoroughly relished every mile. Like his time in New Mexico, the ride in Colorado cemented Jim's love of cycling. Being able to spin up and over towering mountain passes day after day was what the sport is all about.

If you do decide to build your own epic, make sure days 1 and 2 are relatively easier rides. Your "queen stage," a bike racing term for the hardest day in a stage race, should come no sooner than day 3. By then, you'll have settled into the routine of riding long hours each day. Your queen stage will still be hard, but your body will bounce back from it sooner and leave you in shape to face the next day. If you put the hardest ride on day 1 or 2, you will likely ride well but wake up the next day feeling completely thrashed and suffer through that day's miles. And if you had planned to finish off your week-long trip with a big finale, a hard day early on will leave you too exhausted to have fun all the way to the final miles.

9

THE COMMUTER'S PLAN FOR RACE-READY FITNESS

ALMOST IMMEDIATELY AFTER PUBLISHING the first edition of this book, I started getting questions about commuting, which for our purposes refers to riding one's bike to and from work. The questions came from two distinct perspectives: the committed commuter who was already riding 4 to 5 days per week, and the athlete who was so busy that commuting a few times per week was the only way to fit in any training time whatsoever. For the sake of convenience, I'll call the latter group "occasional commuters."

Committed commuters have always faced a problem when it comes to effective training. Riding 4 to 5 round trips to work each week can generate a significant amount of fatigue, making it difficult to commit to additional training-focused rides. To evaluate the workload of commuting, we put a power meter on a coach's commuter bike in Colorado Springs, Colorado. His commute is 4.5 miles, generally flat (about 100 feet of climbing each way), and 80 percent is on a bike path. On average, he accumulates 170 kilojoules of work during his commute, which means 1,700 kilojoules a week if he commutes all 5 days. Assuming 20 workdays in a month, that's 6,800 kilojoules a month. Remember, kilojoules accumulated on the bike are roughly equivalent to the calories burned to accomplish that work, and 1,700 calories a week—nearly 7,000 calories a month—is a lot of energy.

Of course, you can look at the energy expenditure of commuting in two ways. From a training perspective you have to consider that 1,700 kilojoule commuting workload when you plan for your total weekly workload. Too often, committed commuters underestimate the impact that their commute will have on their training. They disregard the commute because it feels too short and too easy. But if you were just training and not commuting, and I put an extra 1,700 kilojoules of work into your training plan every week, there's a good chance your training performance would suffer. That's why it's difficult to just add your training on top of a 4- or 5-day-a-week commuting plan.

The other way to look at the energy expenditure of commuting is from a weight management standpoint. Even though you're only burning energy in 170-calorie chunks, the cumulative monthly total can be very significant. There's also something to be said for burning calories on a frequent basis instead of one weekly 3-hour ride that burns 2,000 calories. Short commutes burn energy but are less likely to trigger the pre- or post-workout eating habits that often overcompensate for your actual energy expenditure. In other words, for commutes lasting 20 minutes or less, most people just get it done and go on with their day without adding extra calories to their meals and snacks.

Occasional commuters, however, have a much easier time integrating training into their commutes. Since the primary purpose of commuting is to find time for training, their commuting days during the week can be scheduled for maximum effectiveness and optimal recovery. You can essentially follow the training plans in Chapter 6 by commuting on Tuesday and Thursday and driving to work Monday, some Wednesdays, and Friday. Complete the workout for the day by extending one of your commutes if necessary. It doesn't really matter if you do the workout during your morning or evening commute, but if your workout is going to be in the evening, focus on keeping a lighter resistance and a higher cadence in the morning. Think of that ride as a chance to loosen up for the evening workout. If your workout is during the morning commute, treat the evening commute as a recovery ride or an endurance-paced ride.

SHOULD BIKE RACERS BE COMMUTERS?

For bike racers, there is an argument against commuting that goes something like this: The limited time you spend on your bike should be focused entirely on intensities that will enhance your fitness and performance. Therefore, commuting is a bad option because the intensity level is generally too low and the duration is often too short to lead to any productive training stimulus. As a result, you're better off driving your car to work because you're not wasting energy that you could use the next time you get on the bike for actual training.

When it comes to high-volume trainers, I absolutely agree with the above argument. To take it to an extreme, consider the case of the bike messenger/racer. Electronic documents and other factors have largely gutted the bike messenger industry, but they can still serve as an example. Back in the 1980s and '90s, I knew a lot of up-and-coming bike racers who thought that working as a bike messenger would be the best of both worlds: They'd get to train while earning money! Invariably, after one month they were worthless as bike racers. They were on their bikes all day doing short runs as messengers, and then they'd go training. Some reversed it and trained in the morning and then spent the rest of the day being a messenger. Either way, they ended up exhausted, burned out, and miserable.

A more common example is the Masters or Cat. III racer who trains at least 12 hours a week. For these athletes I don't recommend a commute that's more than 10 minutes. If they live a relatively flat 2 miles from work, then go ahead. But a 30- to 45-minute commute each way, on top of a 12-hours-per-week training load, is frequently too much. The additional workload from the commute takes away from much-needed recovery more than the extra miles enhance training.

On the other hand, time-crunched athletes who have relatively short (under 5 miles) commutes should really consider commuting at least 3 times per week. The additional workload will not be high enough to knock your training out of balance, but the extra time on the bike—and, more important, the increased frequency on the bike—will help you have high-quality workouts when it is time to train.

Assuming you have a safe route to ride to your office and back and a secure place to store your bike at work, you can make commuting work for you. And as roads become more congested, the financial and stress-relieving benefits of bicycle commuting will become even greater.

THE CASE FOR COMMUTING

According to a US Census report published in 2011, the average American (across all methods of travel) spends a little over 50 total minutes a day commuting to and from work. That's more than 4 hours a week that these people could be riding their bikes and growing fitter and faster.

Then there's the financial benefit of commuting. It's not like you're going to sell your car and only commute, but calculate how much fuel you'd save by commuting 3 days a week. That tank of gas in your car is going to last a lot longer, right? Gas prices are never going back to the days of $1/gallon, so the surest way to reduce fuel costs is to use less fuel. Fewer miles on the car means fewer maintenance costs, too. About the only way you won't save money is on your taxes. You'll still have to pay the registration on your car, and your insurance, and you'll have a lower annual mileage to put on your tax return as a deduction.

Perhaps the best case to be made for commuting has nothing to do with economics, athletic performance, or cardiovascular fitness. Commuting feels good; it's a blast of crisp morning air to wake you up and a relaxing way to spin away the stress of the day on the way home. That's not to say it's all sunshine and roses—sometimes you get caught in the rain or it's ridiculously hot for the ride home. Then again, there are no traffic jams on bike paths (though there can be lots of foot traffic to watch out for).

Understandably, commuting doesn't make practical sense for everyone. If you normally commute 30 miles each way at highway speeds, you could drive it in about 30 minutes door-to-door if traffic is light, but it's going to be 90 minutes each way on the bike even if you can average 20 mph. On a regular basis, 3 hours of bike commuting per day is too much for almost anyone to take on, especially anyone who has a family. For an 8-to-5 workday, you'd have to leave the house before 6:30 a.m. and return after 6:30 p.m. We all have days like that sometimes, but most families wouldn't be very happy to adopt that schedule as the norm.

THE COMMUTING LIFESTYLE

Once you commit to cycling to work, you'll need to be aware that you're making a lifestyle change that affects your family life and your work life. You won't be able to rush out of the office to pick up a sick kid from school, snag some groceries on your way back home, or dash off to a business meeting across town. You'll need to set up fallback options with your spouse or significant other, as well as your boss. I've found that as long as you communicate your plans well in advance, you can make it work.

For instance, you could let your boss know that on Mondays you'll drive to the office, and that you'll schedule your offsite meetings for those days. Or you'll schedule the kid's doctor appointments—or your own—for Fridays when you take the car. The TCTP Commuter plan is flexible like that.

The hardest part about commuting is getting started and setting up the scenario that works for you. There are solutions to almost any perceived obstacle. Here are a few; with luck, you will only need one or two to make your commute work.

Problem: I live too far from work.

 Solution: Park-and-Ride (only different). Instead of driving to the train station, drive part way to work, park the car, and ride your bike the rest of the way. Sounds silly, right? Not to people who live far out in the 'burbs. The initial part of the drive is fast; traffic only gets really slow when you get into the city. So drive the fast part, park near a bike path, and ride into the city. You might actually beat your normal commuting time!

 Problem: I'm a professional; I can't show up looking like a bike messenger.

Solution: Drive to work on Mondays and Fridays to drop off and pick up the work wardrobe you'll need for the week. You can also use these driving days to take care of other errands that are inconvenient on a bike. Another option is to leave 2 or 3 pairs of shoes at the office (they're the bulkiest and heaviest item of clothing to carry) and haul the rest of your work clothes in a backpack.

Problem: I don't want to start my workday sweaty.

Solution: Having a shower at your workplace makes commuting a lot easier, and many career professionals who commute will actually skip shaving before they leave the house (more time saved) and shower and shave at work instead. If you don't have a shower at your workplace, see if there's a gym within walking distance. Some will accommodate commuters with special memberships that are essentially for locker room use only. Even though we have showers at CTS offices, I often use BYOT (Bring Your Own Towel) from Zevlin when I commute. It's a rinse-less body wash you apply to a towel when you need to freshen up without taking the time for a full shower.

Problem: Where am I going to put my bike?

Solution: More and more businesses and office buildings are recognizing the need to provide safe parking areas for bikes. In some cities there are bike lockers in parking garages, and there are bike shops that cater to commuters by allowing them space in the shop to store their bikes.

Why go to this much trouble? Because in the big picture, even adding 15 to 20 minutes each way to ride is a better use of your time during the week, and it'll allow you to enjoy more quality time with friends and family in the evenings and on weekends.

How will commuting by bike give you more time to spend with your family? Check out the training plans in this chapter. Because the Committed Commuter is riding to work at least 4 times per week, there's only one weekend training ride instead of two. This may seem counterintuitive because the whole point of training is to enjoy weekend rides and races. In the later portion of the program, around weeks 7 through 11, you'll have the fitness to be racing and participating in events. During this period, by all means ride both days of the weekend if you have the chance (although if you do that you may want to skip your Friday commute). But during the earlier portion of the program, you need the rest in order to recuperate from the workload induced by training and commuting.

During the week, instead of trying to schedule two 60- to 90-minute training sessions before or after work, you're adding 15 to 30 minutes to your commute 3 to 5 times a week. Of course, how much time you save depends on how far you have to ride and what terrain and surface streets you need to navigate. What's great about incorporating the TCTP into a commute is that it works whether you ride 2 miles to work or 20. On training days, you'll simply take the long route to and from work, enough to get in 45 to 60 minutes of riding each way.

Physiologically, bike commuting keeps your body primed to ride all week long and will make your weekend rides or races better. Even a daily 4-mile round-trip commute will produce a difference in your Saturday rides. This is because those midweek miles preserve joint mobility and counter the impact of being sedentary most of the week. The body is always adapting to recent stimuli (or lack thereof). Waking up from a good night's sleep, you're rested but not invigorated, and it can take a strong cup of coffee to wake up your senses. A 20-minute ride to work in the morning gets the blood flowing through the muscles (and the brain), warms up joints, and leaves you firing on all cylinders by the time you wake up your computer. This is your body responding to the stimulus of your ride. The ride home undoes your body's subtle adaptation to sitting in an office chair all day.

Without these twice-daily aerobic efforts, the body will start adapting to a sedentary life of sleeping and sitting. But by riding twice a day, you've elevated the baseline from which you'll start your high-intensity workouts. As a result, you'll be able to work harder, go faster, and recover more quickly.

Back in Chapter 2 I pointed out a study (Burgomaster et al. 2008) that found no difference in the metabolic adaptations between cyclists who did 6 weeks of 30-second sprints 3 days a week and those who rode 40 minutes a day for 5 days a week at an easy aerobic pace (kinda like a bike commute, right?). The TCTP Commuter programs take the commuter's base mileage and fitness and build on them.

If you've read through this book up to now, you might be scratching your head: "But, Chris, you've told me that the TCTP is so intense that I need to take full days off the bike to recover. Yet here you're saying it's OK to ride 6 straight days a week." That's true, but remember that the original TCTP was designed to produce maximum results with as little riding as possible in a given week. It was for people who couldn't spare more than an hour to an hour-and-a-half, twice during the workweek, to train.

This chapter is for dedicated commuters—and that should be all of us—who want to fold a high-results training program into the task of traveling to and from the office. That work/recovery balance is still very important, however, and to manage it you'll still need at least one day off per week (Sunday and/or one workday), and you'll need to commit to riding very easy on some of your commutes.

THE COMMUTER BIKE

Ideally, you'd ride your high-performance road bike to and from work, especially if that bike is the one with a power meter. And you can do that if you live in a relatively warm and dry year-round climate. Throw your work clothes in a backpack, install lights for those pre-dawn or post-sunset rides, and you're good to go.

Those of you who face rain and snow throughout the winter will want a bike with fenders and beefier, knobby tires. Fortunately, the popularity of gravel and "all-road" cycling has prompted the bicycle industry to produce a wide variety of bicycles with disc brakes, clearance for larger tires, and mounts for fenders.

For cyclists who want to commute and train at the same time, it's helpful for your riding position on the commuter to be as close to your racing position as reasonably possible. You might ride on the tops instead of in the drops, but at least the saddle position should be consistent. Cycling is a very repetitive motion, and if you want to gain power in your race position, you need to ride in that position.

Cyclocross bikes offer a good compromise if you can't or won't ride your primary road bike to work. You can typically set them up in a riding position similar to your road position (although the bars might be a little higher), but the frame allows for larger tires, there's room for fenders, and you might be able to get a rack on the back.

If a new bike isn't in your budget, but you've already got a mountain bike, you can make it work. Swap out your off-road tires for hybrid road/dirt tires, and, at a minimum, make sure your saddle position and height in relation to the pedals, and your handlebar height in relation to the saddle height, are the same as they are on your road bike.

Whether you decide to carry your gear in a backpack or in panniers is a matter of personal preference. The pros to using a backpack: It's the least expensive and most versatile option because you can ride your racing bike. If you have to carry your laptop home with you, it's the safest option because your back offers a smoother ride for fragile electronics. And in the winter, the pack acts like a heat trap on your back and keeps you a little warmer. The cons: Wearing a backpack in a road-cycling position isn't always comfortable, and on hot days the pack prevents heat from escaping, which makes it harder for your body to regulate its temperature.

With panniers, the bags that attach to bike racks, you can shove more gear inside and you don't have to worry about strapping a hot and heavy backpack onto your shoulders. The downside is that racing bikes aren't built for racks, and the added weight over the rear wheel can affect your bike's handling. For the out-of-the-saddle PowerIntervals prescribed in the training plans, you'll need to take more care to control your bike.

Whether you use a backpack or panniers, I recommend a supply of dry bags—if you don't have dry bags, try plastic shopping bags—to protect your clothes, work files, or laptop from sweat, rain, slush, or puddle splashes.

HYDRATION AND NUTRITION FOR COMMUTERS

On days when you're only commuting and not adding workouts to your commute, there is really no dietary adjustment needed. You'll burn a few hundred calories commuting, but it's nothing that requires specific fueling to get through. Personally, I like to eat a very small snack with a cup of coffee before

I commute, and then I'll eat something more substantial at the office. It works better for me than commuting with a full stomach. Similarly, in the afternoon I don't change my eating habits if I'm commuting home. After all, I'm going home for dinner.

The times when you might need to account for your commute are when you're going to include a hard workout in the ride to or from work, and when you're commuting in very high temperatures. The individual workouts in this chapter may be short, but they'll still take a lot out of you. For this reason, you'll want to pay close attention to what you eat before and after those rides.

If you're training in the mornings, eat a simple breakfast of fruit, yogurt, and whole-grain cereal or toast and drink a tall glass of water. Eat as soon as you get out of bed to give your stomach time to digest the meal before heading out. Consider an electrolyte drink for very long or hot rides.

As mentioned in Chapter 11, recovery drinks are typically not necessary following rides with caloric expenditures less than 1,500 kilojoules. The exception to this recommendation is when you will be riding or training twice in a single day, as you will when you're commuting a substantial distance. If that's the case, once you get to work, mix yourself a bottle of recovery drink and consume it before your first cup of coffee (keep a container of drink mix at your office). The quick calories and electrolytes will help you bounce back from the morning commute and start your day alert.

If you're going to turn your evening commute into a training ride, then at least an hour before your ride home—and especially on hot summer afternoons—down one water bottle full of an electrolyte-rich drink. If it's been a few hours since lunch and you're really hungry, a light snack can be a good choice. It's not so much that you need even more energy than the fact that being really hungry makes it difficult to focus on your training. You can suck down a gel or a small granola bar or something similar right before you change into cycling clothes.

MONITORING PERFORMANCE WHILE COMMUTING

One thing you'll immediately notice when you start commuting with the weight of your work, clothes, and lunch strapped to your back or bike is that you go slower. That's expected and nothing to worry about. In fact, if you're on your road bike outfitted with a power meter, you'll see that even though you're moving slower, you're still producing the same amount of watts at the same perceived effort. What you don't need to do is redline your power output to maintain what you perceive to be an "acceptable" speed.

Speed is the least relevant measure of performance, even though being fastest from point A to B is how you win races. When you add 12 pounds of gear (computer, clothes, etc.) to your back, your power-to-weight ratio drops substantially. As a result, at any given power output you'll go slower up hills and you'll accelerate more slowly on flat ground. A headwind will reduce your speed even further.

One of the first things new commuters need to do is completely dissociate their unweighted training speeds from their commuting speeds. You're going to be slower, but it doesn't matter. What matters are the power output and energy expenditure, because they provide a reality check and keep you from overexerting yourself in an effort to maintain "normal" training speeds.

Make sure you have a full water bottle of an electrolyte mix for the ride home, and after you walk in the front door, make sure to down another water bottle's worth of fluids to rehydrate and speed recovery. Three bottles associated with a 1-hour workout may seem like a lot, but it can be difficult to keep up with the hydration demands when it's hot outside and you're commuting over multiple days.

THE COMMUTER TCTP PLANS

The core of the Intermediate and Advanced Commuter training plans in this chapter are the Tuesday–Thursday workouts (see Tables 9.1 and 9.2). Compared to the Competitor programs found earlier in this book, the individual workouts themselves are shorter and somewhat simpler. The main difference is that during the build-up to week 8, when you switch to weekend racer mode, you'll be doing high-intensity work going to the office and on your way home. This allows you to get in up to 2 hours of productive work in a day, a full 30 minutes more than the longest Competitor midweek workout.

On these days, I'm assuming that you've mapped out a route that'll take you between 45 and 60 minutes to complete. If your commute is always greater than 45 minutes each way, you can skip the rides on Mondays and/or Fridays because you're getting plenty of miles in to set you up for a strong weekend performance. If you do ride on those days, just make sure your riding on Friday is very easy. You'll need to conserve your energy for Saturday or Sunday (the plan lists workouts on Saturdays and rest days on Sundays, but you can flip the order if necessary).

Outside of the prescribed workouts' specific time needs (i.e., 45 minutes), just ride your normal commute even if it's only 2 to 3 miles each way. On some days, you'll take the long way to the office to complete your training and then take the short route home. During the two recovery weeks, weeks 4 and 8, you'll have a couple of days of no riding at all. This is sometimes hard for the committed commuter because it breaks up the routine and timing of being a commuter. But the extended recovery is important during the training progression, so the disruption is worth it.

A big part of the strategy behind this mix of workouts and distances is to break up your commute and prevent you from falling into the trap of the "same-ride/same-speed" routine. In short, your body becomes very efficient at traveling the same route to and from work each day and stops adapting.

TABLE
9.1

Intermediate Commuter

WEEK		MONDAY	TUESDAY	WEDNESDAY
1	a.m.	Easy commute	45–60 min. EM commute with 2 × 8 min. SS (4 min. RBI)	45–60 min. EM commute with 3 × 6 min. SS (3 min. RBI)
	p.m.		45–60 min. EM commute with 2 × 8 min. SS (4 min. RBI)	Regular EM commute
2	a.m.	Easy commute	60 min. EM commute with 2 × 10 min. SS (4 min. RBI)	45–60 min. EM commute with 2 × 8 min. SS (4 min. RBI)
	p.m.		45–60 min. EM commute with 2 × 8 min. SS (4 min. RBI)	Regular EM commute
3	a.m.	Easy commute	60 min. EM commute with 2 × 12 min. SS (5 min. RBI)	60 min. EM commute with 2 × 10 min. SS (4 min. RBI)
	p.m.		45–60 min. EM commute with 2 × 8 min. SS (4 min. RBI)	Regular EM commute
4	a.m.	Rest day	Easy commute	Regular commute with 3 × 2 min. FP at 100–110 rpm (2 min. RBI)
	p.m.			Easy commute
5	a.m.	Easy commute	45–60 min. EM commute with 5 × 2 min. PI (2 min. RBI)	Easy commute
	p.m.		45–60 min. EM commute with 10 × 1 min. PI (1 min. RBI)	
6	a.m.	Easy commute	45–60 min. EM commute with 6 × 2 min. PI (2 min. RBI)	Easy commute
	p.m.		45–60 min. EM commute with 10 × 1 min. PI (1 min. RBI)	
7	a.m.	Easy commute	45–60 min. EM commute with 7 × 2 min. PI (2 min. RBI)	Easy commute
	p.m.		45–60 min. EM commute with 10 × 1 min. PI (1 min. RBI)	
8	a.m.	Rest day	40–60 min. EM commute	Easy commute with 5 × 2 min. FP (2 min. RBI)
	p.m.		Easy commute	Easy commute
9–11	a.m.	Easy commute	45 min. EM commute with 2 × [5 × 1 min. PI (1 min. RBI)] (5 min. RBS)	60 min. EM commute with 3 × 8 min. SS (4 min. RBI)
	p.m.		45–60 min. EM commute	Easy commute

RBI: Rest between intervals; **RBS:** Rest between sets; **Week 8:** End of progression, really good weekend to race; **Weeks 9–11:** Holding on to the fitness; **CR:** ClimbingRepeats; **EM:** EnduranceMiles; **FP:** FastPedal; **PI:** PowerIntervals; **SS:** SteadyState; **TL 2/4/6:** ThresholdLadders = 2 min. PI, 4 min. CR, 6 min. SS.

THURSDAY	FRIDAY	SATURDAY	SUNDAY
45–60 min. EM commute with 3 × 6 min. SS (3 min. RBI) Easy commute	Easy commute	120 min. group ride or EM	Rest day
45–60 min. EM commute with 3 × 6 min. SS (3 min. RBI) Easy commute	Easy commute	120 min. group ride or EM	Rest day
45–60 min. EM commute with 3 × 6 min. SS (3 min. RBI) Easy commute	Rest day	120 min. group ride or EM	Rest day
Regular EM commute Easy commute	Rest day	60–90 min. EM	Rest day
45–60 min. EM commute with 5 × 2 min. PI (2 min. RBI) 45–60 min. EM commute with 2 × [8 × 30 sec. PI (30 sec. RBI)] (5 min. RBS)	Easy commute	120 min. group ride or EM	Rest day
45–60 min. EM commute with 5 × 2 min. PI (2 min. RBI) 45–60 min. EM commute with 2 × [8 × 30 sec. PI (30 sec. RBI)] (5 min. RBS)	Easy commute	120 min. group ride or EM	Rest day
45–60 min. EM commute with 5 × 2 min. PI (2 min. RBI) 45–60 min. EM commute with 2 × [8 × 30 sec. PI (30 sec. RBI)] (5 min. RBS)	Easy commute	150 min. EM with 3 × 12 min. TL 2/4/6 (5 min. RBI), or fast-paced group ride	Rest day
45–60 min. EM commute Easy commute	Easy commute	Race, or fast-paced group ride	Rest day
Easy commute with 3 × 2 min. FP (2 min. RBI) Easy commute	Easy commute	Race, or fast-paced group ride	Rest day

TABLE
9.2

Advanced Commuter

WEEK		MONDAY	TUESDAY	WEDNESDAY
1	a.m.	Easy commute	45–60 min. EM commute with 3 × 8 min. SS (4 min. RBI)	45–60 min. EM commute with 2 × 10 min. SS (4 min. RBI)
	p.m.		45–60 min. EM commute with 2 × 8 min. SS (4 min. RBI)	EM commute
2	a.m.	Easy commute	60 min. EM commute with 3 × 10 min. SS (4 min. RBI)	45–60 min. EM commute with 3 × 8 min. SS (4 min. RBI)
	p.m.		45–60 min. EM commute with 2 × 8 min. SS (4 min. RBI)	EM commute
3	a.m.	Easy commute	60 min. EM commute with 2 × 15 min. SS (5 min. RBI)	60 min. EM commute with 2 × 12 min. SS (4 min. RBI)
	p.m.		45–60 min. EM commute with 2 × 8 min. SS (4 min. RBI)	EM commute
4	a.m.	Rest day	Easy commute	EM commute with 5 × 2 min. FP at 100–110 rpm (2 min. RBI)
	p.m.			Easy commute
5	a.m.	Easy commute	45–60 min. EM commute with 6 × 2 min. PI (2 min. RBI)	EM commute
	p.m.		45–60 min. EM commute with 10 × 1 min. PI (1 min. RBI)	Easy commute
6	a.m.	Easy commute	45–60 min. EM commute with 7 × 2 min. PI (2 min. RBI)	Regular EM commute
	p.m.		45–60 min. EM commute with 10 × 1 min. PI (1 min. RBI)	Easy commute
7	a.m.	Easy commute	45–60 min. EM commute with 8 × 2 min. PI (2 min. RBI)	Easy commute
	p.m.		45–60 min. EM commute with 10 × 1 min. PI (1 min. RBI)	
8	a.m.	Rest day	Easy commute	Easy commute with 3 × 2 min. FP (2 min. RBI)
	p.m.			Easy commute
9–11	a.m.	Easy commute	45 min. EM commute with 2 × [5 × 1 min. PI (1 min. RBI)] (5 min. RBS)	60 min. EM commute with 2 × 12 min. SS (4 min. RBI)
	p.m.		45–60 min. EM commute	Easy commute

RBI: Rest between intervals; **RBS:** Rest between sets; **Week 8:** End of progression, really good weekend to race; **Weeks 9–11:** Holding on to the fitness; **CR:** ClimbingRepeats; **EM:** EnduranceMiles; **FP:** FastPedal; **PI:** PowerIntervals; **SS:** SteadyState; TL 2/4/6: ThresholdLadders = 2 min. PI, 4 min. CR, 6 min. SS.

THURSDAY	FRIDAY	SATURDAY	SUNDAY
45–60 min. EM commute with 2 × 8 min. SS (4 min. RBI) — Easy commute	Easy commute	120 min. group ride or EM	Rest day
45–60 min. EM commute with 2 × 10 min. SS (4 min. RBI) — Easy commute	Easy commute	120 min. group ride or EM	Rest day
45–60 min. EM commute with 2 × 10 min. SS (4 min. RBI) — Easy commute	Rest day	120 min. group ride or EM	Rest day
EM commute — Easy commute	Rest day	60–90 min. EM	Rest day
45–60 min. EM commute with 6 × 2 min. PI (2 min. RBI) — 45–60 min. EM commute with 2 × [8 × 30 sec. PI (30 sec. RBI)] (5 min. RBS)	Easy commute	120 min. group ride or EM	Rest day
45–60 min. EM commute with 7 × 2 min. PI (2 min. RBI) — 45–60 min. EM commute with 2 × [8 × 30 sec. PI, (30 sec. RBI)] (5 min. RBS)	Easy commute	120 min. group ride or EM	Rest day
45–60 min. EM commute with 8 × 2 min. PI (2 min. RBI) — 45–60 min. EM commute with 2 × [8 × 30 sec. PI, (30 sec. RBI)] (5 min. RBS)	Easy commute	150 min. EM with 3 × 12 min. TL 2/4/6 (5 min. RBI), or fast-paced group ride	Rest day
45–60 min. EM commute with 4 × 1 min. PI (1 min. RBI); 6 min. recovery, then 9 min. TL 1/3/5 — Easy commute	Easy commute	Race, or fast-paced group ride	Rest day
Easy commute with 3 × 2 min. FP (2 min. RBI) — Easy commute	Easy commute	Race, or fast-paced group ride	Rest day

We're adjusting the workload of the commutes to focus some rides on being hard enough to stimulate adaptation, and others easy enough to allow those adaptations to take place.

In some of the higher-intensity weeks, I'll have you doing three hard workouts on three consecutive mornings with the afternoon commutes serving as easier recovery or EM rides. The key to these blocks of training is that afternoon ride. Having the opportunity to spin the legs out, increase your heart rate slightly, and increase circulation to fatigued muscles is actually an advantage you have over cyclists who train but don't commute. You get to benefit from an active recovery activity while they are sedentary.

The difference between the Advanced and Intermediate Commuter plans is in the number of intervals assigned on a given day. The timing of the two plans is pretty much equal, but the Advanced plan has more workload because of the increased number or duration of intervals. I recommend new commuters start with the Intermediate plan, as should experienced commuters who are new to bike racing or serious training. Experienced commuters who have already been racers for more than two seasons will probably want to start out with the Advanced plan. Similarly, racers who are Cat. III or higher and/or have many years of racing experience can typically handle the workload in the Advanced plan.

And do yourself a favor on mornings that call for high-intensity workouts by starting the interval sets right after you complete a 10-minute warm-up. This way you'll give yourself a few miles to cool down and stop sweating before you reach the office. Nothing's worse that steamrolling to the office, still out of breath from your last SteadyState interval, and quickly changing into your work clothes only to soak them through because you're still overheated from the ride in.

PART III

Weight Loss, Nutrition, Hydration, and Heat-Stress Management

Time-crunched athletes are a unique population. If you have read this far, you are obviously okay with hard work. You just don't have a lot of time to commit to it. That presents a challenge for maintaining or reducing body weight because despite the increased intensity of your workouts under the program, your total caloric expenditure from training 6–8 hours a week is still far lower than it was when you were training 12-plus hours a week.

In the years since the first edition of this book was released, tens of thousands of athletes have improved their fitness, and many initially lost weight as well. But as athletes repeated the programs over and over again, their weight plateaued. In some cases, athletes started regaining weight they had lost. One of the truths that became apparent was that athletes using the Time-Crunched Training Program cannot simply ride off the pounds.

To continue making progress, we had to address the dietary side of the calories in/calories out equation. In previous editions of this book I focused on effective fueling for high-intensity training. In this edition I have taken sports nutrition to the next step in order to directly address weight loss.

The challenge with weight loss for time-crunched athletes is that the vast majority of you already eat an athlete's diet. When we perform dietary analyses on athletes in our program, we find diets rich in fruit and vegetables, high-quality proteins, heart-healthy fats, and whole grains.

We don't typically see an excess of packaged foods, fast food, or added sugars. There's not a lot of junk to cut. As you'll see in this section, the solution to achieving weight loss is not centered on eliminating food groups or cutting out junk food. Instead, it is focused on changing eating behaviors.

By modifying the way you interact with food, you can train at a high level while eating less, without feeling deprived. And to help in that pursuit I have worked with renowned chefs Michael Chiarello and Matthew Accarrino to provide easy-to-prepare, nutrient-dense, and immensely tasty recipes. They are both time-crunched cyclists and CTS athletes, so they are uniquely qualified to translate the concepts in this section into recipes you will crave!

10

WEIGHT LOSS FOR THE TIME-CRUNCHED ATHLETE

WHEN WE PUBLISHED THE FIRST EDITION of *The Time-Crunched Cyclist*, the notion of high-intensity, low-volume training was relatively new. Athletes transitioning from traditional endurance training programs experienced immediate and substantial improvement in their fitness and performance and rediscovered their love for cycling. Year after year those athletes cycled through the programs and made incremental gains, moving from the New Century program to Experienced Century and then on to the Competitor programs as their fitness improved. But for many athletes, that progress eventually started to plateau, which led me back to the drawing board to find a new way for them—and you—to move forward.

The beauty of the Time-Crunched Training Program is that it dramatically cuts down the weekly training hours necessary for a cyclist to develop and maintain high-performance fitness. But its greatest strength is also is biggest weakness: time. Athletes who had been through the TCTP several times and were seeing diminishing returns had maximized the workload they could pack into the time they had available. With only 6 hours a week available to train, there is a ceiling to the work you can do.

In the beginning, time-crunched athletes were operating so far below this performance ceiling that focusing primarily on the training component of the TCTP yielded huge improvements. It was only years later, when athletes had maximized the training workload they could accumulate in the time available, that it became apparent that further improvement would need to come from a different avenue.

If you can't pack in more work, where do you turn to get more improvement? The answer is staring you in the full-length mirror every day: You have to optimize weight.

HEALTH, BODY IMAGE, AND PERFORMANCE

Let me make one thing perfectly clear: I am an endurance sport coach. When I say someone should optimize weight—which typically means losing weight—in order to be a faster cyclist, I am telling you what it will take to improve athletic performance. I'm not telling you to lose weight to improve your health (although that will likely happen as well). I don't care how you look in a bathing suit, and I really don't care what you look like naked. I care what you look like standing on top of a podium!

Weight management can be a thorny issue, however, because it is so closely tied to health and body image. It will come as no surprise to athletes reading this book that the United States has an obesity epidemic. According to the Centers for Disease Control, one-third of adult Americans were obese in 2014. That's 78 million people! There was no state in the United States where adult obesity rates were lower than 20 percent, and Arkansas, Mississippi, and West Virginia had adult obesity rates of 35 percent or higher. Obesity is a serious threat to health, increasing risk factors for heart attack, stroke, Type II diabetes, and a long list of acute and chronic illnesses. It is understandable, then, that there are massive efforts in the research communities devoted to better understanding the complexities of helping overweight and obese individuals lose excess body fat, become more active, and improve cardiovascular health.

One reason a statement like "You need to lose weight" is problematic is that you cannot simply tell an obese person he or she needs to lose weight and expect it to happen. Eating habits, food choices, and activity level contribute to overweight and obesity, but many of these aspects are heavily influenced by the environments people live in, the traditions that were maintained in their homes, the relationships in their lives, their economic condition, and the ways they cope with stress and social pressures. When you ask people to change how and what they eat, and add more physical activity to their days and weeks, you're asking them to work against all the influences—social, economic, psychological—that have led them to their current lifestyle. If your family and social group are primarily overweight and sedentary, and the foods prepared in the home and available at social events are unhealthy, attempting to change your own habits in the midst of that environment is very difficult, can be very stressful, and can strain relationships with family and friends.

The complexity of obesity makes people avoid talking about weight loss, because from person to person it is difficult to determine the underlying causes of their current weight. Advice that might motivate some people is totally unrealistic and psychologically hurtful to others. The same is true when it comes to body image.

When you start putting out messages via magazine columns, blog posts, and social media saying "Cyclists need to lose 10 pounds" and providing tips to accomplish that weight loss, you get a mixture of responses. A lot of people will thank you for providing motivation and actionable tips while others will accuse you of fat shaming, encouraging eating disorders, and promoting an unrealistic body image. Those are serious issues influenced by a wide range of psychological and sociological factors.

The fact that health, body image, and performance are intertwined in any conversation about diet and weight management makes the subject of sports nutrition confusing for a lot of athletes. When we talk about consuming carbohydrate versus fat, are we talking about it from the perspective of cardiovascular health, insulin sensitivity, or supplying energy for workouts? Which of these outcomes is most important?

After working with more than 17,000 athletes, my view is that performance is the top priority for an athletic population. I say this not because the other aspects are not important, but because focusing your dietary choices and habits on the pursuit of improved performance almost always achieves or maintains the positive health outcomes sedentary populations seek through dietary changes. As a result, in the following discussion of weight management for time-crunched athletes, the primary focus is on improving your performance.

WHY WEIGHT LOSS IS DIFFICULT FOR TIME-CRUNCHED ATHLETES

Any athlete who has experienced a period of significant weight gain understands that there's a difference between losing the first 10 pounds and losing the last 10 pounds as you return to your goal weight. Weight loss for time-crunched athletes is difficult for two reasons: diminishing returns and diet. Let's look at those two components.

You Don't Have That Much Weight to Lose

Significant and rapid weight loss is relatively easy to achieve when there is a lot of weight to be lost. This is a big factor in the short-term success of named diets like Atkins, Paleo, and even ketosis. Although these and similar diets use different methods for changing the way people eat, they all achieve weight loss results the same way: caloric restriction. If someone adds exercise to the equation, the initial weight loss is even faster and more significant. But after a while, weight loss slows or stops altogether because the process of constantly counting calories and cutting calories is hard. For people who are only pursuing weight loss (and not improved performance), the absence of continued progress is discouraging and they almost always loosen up on the dietary restrictions they were previously committed to. As a result, they gravitate back toward the eating habits and food choices they made before and regain the weight.

Athletes pursuing improved performance also experience rapid initial weight loss through caloric restriction, and they combine it with an increase in caloric expenditure. Despite the addition of exercise, however, athletes also reach a point of diminishing returns where their weight loss stagnates. In order to maintain high-quality training, you have to eat to support your workouts, which limits your ability to create a caloric deficit through restricted eating. And time-crunched athletes can't increase their training workload because of their limited training time.

Your Diet Is Already Pretty Good

If all I had to do was teach you to make good food choices—eating more fruits and vegetables, eating fewer heavily processed and refined foods, and eliminating sugary sodas—this weight loss thing would be pretty easy. But 17 years of dietary recalls (food journals) with athletes proves you already know that. It is rare to find an athlete who is motivated to improve athletic performance who hasn't already adopted a balanced nutrition strategy featuring fresh, whole foods and leaner proteins while reducing intake of junk food. The dietary recalls we see from time-crunched athletes make clinical dietitians working with obesity patients swoon.

This is a good news/bad news scenario. The good news is that you are most likely making good choices for your overall health. The bad news is that because your diet is already pretty good, there isn't much room for major improvements in nutritional quality. There is some room, and we'll talk about ways to make those adjustments later, but I think it's important to recognize that one of the things that separates you from the general population is that your food choices are not the biggest part of the problem. It's not what you're eating; more likely, it's how you're eating, when you're eating, and how much you're eating.

THERE IS NO PERFECT WEIGHT

Athletes frequently ask, "How much should I weigh?" The truth is, there is no perfect weight that will predict optimal performance. Being lighter reduces the energy cost of moving from point A to point B, in any sport and over any terrain, but being as light as possible is not always ideal.

When you are too light, you do not have the muscle mass to produce the power necessary to perform optimally. In order to achieve and maintain an especially low body weight, you have to create significant energy deficits (burn more than you consume), which hinders training performance. You're lighter but less powerful. Failing to support your activity level with sufficient energy also hinders recovery and places undue stress on your immune system, which means athletes who are too lean suffer from more frequent illnesses and injuries.

Your ideal weight is also governed by your goals and the level of effort you are willing to devote to weight management. Let's say you currently weigh 175 pounds. From experience you may know that your best competition weight was 155 pounds, but that was 15 years ago when you had an entry-level job, no family, and all the time in the world to devote to training. You could get back to 155 pounds now, but the level of focus and effort required may not be worth the increase in performance. It may be more realistic and maintainable for you to reach 160–165 pounds.

Could you achieve greater performance improvements by getting all the way down to 155? Yes, but 155 pounds may no longer be your ideal weight because it is out of balance with your priorities. So while it is good to set a target weight, be careful not to get too hung up on the exact number. Initially, the number you choose is somewhat arbitrary; it gets you moving in the right direction. When you hit your initial performance goals, you can take a fresh look at your weight and decide whether you want to pursue further weight loss.

KEY CONCEPTS IN SPORTS NUTRITION

After publishing an entire book on sports nutrition and nutrition periodization (*Chris Carmichael's Food for Fitness*) and writing extensively on the importance of proper nutrition in optimizing health and fitness (*5 Essentials for a Winning Life*), it's difficult for me to resist the temptation to write an exhaustive treatise on sports nutrition for this book as well. But because this is a book for athletes who are short on time, I'm going to do my best to cut to the chase.

Just to make sure we're all on the same page, let's quickly review the basics. First of all, all the calories you consume come from three macronutrients: carbohydrate (4 calories per gram), protein (4 calories per gram), and fat (9 calories per gram). (Note: To avoid confusion, I use the more common spelling of food calories using a lowercase "c," even though the scientifically accurate terminology would either be kilocalories or Calories with a capital "C." If in your reading you come across references to kilocalories, these are the same as what we and the chefs and nutritionists we work with call "calories.")

The macronutrients you take in directly and indirectly provide all the energy you use to build and maintain your body, perform all your normal bodily functions, and complete all your voluntary tasks, including exercise.

On top of these macronutrients, there are three other items you need to consume to stay alive and healthy: water, vitamins, and minerals. Despite delivering zero calories, water is sometimes referred to as a fourth macronutrient because of its overwhelming importance. In fact, water is probably more important than anything else you consume, because dehydration can kill you in days, whereas you can survive quite a while without food. Vitamins and minerals, known as micronutrients, also deliver zero calories but are necessary in varying amounts for completing the biochemical reactions that keep your body functioning properly.

Your body burns calories every minute of every day, and you are constantly deriving that energy from a mixture of carbohydrate, protein, and fat.

The relative percentage of energy coming from each depends on many factors, but for the purposes of this book, I concentrate most on the impact of exercise intensity on fuel utilization. Of the three macronutrients, you rely on protein for a relatively low and constant amount of energy during exercise. Protein is an important component of an athlete's nutrition program and performance, but under normal conditions a healthy individual derives 10 to 15 percent of his or her exercise calories from protein, regardless of exercise intensity. As a result, and for the sake of simplicity, I will set aside protein from the equation and focus on the relative contributions from carbohydrate and fat during exercise.

As I explained in Chapter 2, during exercise your muscles process carbohydrate and fat to produce energy using aerobic metabolism and glycolysis. Your exercise intensity and fitness directly affect the relative amount of energy being produced by each method. At rest, your body relies on fat for 80 to 90 percent of its energy needs (breathing, digestion, pumping blood, etc.). At very low exercise intensities (20 to 25 percent of VO_2max), you're still relying on fat for about 70 percent of your energy. As you reach 40 to 60 percent of VO_2max, your fuel utilization reaches about a 50–50 balance between fat and carbohydrate. Athletes with greater aerobic fitness will reach and maintain this 50–50 balance at a higher relative workload than will athletes who are less fit.

As your exercise intensity rises beyond 60 percent of VO_2max, the relative contribution from carbohydrate increases dramatically because of the increased reliance on glycolysis. But remember, even when you're burning a lot of carbohydrate at higher exercise intensities (glycolysis burns carbohydrates exclusively), you are still processing fat and carbohydrate using aerobic metabolism. Once you exceed your lactate threshold intensity (70 to 90 percent of VO_2max, depending on your fitness level), more than 80 percent of your energy is being derived from carbohydrate.

The fact that the TCTP features a lot of high-intensity interval workouts means you will burn carbohydrate quickly, and for many years endurance athletes have relied on high-carbohydrate diets to fuel performance. In recent years, this notion has been challenged by proponents of a wide variety of nutrition strategies and named diets, including Paleo and a range of high-fat/low-carb strategies that cut carbohydrate to anywhere from 5 to 40 percent of total calories. As a time-crunched athlete, it is important to look at these dietary strategies from both weight loss and athletic performance perspectives, so let's do that next.

THE PERFECT DIET MYTH

One reason athletes are so confused about nutrition is because the vast majority of the dietary information we see is aimed at weight loss and not performance. For decades, scientists and marketers have been trying to pin down the perfect macronutrient composition for humans. However, there was very little said on this topic before the 1960s, which is about the same time heavily processed foods entered the food supply in developed countries and we started to see dramatic increases in the number of people who were overweight, obese, and/or suffering from heart attacks, hypertension, Type II diabetes, and so on. The implication is that if we can just get the macronutrient composition correct, these problems would go away and people would be healthier.

Over the past 50 years, popular diets and dietary strategies spanning the entire spectrum of macronutrient ratios have emerged and faded. On one end you have the Ornish diet, which is extremely high in carbohydrate (CHO) and extremely low in fat. On the other end of the spectrum is nutritional ketosis or the ketogenic diet, which is extremely high in fat and extremely low in carbohydrate. Interestingly, across the spectrum of these named diets and dietary strategies, protein intake stays relatively consistent: about 20 to 30 percent of caloric intake.

There are pros and cons to every macronutrient ratio and dietary strategy in Table 10.1. The Ornish diet, for example, is initially great for reducing cardiovascular risk factors, but it is so restrictive that people rarely stick with it. Promoting a low-fat diet (less than 30 percent of calories from fat with less

TABLE
10.1

Macronutrient Levels in Popular Diets

DIET TYPE	EXAMPLE	CARBOHYDRATE	PROTEIN	TOTAL FAT
Extreme high carb	Ornish	74%	18%	8%
High carb	Standard U.S. Diet	60%	20%	20%
High protein	Zone Diet	40%	30%	30%
High fat, high carb	Mediterranean	40%	20%	40%
High fat, high protein	South Beach Diet & Paleo	28%	33%	39%
High fat, low carb	Atkins Diet (induction phase)	<15%	30–35%	55–60%
Extreme high fat	Ketosis	<10%	20–25%	70–75%

than 10 percent of calories from saturated fat) in the United States contributed to massive increases in the amount of sugar Americans consumed in pursuit of satiation, and subsequent increases in obesity and Type II diabetes. Reducing the fat intake isn't necessarily bad, but replacing it with excess sugar and heavily processed foods certainly is.

In an effort to mediate the damage from excess sugar, the pendulum swung the other way to high-fat and/or high-protein diets. Proponents argue that there are benefits from both the reduction in carbohydrate/sugar intake and the increase in fat intake. But as with the extremely high-carbohydrate diets, people struggle to stick with the alternatives and tend to gravitate back toward the middle. And perhaps that's the most revealing fact: people gravitate to the middle.

High-fat, low-carbohydrate (HFLC) diets have become a hot topic for athletes in the past several years. As with any diet that significantly restricts food choices, weight loss is driven through caloric restriction rather than the macronutrient composition, but proponents of this nutritional strategy sell it to athletes based on the idea that a "fat-adapted" athlete will perform better than an athlete who is more dependent on a steady consumption of carbohydrate. I'll discuss these HFLC diets for athletes in greater detail later, but my reason for bringing them up here is that when you examine dietary analyses of athletes who report that they consume a HFLC diet, their carbohydrate intake is often substantially higher than they think. They may have started out with a very low percentage of energy coming from carbohydrate, but many gravitate back toward the middle and consume at least 45 percent of their calories from carbohydrate.

There is no perfect macronutrient composition for weight loss or performance. There are no perfect foods that must be consumed or terrible foods that must be avoided. Intuitively this makes sense to most athletes, and you need only look to elite athletes to illustrate this point clearly. There are very few athletes operating at the extremes of either very high carbohydrate or very high fat. Like dieters, many athletes have tried the extremes and gravitated back toward the middle. But even in this middle ground, there is nothing magical about a 55/20/25 or 60/20/20 or even 45/20/35 carbohydrate-protein-fat ratio. Instead, the keys are to consume enough total energy to support your activity level and enough of specific nutrients to fuel high-quality training while avoiding overconsumption of anything.

THE PROBLEMS WITH THE WAY WE EAT

Here's the challenge: There is no perfect diet and no ideal weight. You don't have a ton of weight to lose to begin with. And moreover, as a time-crunched athlete, your overall food choices are probably pretty good. So how are you supposed to achieve modest but meaningful weight loss and improve performance? This is the scenario we confront every day, and what works is a series of behavioral changes that focus more on altering *the way* athletes eat and less on *what* athletes eat (since it's already nutritious). To start with, we need to take a look at how time-crunched athletes typically eat.

We Eat What's in Front of Us

If I put a plate of food in front of you, you will most likely eat everything on the plate. Culturally, we have been raised this way from childhood. Whether it was our parents' desire to make sure we actually consumed enough energy to grow or our learned desire not to waste food, there is a strong cultural drive to clean your plate. When you order food in a restaurant, there's an added financial motivation to eat what you paid for.

As you can probably guess, this gets back to the idea of portion control, but my point is that even though you intuitively know that eating smaller portions would reduce caloric intake and aid in weight loss, you don't do it. You eat what's in front of you, and what you're putting in front of yourself—or what is being put in front of you—has been getting progressively larger. Today's salad plate was big enough for an entrée in 1950. A set of normal dishes from 100 years ago looks like a child's toy tea set today. Yes, you could eat a small portion on a giant plate, but you're less likely to because the giant plate changes your perception of how much you're eating. Your expectation is that you're not eating very much, not eating enough, because visually the proportions are off.

What's in front of us also makes a difference. Long-standing advice from clinical and sports dietitians is to include a wide variety of foods in your diet. The main idea is that doing so increases the spectrum of nutrients you consume. Typically this strategy minimizes the impact of calorie-dense processed foods by balancing them with more nutrient-dense whole foods. That's very positive, but variety also changes the way we eat. A buffet is the classic example. With more possibilities of what you can eat, you will choose to eat more items and more total calories. And the same thing happens when you have more variety on a plate of food at home. Now, that's not necessarily a bad thing, because eating a variety of foods typically increases the nutritional quality of your diet, but it is nevertheless an eating behavior athletes need to be aware of.

We Eat Quickly

Eating too fast is one of my biggest challenges. When I am thinking about a project at work or moving between appointments, I eat very quickly. I never really thought much about it until I went to lunch with another CTS coach and he ordered his food to go. We were at a place where you order at the counter and they deliver the food to the table, and I placed my order as "eat in." A few moments later, the other coach ordered his to go. From experience he knew my mind was racing with everything except what I was eating, so I was going to shovel in the food and be ready to get back to the office quickly. Rather than feel compelled to race through his meal, he ordered his food to go, and true to form by the time his order arrived at the table I was already halfway through mine.

Part of the reason you're a time-crunched athlete is that you're time-crunched in everything you do. You have a lot to do every day. You might enjoy lingering over a meal sometimes, but there are times when athletes appreciate great food and times when you feel compelled to just eat and get on with your day. It's the latter circumstance that typically leads to speed eating.

A faster eating rate has been shown to increase the energy intake from a meal, and a slower eating rate has been shown to reduce energy intake—particularly in normal-weight individuals (Shah et al. 2014). In the context of nutritional research, the time-crunched athlete audience would typically be considered a normal-weight audience. You're certainly not obese, and even if your body mass index (BMI) is on the high end of normal for your height, or indicative of being overweight for your height, you're carrying more muscle and are more active than a sedentary individual with the same BMI.

There are a few reasons speed eating leads to greater energy intake. The first is that humans are not very good at estimating the energy content of food based on what it looks like. If I put a plate full of food in front of you, or even in front of a registered dietitian, it would be difficult for either of you to estimate the total calories on the plate within 10 percent. It gets more difficult and less accurate when you add more variety to the plate. It gets even more difficult when you're not preparing the food yourself. Misjudging the energy content of a plate of food by 10–20 percent might not seem that bad, but if you think you're putting about 500 calories on a plate and it's closer to 600, that adds up over the course of a day and week.

How does misjudging the energy content of food relate to speed eating? When you eat faster, you consume calories more quickly than your brain can register feelings of fullness. You can easily shovel in 1,000 calories in 5 minutes and not feel particularly rushed doing so. Ten minutes later your brain is telling you that you're overfull, you're telling your buddy, "Man, I shouldn't have eaten that much," and your body is trying to figure out where to put it all. If you underestimated the energy content of the meal to begin with, consuming it quickly compounded the error by overriding the normal feedback mechanisms that would have otherwise signaled you to stop eating when you were appropriately satiated. But, as I explained in the previous section, we eat what's in front of us, so even with signals of fullness and satiety, you probably would have finished it anyway.

Time-crunched athletes benefit from slowing down at the table, but I'm not going to recommend something like chewing each bite of food 30 times. No one sticks to that recommendation. Yes, it slows your eating rate, but in many cases it's unpleasant to keep food in your mouth that long. Rather, later in this chapter I'll give you some reasonable and actionable techniques for eating more slowly.

We Overcompensate for Exercise Expenditure

Eating too fast and eating what's in front of us are not problems unique to athletes or time-crunched athletes. But overcompensating for caloric expenditure is definitely something that affects athletes—particularly time-crunched athletes—more than other populations.

In overweight and obese populations, high-intensity exercise may blunt feelings of hunger and actually reduce caloric intake for up to 36 hours following the exercise session (Sim et al. 2013). But for moderately trained individuals and time-crunched athletes, strenuous exercise can lead to increased compensatory eating, or caloric overcompensation.

Following a hard exercise session, many athletes gorge on a high volume of food because they overestimate the calories required to replenish depleted energy stores, and/or indulge in high-calorie foods because they perceive that the strenuous work validates their craving for high-calorie foods ("I earned that donut!"). This compensatory eating, however, is not a physical response. Ghrelin is a hormone secreted by the stomach that signals hunger and drives appetite. Not only has high-intensity exercise been shown to reduce the secretion of ghrelin in the short term, but a recent study indicates that ghrelin was still suppressed even the day after exercise (King et al. 2015). Physiologically, there isn't a compensatory drive to increase appetite or caloric intake in response to exercise. The compensatory drive is behavioral.

Interval training is strenuous, and the workouts in this program are purposefully difficult. But even though your perceived exertion and perception of total energy expenditure are likely to be high, your actual energy expenditure on this program is not very high. The programs in this book range from 6 to 8 hours of training, and even during the hardest interval workouts your hourly expenditure is not likely to exceed 1,000 kilojoules (approximately 1,000 calories). It is far more likely that a moderately fit, medium-sized cyclist on these programs will burn about 600 to 700 kilojoules per hour over the course of a week.

Here's how overcompensation works: When you get off your bike following a 75-minute interval workout and grab a recovery drink (150 calories), and then increase your portion size during your post-exercise meal from 500 calories to 700, you have consumed approximately 850 calories following a workout that probably cost you just about the same amount of energy. But you started that workout with 1,600–2,000 calories of stored carbohydrate in your muscles and liver, and because you burned both carbohydrate and fat during the session, not only did you not deplete those carbohydrate stores, you burned far fewer than 850 calories worth of them.

BUT WAIT, DON'T I NEED CARBS FOR RECOVERY?

Yes, carbohydrates are necessary for post-exercise recovery. Yes, you need some protein in order to build and maintain muscle tissue. And yes, you need adequate total calories to maintain an energy balance that supports your activity level.

Keep in mind, however, that your body recovers from exercise over the course of time, and that while carbohydrate replenishment rate is fastest during the first hour after exercise and gradually declines over time, you will achieve full replenishment within 24 hours regardless. This means you will start your next workout with full glycogen stores and have all the fuel you need for another high-quality workout.

The time when immediate and substantial post-workout carbohydrate is most important is when athletes are training twice a day or competing more than once in a 24-hour period. Similarly, if you are training hard in the evening and planning an early-morning workout the following day, it would be beneficial to focus on a high-carbohydrate meal within the first hour after exercise and consistent intake of fluid and carbohydrate snacks through bedtime.

The bigger problem with caloric overcompensation is that it happens throughout the day, every day, for a lot of people. You eat a bigger breakfast in anticipation of the workout you're going to do. You look at snacks and meals before training as "fueling up" and so you take a bit more than you might otherwise need. After training sessions, you overestimate the calorie and carbohydrate needs for replenishment, as explained above. You take bigger portions or expect to eat bigger portions, and because we eat what's in front of us and finish what we take, you eat it all. And many athletes reward themselves with sweets or alcohol when they do the math in their heads and figure they exercised enough to earn the extra calories. The key to changing this behavior isn't necessarily counting calories but changing the way we eat and using different cues to govern the amount we eat.

Counting Calories Doesn't Work

In the real world, counting calories is not an effective way for people to manage their nutrition long term. I do believe that having a sense of your daily calorie needs and tracking your caloric intake can be useful in the short term to help you formulate a better sense of the relationship between portions and calories. Doing so can also give you a better sense of the overall energy content and macronutrient composition of your diet. But the reality is that very few people will consistently enter information into food logs.

I've tried many different methods using all levels of technology, but even with mobile phone apps that scan bar codes and feature a database of nearly limitless food choices, people rarely stick with counting calories very long. Ironically, keeping track is easiest for people who eat highly processed foods because the packages they come in have bar codes. The people for whom counting calories is most tedious and time-consuming are people eating a wide variety of whole foods. These items don't generally have bar codes, and the amounts used are not in neat little packages. So we estimate, poorly. Did you add third of a cup of broccoli or a half? Maybe it was a quarter?

The bigger question is: Do I really want you to spend the time and effort to get all those calorie counts correct, or do I care more that you're eating a meal comprised of a wide variety of whole-food ingredients? I want you to do the latter, and use behavior cues to govern the amount you eat rather than resorting to a calorie counter. This learning process is similar to what we do when athletes train with heart rate or a power meter. Initially you spend a lot of time focusing on the numbers, but gradually you learn how to gauge intensity by feedback cues rather than by the number on a display.

Cyclists working with power meters can use the kilojoule information from their workouts to obtain a more precise view of how training affects their total daily caloric expenditure. The kilojoules of work you perform during a cycling workout are approximately equal to the number of calories you burned during that time. Sports dietitians and coaches have long used equations and estimates to calculate an athlete's total daily caloric expenditure, and kilojoule data from power meters allow us to replace an estimate with a real measurement, which leads to a more accurate result. If you track the kilojoule information for a few weeks, you'll soon get a reliable picture of the impact that your training has on your energy intake. You can then use that number to plan your daily meals. Don't be surprised if you discover that you've been overeating, even if just a little bit.

Components of Energy Expenditure

Having just read why counting the exact number of calories you consume isn't all that effective, you might wonder why it's important to calculate your daily caloric expenditure. The reason I believe this is a valuable exercise is that it provides an athlete with a ballpark sense for his or her energy requirements. Just as time-crunched athletes—and all athletes—often overestimate the calories they burn during workouts, they also tend to overestimate their overall daily caloric expenditure.

It is easy for athletes to have significant misconceptions about their normal daily caloric expenditure simply because there are a number of variables involved in the calculation. Your total energy expenditure for a day has three main components: resting metabolic rate (RMR), lifestyle, and exercise. Your RMR can be measured directly in a lab, but it is more often derived from one of several calculations. The energy requirement for your lifestyle (work, daily activities) is calculated by multiplying your RMR by a lifestyle factor. The calories you expend during voluntary exercise can be either estimated or measured directly, depending on the exercise and the equipment available.

Use the following steps and equations to calculate your total daily energy expenditure:

1. **Determine your resting metabolic rate (RMR):** Resting metabolic rate (sometimes called basal metabolic rate) represents the number of calories your body needs every 24 hours to complete basic bodily functions and keep you alive. At CTS we prefer the Mifflin-St. Jeor equation, which is a little complicated to calculate but has been shown to be more accurate than other equations. To find your RMR using this equation, you will need to know your weight in kilograms (1 kilogram = 2.2 pounds), your height in centimeters (1 inch = 2.54 centimeters), and your age in years. Input your data into the appropriate equation below:

   Male: RMR = (10 × weight) + (6.25 × height) − (5 × age) + 5
   Female: RMR = (10 × weight) + (6.25 × height) − (5 × age) − 161

2. **Lifestyle factor:** Take the number from your RMR above and multiply it by the appropriate lifestyle factor from Table 10.2. Example: A 37-year-old male who stands 5 feet 10 inches and weighs 150 pounds has an RMR of 1,612 calories. He works at a desk all day and drives to and from the office, so his lifestyle factor is 1.25. Thus his minimum daily need is 2,015 calories (1,612 × 1.25).

3. **Exercise calories:** This is where you get to apply the kilojoules displayed on your power meter. If you're not using a power meter, you can use Table 10.3 to estimate how many calories you burn during your workouts. Once you determine your caloric expenditure from exercise, add that number to the total of your RMR times your lifestyle factor to determine your caloric expenditure for the day. Using the example above, our 150-pound male with a minimum daily calorie total of 2,015 exercises roughly 1 hour a day. Thus he'd need to add 750–800 calories to his diet, for a total of 2,765–2,815 calories burned each day.

TABLE 10.2

Lifestyle Factors

ACTIVITY FACTOR	DESCRIPTION	MULTIPLY RMR BY
Very light	Most of workday is sitting or with some standing—relatively little physical activity.	1.25
Light	Work involves some sitting, mostly standing and walking—for example, retail sales—light recreational activity.	1.55
Moderate	Work involves sustained physical activity with little sitting—for example, UPS or mail delivery person—active recreational pursuits. Walk or bike to work.	1.65
Heavy	Occupation is physical labor—very active recreationally. Few jobs fall into this category.	2

TABLE 10.3

Calories Burned During Workouts

FEMALE BODY WEIGHT, KG (LBS)	CALORIES BURNED PER HOUR OF AEROBIC EXERCISE	MALE BODY WEIGHT, KG (LBS)	CALORIES BURNED PER HOUR OF AEROBIC EXERCISE
54 (120)	572	63 (140)	731
63 (140)	668	72 (160)	835
72 (160)	762	82 (180)	940
82 (180)	857	91 (200)	1,044
91 (200)	953	100 (220)	1,148

It is important to know that the process of calculating total daily caloric expenditure is not perfect. The Mifflin-St. Jeor equation is more accurate than others, but calculations are often less accurate than direct measurements. The lifestyle factor provides a good way to account for the energy demands of your lifestyle, but it's a multiplier, not a direct measurement. Even the one direct measurement you can get from your power meter, kilojoules, doesn't provide a truly accurate accounting of the number of calories you burned, because, as I explained previously, the conversion between kilojoules and calories is close but not perfect. Nevertheless, the process described here, using data from your power meter, is one of the most accurate available outside a laboratory.

Keeping Total Caloric Expenditure in Perspective

As I mentioned earlier when describing how to calculate daily energy requirements, the calculations are most helpful for making sure your energy intake is in the right ballpark. The calculations are usually accurate to within a few hundred calories, and any estimation of intake would most likely be off by a similar amount. As a result, it's difficult—and typically unproductive—to consider either number exact. Rather, these calculations are best used to gain a more accurate picture of how your energy expenditure fluctuates with your training.

Because the kilojoules of work you produce are roughly equal to the calories you burned to produce them, a power meter provides you with a reasonably accurate accounting of your daily exercise caloric expenditure. Now, does that mean you should change your eating habits every day based on your training session? No. You'd drive yourself—and your spouse and kids—crazy in the process, and there's no counter that resets to zero at midnight.

It's better to think about energy balance over a 3-day period. The information from your power meter may tell you that right now you're burning 700 calories during your hard interval workouts and 1,500 calories during your slightly longer weekend rides. After you've gained fitness, these numbers may go up to 900 and 1,800. This is good information to have when you start looking at your eating behaviors and the appetite cues.

EATING BEHAVIORS THAT PROMOTE PERFORMANCE AND WEIGHT LOSS

In the past I have advocated both specific macronutrient ratios and the elimination of specific foods in an effort to help athletes optimize their fueling strategies and lose weight. And while I still think those methods can be useful and effective for some athletes, I have grown to believe that eating behaviors have more impact both on eating for performance and on weight management. As I've explained before, this is partly because, both in my experience and in nutrition research, adherence to either specific macronutrient ratios or food prohibitions tends to be low or only sustainable for a short period of time. And because data from thousands of dietary recalls confirms that time-crunched athletes generally eat a balanced diet with plenty of fresh, whole foods, the largest portion of the audience for this book won't dramatically benefit from recommending prohibitions. Most of you have already removed or minimized your intake of obviously poor nutrition choices. This is why I have evolved my thinking on performance nutrition and weight management to focus instead on improving four key eating behaviors.

Respond to Hunger, Not Habit

As much as we sometimes like to rail against it, humans thrive on structure and routine. There have always been schedules to follow. Long before there was a workday or a project list, there was the natural rhythm of daytime and nighttime, and physiologically our bodies have been following cyclical schedules since the beginning of time. We eat on schedules, too, and one of the key distinctions that time-crunched athletes need to make is the difference between eating based on physiological hunger and eating according to habit.

When we eat according to habit, we may be eating when we are not physiologically hungry. We are responding to social cues, societal norms, and the other scheduling priorities we have built into our daily lives. To focus on eating for performance and change our behaviors to optimize both performance and weight management, we need to break away from eating based on habit and instead focus on eating based on hunger.

Physiological hunger is characterized by physical signals. A rumbling stomach or feelings of hunger pangs are hardwired signals from your body that it's time to seek out food. The clock striking twelve, the sound of the factory whistle, or the three o'clock doldrums are not physical signals; they are cultural or conditioned signals we have adopted. What is interesting is that our conditioned signals for hunger have an impact on our physiological signals for hunger.

The physical signals of hunger are modulated by the hormone ghrelin (Wren 2001). When the stomach is empty, ghrelin levels in the blood increase and signal the hypothalamus to initiate hunger. When you eat on a schedule, ghrelin levels rise according to the schedule, in anticipation of an upcoming meal (Lesauter et al. 2009). This may be part of the reason you feel insatiably hungry at 3 p.m. despite having eaten lunch 2 or 3 hours earlier, whereas you can go from 7 a.m. to noon (5 hours) without feeling similarly hungry after breakfast. In other words, your habits can start to drive your appetite, because the conditioned response to the schedule is stimulating the release of the hormone that tells you it is time to eat. The good news is that conditioning works both ways, meaning that you can also turn it around and change your physiological signals for appetite by changing your habits.

People don't like to feel hungry, but for the vast majority of human history hunger was a constant companion. Logically, how can it be that—generally speaking—despite consuming more calories per day than our grandparents did, and expending fewer calories per day in activities of normal living, we still feel hungry? Our ancestors consumed even less and yet did just as much as we do each day, if not more. They had adapted to a lower calorie lifestyle. We, in comparison, have adapted to a higher calorie lifestyle.

We feel hungry not because we need the calories, but because of the expectation of the amount of food we typically eat. When you reduce caloric intake, initially you will experience feelings of hunger. Over time, though, you will adapt to your energy intake and feeding schedule and your appetite will respond in the same way.

From a practical standpoint, cutting back and responding only to hunger means getting comfortable with being hungry, at least in the short term. Decades of conditioned behavior and easy access to relatively inexpensive food have shifted the drive to eat from a physiological need to a habitual one. While this is not universally true (there are absolutely people who are not consuming enough energy), for the vast majority of time-crunched athletes my

COACHING EATING BEHAVIORS
Max Shute, PhD

If you are reading these words, you are in a unique and arguably lucky first-world position. Your days of hunting and gathering are likely over. You have the luxury of choosing how to spend your energy, including on your bike. But because your food choices are so great and you are surrounded by such an abundance of calories, you need to take ownership of your eating habits. No one else trains for you, and no one else can ensure you eat well. It's up to you. Once you accept that nutrition and sleep are integral parts of your training, you are on your way to a thriving lifestyle.

Eat, sleep, train. Words to live by. The training is the easy part. We love to feel fit and work on goals. So why do we often neglect the other two? American culture guides us to think of needing sleep as a weakness. The irony, of course, is that it is during sleep when we become stronger. When you sleep, you use the nutrients you consume to repair your muscles. To neglect sleep is to not honor your training.

The same holds true for nourishing your body. You may be busy, but that doesn't mean you can't nail down all three aspects of eating, sleeping, and training.

"The art of eating well" is first and foremost learning to slow down. I've been using a holistic approach to training athletes for many years now. It's not enough to simply guide training. Training that isn't supported by thorough recovery and optimal nutrition is not effective. So let's have it all. Once athletes accept sleep and nutrition as the ultimate performance enhancers, they are on their way. No ceiling.

This energy and vitality bleeds over into other areas of life as well. Think you're too busy and stressed at work? Maybe you are just too tired and undernourished to handle it. Change takes time and it is challenging, but I've had spouses of athletes call me and say, "You gave me my husband back! This is the person I married but haven't seen in 10 years." Everything is better when we are nourished and rested. This book is ostensibly about training, but really it is about enhancing every aspect of your life.

How do we slow down when eating? Changing habits isn't easy, and just like training it takes a plan and constant dedication. You are hard-wired to over-eat. Not so long ago it was indeed in our best interest to overeat. The next meal wasn't always coming soon. Now we have the luxury of eating only when hungry and the exotic challenge of stopping when perfectly full. The benefits of abundant food are numerous, not the least of which is more constant daily energy. The downside, which at least in part manifests itself in a worldwide obesity crisis, is that we can so easily consume more calories than we use.

I have a few successful techniques I use with my athletes. The first step is simple. We put the utensil down in between every bite. All the way. Let it go. Fingers off. Then we simply enjoy that bite of food. You will swallow eventually. Once you do you are free to begin this process again. With new athletes I have them eat normally for a day and set a stopwatch to time how long it takes to consume three typical daily meals. The next day we time them again but utilize the fork-down protocol. Usually they take twice as long to consume the same amount of food! However, most important, they always comment on feeling full well before the plate is empty. What changed? They gave themselves a chance to feel full.

The next step is to employ the fork-down approach and now simply stop eating when you feel full. You aren't denying yourself a thing. You feel full. So walk away. You're done eating and you feel great. What's next? You're ready for anything because you are not wasting energy on digesting a huge bolus of food. Congratulations; you have nourished well and without overfeeding or mindless eating. >

I am not a Buddhist monk, but many Buddhist practices are of interest to the time-crunched athlete. Live in the moment and focus on your task at hand. Training is *your* time. Eating is *your* time. Sleeping is *your* time. The rest of your world will be waiting when you finish, and that world demands that you be at your best.

It may seem counterintuitive to slow down with a population that seems to be running short on time. A few things are worth considering. Yes, learning to sleep an additional 30 to 120 minutes does decrease your wakeful hours. But what if this increase in sleep provides you with the energy and vitality to do your job better and more quickly? Sleep-deprived people waste time during the day. They are not efficient and their work is poor. Why live like that? I guarantee that for every additional minute of sleep you will get back 2 more in productive awake time. And, you will enjoy those 2 minutes more as well as be better at what you are doing, whether it be playing with the kids, working, or—yes—training!

Give sleep and nutrition the priority they deserve and they will pay you back ten-fold. Take ownership of your food. Get your butt to bed. Eat less, nourish more. You can't afford not to.

Max Shute has been a CTS coach for many years, and he also teaches nutrition in sport and health for the Kinesiology Department at Valdosta State University. He has a PhD in nutrition in sport and chronic disease. His combined experience as a coach and educator led him to conclude that modifying eating behaviors is the most effective route to weight management for time-crunched athletes.

coaches and I have worked with, people who adapt to eating less feel equally satiated with fewer calories and perform equally well on fewer calories. Some of this can be influenced by the composition of your meals, which I'll cover a little bit later, but the point is that hunger is trainable.

Set Expectations Before Eating

The amount of food you eat is largely governed by the amount of food you plan to eat or think you should eat. If you sit down at a table believing you are there to eat a large meal, then a large meal you will consume. Regardless of your energy balance, how many calories you recently expended, or how recently you previously ate (Callahan 2004), your intentions play a big role in determining how much you're going to eat.

Like plate size, this expectation has to do with portion control. But unlike plate size, which is extrinsic, your expectation for the meal is an intrinsic factor. Expectations play a big role in caloric overcompensation. Your overestimation of the energy expenditure from exercise drives an inflated expectation of the meal you should consume. Suddenly, a burrito that would otherwise look ridiculously excessive now seems reasonable.

The goal you set or the plan you make establishes your measure of success. It sounds overly simplistic, but one of the first steps to changing the way you eat is changing the way you think about your meals.

People consume what's in front of them and will consume more food than they need to feel satisfied simply because it is there. In other words, once the food is on the plate, it's too late. You won't make changes to the amount you eat by preparing and serving food the same way you always have and then eating less of it.

Every time you go out for a workout you have distinct expectations. You are going to perform a set number of intervals, at a specific intensity, and upon accumulating the requisite time-at-intensity, you are going to go home. Similarly, when you complete tasks at work, you approach them with established expectations for what constitutes success. The same should be true for your meals, but it often is not. When you change your eating habits to match your meal to your true energy needs, you are more likely to eat within the expectations you have outlined ahead of time.

Stop Multitasking During Meals

Eating time should be for eating. It makes logical sense that mindlessly eating potato chips or other snacks while watching television leads you to eat more than you need. But that's really not that different than shoveling lunch into your face while typing emails on your phone. In both cases you are eating while paying no attention to what you are eating or that you are eating at all.

As demonstrated in the discussion of eating based on hunger and eating based on expectations, the amount of food you eat is heavily dependent on psychological cues, not just physiological ones. If you are not paying attention to what you are eating, and if you are barely tasting what you are eating, it is not going to be satisfying. It is not going to be fulfilling. It is not going to be filling until the moment you realize that you ate way too much. The more present you are while you are eating, the more accurately you will gauge the amount of food you should consume to be satisfied.

This is a hard ask for time-crunched athletes. You eat on the go. You pride yourself on maximizing efficiency by eating at your desk or using mealtime to catch up on correspondence. What I am encouraging you to do, for the sake of your performance, is to reserve mealtime for eating. Enjoy your food, taste it, think about why you're eating it. And take your time. That doesn't mean you need to chew each mouthful a certain number of times, but it does mean deliberately tasting your food and experiencing your meal, rather than shoveling the food into your mouth with the goal of getting it down your gullet faster so you can get to the next bite.

What about socializing during meals? Does that count as multitasking? No. Eating in a group, whether it's a family dinner or a lunch with coworkers, typically makes the meal take longer. Conversations are a great way to slow down your rate of eating. But you still need to focus on what you are eating and your sensations of hunger and satiety. We have all had the experience of getting up after a great meal with friends to realize we are way overfull. As with meals you plan and prepare for yourself, it is important to pause and set expectations for a social meal as well.

Improve the Quality of Your Choices

Last, even though many years of dietary recalls show that the overall nutrition choices of time-crunched athletes are pretty good, it is still worth taking a look at ways to improve the quality of your individual choices.

Fruits and Vegetables

The big thing with this category of foods is to find ways to increase your consumption of both. They tend to be low in energy density but high in nutrient density, meaning they deliver a relatively low number of calories for the volume of food consumed but that those calories deliver a lot of high-quality nutrients. This should come as no surprise, but even with all the various types of diets and strategies that have come and gone, a diet characterized by low-energy density (foods high in fiber and water content) and high-nutrient density has consistently been shown to help athletes achieve and maintain optimal performance weights (Manore 2015).

Lean Animal Protein and Eggs

In recent years, the scientific understanding of lean versus fatty meats has shifted. For a long time, high-fat meats were thought to cause elevated cholesterol levels, leading to the development of heart disease. More recently, scientists have concluded that genetics play a larger role in the development of high cholesterol levels and subsequent health conditions like atherosclerosis and increased heart attack risk. Does that mean the fat content of your meat choices no longer matters? No. If you eat meat, poultry, fish, and eggs, you are primarily after the protein they deliver. Applying the same low-energy/high-nutrient density concept we talked about with fruits and vegetables, lean

SHOULD I BUY ORGANIC?

From a performance nutrition standpoint, it doesn't matter whether you choose organic or conventionally grown produce. The nutritional profiles have been shown to be similar, and by consuming a relatively high volume of food and a wide variety of fruits and vegetables, you will consume all the micronutrients you need. There may be some differences in the nutrient profiles of grass-fed meat compared to animals fed in feedlots, as well as wild-caught fish compared to farmed fish. But even with these foods, it is difficult to show that consuming one versus the other results in improved training or competitive performance.

Again, my focus is on fueling athletic performance. From health and ethical perspectives, I prefer organic fruits and vegetables and meat from grass-fed animals that have not been treated with antibiotics or subjected to miserable conditions on factory farms. You may feel the same way, or not.

Part of preparing athletes for competition is preparing them to handle adversity. Sometimes you will travel to a bike race and the food choices will not be what you want. If you are convinced your optimal performance depends on organic spinach, grass-fed beef, or free-range eggs, what are you going to do when those aren't available? Go home?

I have frequently said that there are racers who could be world champion if the race was held in Boulder, Colorado, on a warm, sunny, windless day on a course they've ridden for years, as long as they could sleep with their special pillow the night before and have their latte just so in the morning. But that's not how racing works, and that's not how life works. Things are rarely, if ever, perfect, and that is also true with food choices.

Whether you choose to purchase conventional, organic, non-GMO, sustainably harvested, grass-fed, cage-free, local, or any combination of these is up to you. From a performance fueling perspective, though, they all work.

animal proteins (less than 10 percent fat) provide the protein you're after with lower energy density, compared with high-fat meats.

Plant Proteins

Nuts, seeds, beans, and legumes are huge assets to time-crunched athletes. Nuts and seeds make great snack substitutions for sweets that are high in refined sugar, and they supply valuable protein and vitamins for athletes who eat few or no animal products. One way to improve the quality of your choices is to switch to reduced-sugar or no-sugar-added nut butters and consume nuts and seeds that are raw, dry roasted, and/or salted/spiced, but not prepared with added sugar.

Whole Grains

In the years since the first edition of *The Time-Crunched Cyclist*, both gluten-free and high-fat, low-carb diets have surged in popularity, the former with the general population and the latter with athletes. As with many dietary manipulations, the question is not whether it is possible to be a successful athlete without consuming grains, but rather whether eliminating grains will enhance performance.

For people with celiac disease, the answer is yes. But non-celiac gluten sensitivity appears to be a sensitivity of the mind rather than the gut (Biesiekierski et al. 2013). In a randomized, double-blind, crossover-controlled feeding study, subjects with non-celiac gluten sensitivity had a run-in period featuring a reduction in fermentable, poorly absorbed, short-chain carbohydrates. During the run-in period their symptoms virtually disappeared. They were then fed either a high-gluten, low-gluten, or placebo diet for 7 days. Subjects in all three groups reported worsening symptoms. The 7-day trial was followed by a washout period, and then the subjects were fed one of the three diets again for 3 days. Again, the results failed to show a dose-dependent connection between gluten and symptoms of non-celiac gluten sensitivity.

If you want to go gluten-free, there's no real harm in doing so as long as you are still able to get the carbohydrate you need to support your training and active lifestyle. But if you do not have celiac disease, don't expect a performance boost from purging gluten from your diet.

Whole grains are already a concentrated, energy-dense source of carbohydrate (compared to watery fruits and vegetables). The more refined the grains, the more energy-dense the products made from them become (there's more energy in a pound of cornmeal than a pound of corn kernels). However, products with more refined grains also tend to include a lot of other highly processed ingredients. So it is preferable to stick with whole grains as much as possible.

Reducing intake of a concentrated, energy-dense carbohydrate may be a good idea for sedentary, overweight individuals. This is part of the reason popular diets that reduce carbohydrate intake target whole and refined grains for reduction or prohibition, and one of the reasons that people initially lose weight when they go gluten-free. For active athletes, however, a concentrated and energy-dense source of carbohydrate can be a great asset to a nutritional program, because carbohydrate is still the preferred fuel for high-intensity exercise.

In the context of performance nutrition and weight management for time-crunched athletes, my views on grains have changed somewhat since the first edition of this book. I used to basically believe that during periods of intense training athletes needed to consume as much carbohydrate as they could, and make room for it by reducing fat intake and consuming only the required amount of protein (1.2–1.7g/kg for endurance athletes, which is higher than the 0.8g/kg recommended daily allowance). During periods of lower training volumes and intensities, I dialed the carbohydrate intake back and increased both fat and protein intake.

But my thinking has evolved. While carbohydrate is necessary for supporting high-quality workouts and promoting optimal recovery, extremely high carbohydrate intakes (more than 60 percent of calories from carbohydrate), primarily made possible by consuming a lot of whole grains and/or rice, aren't necessarily beneficial for time-crunched athletes. When you eat a lot of fruits, vegetables, and grains, your total carbohydrate intake can grow quickly because grains are so energy-dense. Similarly, when you focus on maintaining or increasing your fruit and vegetable intake while modestly reducing grain intake, total carbohydrate intake may come down significantly and allow you to make a caloric reduction while retaining your more nutrient-dense carbohydrate sources.

How much of a reduction you should make depends on the athlete. I encourage athletes who cut back on grains to monitor their training performance to make sure they are still consuming enough carbohydrate energy for high-quality training sessions.

Dairy

If you like and are able to tolerate dairy, it can be a great component of your time-crunched athlete diet. And because the science on cholesterol and the links between fat and heart disease have changed in recent years, it doesn't make sense to place prohibitions on full-fat dairy products. However, keep in mind they are obviously a lot more energy-dense than reduced-fat (2 percent milkfat) or low-fat (1 percent milkfat) products.

The good news is that the fat and protein in full-fat and reduced-fat dairy products make them filling, rich, and satisfying, which may help you feel full without necessarily consuming a ton of calories. The downside is that they are very energy-dense and easy to over-consume, and many dairy products (including a lot of yogurts) are loaded with added sugar.

Fats

I've said a few times already that the newer science on cholesterol has made some previously "bad" foods not so bad anymore, including some cuts of meat and full-fat dairy products. That doesn't mean that all fat is the same or that bacon is good for you. Unsaturated fats from nuts, vegetables, and fish are still preferable to saturated fat, if not for health reasons related to the fat itself then due to the total nutritional quality of the foods containing that fat. Maybe bacon won't kill you, but there are still better sources of fat and protein that are more nutrient dense and less energy dense.

Quick Tips

Start meals with a low-energy-density food/drink. Your sensation of fullness and satiety are partly governed by the volume of what enters your stomach, independent of calorie content. So have a big glass of water when you sit down, or choose the soup or salad with your meal and eat it first, entirely.

Put your utensils down. This is a tip CTS coach Max Shute uses with his time-crunched athletes as an exercise to help them slow down and focus on their food (see "Coaching Eating Behaviors" earlier in this chapter). After each bite of food, he asks them to return their utensils to the placemat (or set down their sandwich) and take their hands off them completely until they are done chewing and swallowing. Obviously, the added steps in the routine slow the eating rate a bit, but he also emphasizes this exercise as a means of using that time to focus on the food as you're eating it, rather than focusing that time on the process of acquiring the next bite.

Clean out the cupboards. You eat what's in front of you, not only when you sit down to a meal but when you open the cupboards and refrigerator. This is an easy tip for athletes who live alone, but a much harder one for athletes with families. Throwing out the cookies just because you don't want to eat them isn't going to score you any points. One solution to this delicate situation is to find alternatives the family enjoys but you don't. For instance, if ice cream is an unavoidable temptation for you, see if there's a flavor the kids like that you're not interested in.

Stop eating in front of a screen. This is an extension of the "stop multitasking while eating" recommendation for eating behaviors, but I mention it here specifically to address mindless eating in front of the television or whatever device you're using for streaming entertainment. Remember, when you focus on what you're eating you are more aware of when you have consumed enough food and are less likely to overeat. Even if you maintain good portion control (the same meal you would have eaten at the table), you are more likely to still feel hungry after consuming that meal when you are eating it while distracted by entertainment.

Stock up on a variety of snack foods. Once you clear the sweets and junk from the cupboards and fridge, you are still going to need some convenient, go-to snacks you can reach. The key to stocking up on snacks is to cover your bases: Make sure you have something salty, something sweet, and something savory. A lot of people decide they'll stick with salty snacks, but then when you get a craving for something sweet the only snacks available are the ones you don't really like but are around because other family members like them. In a pinch, you'll eat them, too. To avoid this, make sure you have good choices that cover the range of your cravings.

HIGH FAT VERSUS HIGH CARBOHYDRATE FOR TIME-CRUNCHED ATHLETES

The debate about high fat, low carb (HF) versus high carbohydrate, low fat (HC) diets has gotten a lot more intense in the past several years. As with other areas of nutrition, it's important to realize that there's a difference between talking about HF or HC and their impact on cardiovascular health, diabetes, and so on, and thinking about them in terms of sports performance. And while there are extremists on both ends of the spectrum when it comes to the HF-HC argument, from my perspective as an endurance coach working with real people, there's a sweet spot in the middle that leverages recent research to optimize performance and body weight for athletes in the real world.

For athletes, the case for an HF diet mentioned earlier in this chapter ("The Perfect Diet Myth") goes like this: You have a virtually unlimited supply of calories from stored fat, whereas you can only store 1,600 to 2,000 calories of carbohydrate in your muscles and liver. During prolonged exercise, glycogen depletion hastens time to exhaustion, so athletes supplement with exogenous carbohydrate during training sessions and competitions to supply working muscles with carbohydrate. The idea behind HF is that by dramatically reducing the amount of carbohydrate in the diet, athletes will adapt to produce more energy via fat oxidation, use less carbohydrate at any given intensity, and therefore maintain their power and pace longer and increase time to exhaustion.

The case for an HC diet is that carbohydrate can be burned for energy at all intensities, whereas the oxidation of fat is more limited to lower and moderate intensities. Breaking carbohydrate down for energy is a two-stream process. You can break it down through normal aerobic metabolism, or you can utilize a metabolic shortcut called glycolysis to produce energy faster when demands are higher. The idea behind HC diets is that you are supplying muscles with the high-octane fuel needed to perform at high intensity.

The Dietary Spectrum

In order to talk about whether someone is on an HC or HF diet, we have to define what that means. A convenient way to do this is to revisit our table of popular diet methods as a reference (repeated here as Table 10.4).

The starting point for low-carb diets is anything under about 40 percent of daily calories coming from carbohydrate. Some of these named diets get there by food or food group restriction (South Beach and Atkins), whereas Paleo restricts food choices by origin or preparation (you can only consume foods that our hunter-gatherer ancestors would have had access to). At the extreme low-carb end is a ketogenic diet, which aims to put the body into a state of nutritional ketosis and thereby use ketones derived from fat to fuel

Macronutrient Levels in Popular Diets

TABLE
10.4

DIET TYPE	EXAMPLE	CARBOHYDRATE	PROTEIN	TOTAL FAT
Extreme high carb	Ornish	74%	18%	8%
High carb	Standard U.S. Diet	60%	20%	20%
High protein	Zone Diet	40%	30%	30%
High fat, high carb	Mediterranean	40%	20%	40%
High fat, high protein	South Beach Diet & Paleo	28%	33%	39%
High fat, low carb	Atkins Diet (induction phase)	<15%	30–35%	55–60%
Extreme high fat	Ketosis	<10%	20–25%	70–75%

muscles and the brain. In order to achieve ketosis, you have to deprive the body of carbohydrate for a substantial period of time, from a few days to a few weeks.

Should Time-Crunched Cyclists Go Keto?

Ketosis sounds like an endurance athlete's dream: endless energy, freedom from bonking, and efficient weight loss. So is it time to go Keto?

To achieve dietary ketosis, you need to severely restrict carbohydrate intake (fewer than 50 grams per day) so your body transitions to using ketones for fueling muscles and the brain. Ketones are produced from fat, so ketosis appeals to athletes because we have virtually unlimited fat reserves. And because bonking results from low blood glucose, an athlete fueled by ketones would be theoretically "bonk-proof."

Dietary ketosis for athletes is a hotly contested subject. Proponents point to the metabolic advantage of relying on fat instead of carbohydrate. Critics point out the physiological limitations of eliminating carbohydrate as a fuel for performance. You'll find bias in both groups. Some scientists and coaches (including me) have long been in the high-carbohydrate camp, but there's also money to be made from creating new supplements. As mentioned earlier, my views on carbohydrate have evolved, and I think many athletes can achieve high performance with less carbohydrate. So while I recognize my historical bias toward carbohydrate, I have tried to look at the science objectively.

Briefly, my conclusion is that while exogenous ketones may have promise as an additional fuel source for endurance athletes (see below), dietary ketosis has limitations that make it difficult to recommend to most athletes. I believe athletes are better served by periodizing carbohydrate availability in order to maximize training quality and performance outcomes. Here's why:

Ketosis Doesn't Improve Endurance Performance

If you do everything right, you may achieve similar performance levels during steady-state endurance exercise following a high-carb (50–65 percent) diet or a high-fat (HF) diet (70–80 percent fat and less than 5 percent carbs). This means you may be able to sustain a submaximal pace equally well using either strategy. The HF strategy may increase the use of fat for energy, especially in long-term (20 months) fat-adapted athletes (Volek et al. 2016). However, the energy cost of locomotion increases on an HF strategy (Burke et al. 2016). This isn't necessarily a problem, because you have a large supply of energy to burn, but these findings don't indicate an improvement in endurance performance. Athletes don't go faster on HF, which is why elite athletes utilize HF during specific periods and then complete high-intensity training and competitions with high carbohydrate availability (more on that later).

Ketosis Is Physiologically Limiting

Without stored and exogenous carbohydrate during exercise, you have very little fuel available for anaerobic glycolysis (you'll make a little in the liver via gluconeogenesis). Ketones can be converted to acetyl-CoA and metabolized aerobically in mitochondria, but you miss out on the energy boost from anaerobic glycolysis and have limited capacity for high-intensity efforts that rely on carbohydrate for fuel.

Almost all endurance sports are intermittent-intensity sports rather than steady-state activities. Hard efforts are required to stay in the group, drop rivals, and build winning margins, whether the events are short or ultradistance. You will achieve your best performances in events featuring intermittent high-intensity efforts by optimizing your ability to use all fuels.

Ketosis May Prevent Gastric Distress

Athletes in ketosis can perform well at a steady endurance pace, and can do so for many hours while consuming far fewer calories than carbohydrate-dependent competitors. As a result, ketosis may be a good solution for athletes who struggle with gastric distress during ultradistance events. During exercise lasting 9 hours or more, changes in blood volume, heat stress, and hydration status can slow or halt gut motility. Consuming large amounts of energy and fluid is problematic because food that stays in the gut too long creates the gas, bloating, and nausea that make athletes drop out of races. Preventing that gastric distress could make dietary ketosis a reasonable solution for some ultradistance athletes, but most Time-Crunched athletes do short, high-speed events where this is not an issue.

Ketosis Disrupts Training

Carbohydrate is the go-to fuel for muscles and the brain. Only in carbohydrate's absence will the body transition to producing and using more ketone bodies for energy.

Initially on a ketone diet, you'll have neither enough carbohydrate nor ketones to fuel your brain. While you are always producing ketones, it takes 2 to 3 weeks to increase production to the point they can be your primary energy source. During this period, performance suffers. Power output diminishes. Perceived exertion goes up at all intensities, and recovery is hindered.

Once adapted to fueling with ketones day-to-day, you still need to adapt to performing as an athlete. This can take months, during which time your only progress will be in fat adaptation, not aerobic development or the ability to produce power. If you want to try ketosis, the best time would be a period of general endurance training. It would be a mistake to go keto during focused, high-intensity training.

Dietary Ketosis Alone Does Not Cut Weight

Exercise studies of athletes adapted to ketosis show they burn more fat than when they were carbohydrate-fueled, but not that they produce more work (Zajac et al. 2014). When athletes get faster after adapting to ketosis, the increased speed is largely due to weight loss. From a performance standpoint, weight loss increases VO_2max, improves power-to-weight ratio, and lowers the energy cost of locomotion. Even if fitness doesn't improve, you are faster and more economical when you lose weight. That's good, but the weight loss is primarily a result of caloric restriction. Diets that severely restrict or eliminate food groups cause people to pay attention to all food choices. Increased focus reduces mindless eating and consumption of junk food, alcohol, and excess sugar. It typically increases consumption of fresh, whole foods. With ketosis, it increases consumption of protein, fat, and vegetables. That's a good outcome, too, but weight loss is still primarily due to caloric restriction.

Compliance Is a Major Barrier

Advocates of ketosis paint a picture of a glorious carbohydrate-free lifestyle where you're never hungry nor suffer from energy fluctuations. From a health perspective, claims include increased insulin sensitivity, lower blood pressure, slower growth in cancerous tumors, improved cognitive function, and more. But will vulnerable populations that would benefit most stick with it? If the original Atkins diet (more protein, fat, and fresh vegetables; less sugar and processed food) was too hard to stick with and rapidly corrupted by packaged food manufacturers, how is it realistic to expect the overweight and/or chronic disease populations to adopt and stick with a much more restrictive strategy?

I have worked with committed, goal-oriented athletes for more than 20 years. Motivated athletes barely stick with an organized nutrition plan—inclusive of all macronutrients—for more than 6 months. In the general population, even people who experience great results with diets like Atkins, Paleo, or The Zone gradually move back toward 45–55 percent carbohydrate, 15–20 percent protein, and 25–30 percent fat within 12 to 24 months. Perhaps the negative feedback of feeling sick after eating sugar and getting kicked out of ketosis could be motivating for some people, but for most athletes ketosis is too restrictive for long-term compliance, even with good results.

Ketosis Will Be Corrupted

Experience also tells me nutritional ketosis will be corrupted by supplement and packaged food industries the same way Atkins, Paleo, and Zone have been. The pattern linking the rise and fall of named diets begins with a strategy that focuses on whole foods and somehow restricts energy intake. The strategy works, people feel great and lose weight. Foods and supplements are developed to make compliance more convenient, but these shift people back to old habits of consuming fewer whole foods. The packaged foods and supplements contribute to increased caloric intake, people regain weight, and once the positive results have disappeared their compliance diminishes and they return to their normal food choices and eating behaviors. As soon as you see "keto-cookies," it's over.

Ketosis is a Competitive Disadvantage

If eating a banana during a competition will diminish your performance, there's something wrong with your nutrition strategy. That's not my bias toward sugar, but rather an observation based on race experience that shows me the most adaptable athletes are the most prepared. To be successful you have to perform using the fuel available and the equipment you have, in the environment provided. Courses change, aid stations run out foods, support crews get lost, food falls out of pockets. If you can't change your strategy to match your situation, you're at a competitive disadvantage.

Exogenous Ketone Supplementation

Exogenous ketone supplementation may be the most promising development from this round of high-fat science. Ketone esters have made it possible to consume ketones in a drink and reduce the time necessary to achieve ketosis. They make the idea of "dual fueling" compelling, wherein an athlete could potentially supplement with exogenous ketones and thereby conserve limited carbohydrate stores for high-intensity efforts (Cox 2014). This supports the fundamental tenet of using training, nutrition, and recovery to maximize your body's capacity to do work. I'm not sold yet, but it has promise.

In summary, based on current science, ketosis works if you want to lose weight in the short term. If you want to train effectively, go with a mixed diet that includes carbohydrate, and look into manipulating carbohydrate availability (discussed next).

Carbohydrate: High-Octane Fuel for Performance

Fat helps you keep going; carbohydrate helps you go fast. I often listen to National Public Radio, and that means I learned a lot from Click and Clack (Ray Magliozzi and his late brother Tom, former hosts of "Car Talk") when they were on the air. Over the years, they answered many questions about the difference between regular and premium gasoline, particularly who needs it and who's wasting money on it. My interpretation of their advice was that it basically comes down to the engine in your car. High-performance cars are built with engines that create higher levels of compression in the cylinders, which produce a bigger bang (literally) every time the cylinder fires. That in turn leads to greater horsepower and more speeding tickets. High-compression engines perform better on high-octane fuel because the fuel burns better at higher temperatures and pressures. Most cars, though, are designed with lower-compression engines that run well on regular gas and don't really benefit from premium fuel.

In some ways, you can look at your body as having two engines that power your training. Your aerobic engine is the smooth and steady motor you'd find in the family minivan, and your glycolytic system is the turbo-charged, smoke-the-tires, 500-horsepower fire-breather in your sports car. Ideally, you'd take great care of both, but the minivan will be more forgiving of poor fuel while the sports car needs premium fuel to deliver top performance. Because the high-intensity efforts in the TCTP rely heavily on the glycolytic system, your success using the program depends on providing your muscles with high-octane fuel.

Carbohydrate is your body's high-performance fuel. As we've already talked about at length, fat is a great fuel for endurance athletes, but it has limited value when it comes to high-performance training and mixed-intensity competitions. There are some people who push protein as the preferred fuel, because high school biology taught us that muscle is made of protein, and therefore you must eat protein if you want to use your muscles. Protein is indeed necessary for building and maintaining muscle tissue, but it's not a very good fuel for intense exercise. For the most part, it has to be transported to the liver and be converted into carbohydrate (a process called gluconeogenesis, literally "creating new glucose") so it can be transported back to muscles and be burned as fuel. Protein plays important roles in sports nutrition (muscle maintenance, immune function, enzymes, etc.), but those roles don't include being a primary fuel source for high-intensity, high-performance efforts.

Carbohydrate is your high-performance fuel because it can be used to power aerobic metabolism and is the primary fuel for high-intensity efforts. When you hit the throttle and demand energy for accelerations, attacks, strenuous climbs, or hard pulls at the front of the group, you call on the glycolytic system for a lot of that energy. The glycolytic system only burns carbohydrate, which means you'd better have it on board if you want to continue pushing the pace.

The crucial determinant of whether you are consuming enough carbohydrate in your overall diet is whether you are able to fully replenish your carbohydrate stores before your next training session. This is crucial because you want to begin each training session with full stores of glycogen (the storage form of carbohydrate in muscles and your liver). Starting training sessions with full glycogen stores increases your time to exhaustion, which is to say that you'll be able to exercise longer before fatigue significantly hurts your performance.

In the context of the relatively short workouts in the TCTP, having full glycogen stores means you'll be able to complete more high-quality efforts before you fatigue to the point that you should stop. Completing more efforts at higher power outputs leads to a greater training stimulus and bigger gains.

The problem, of course, is that there is no gauge that automatically tells you when your carbohydrate stores are replenished. For a long time, we got around this inconvenient fact by promoting very high carbohydrate diets. When you consume 55 to 65 percent of your calories from carbohydrate and are consuming enough total energy to support your caloric expenditure, you are virtually guaranteed to have 100 percent replenished glycogen stores within 24 hours after exercise of any duration or intensity. When you reduce that carbohydrate intake substantially, full replenishment in 24 hours is likely but not guaranteed.

If you choose to go lower in carb intake, it will be important to monitor your training performance. You will need to increase your intake of carbohydrates if your power output during intervals is lower than expected, if your power outputs during interval workouts decline faster than expected, or if you are struggling to recover in time for your next high-quality training session.

Train Low/Train High: When Low Carb Makes Sense for Time-Crunched Athletes

Although I don't recommend HF or ketogenic lifestyles to maximize performance for endurance athletes, the focus on this area of sports science has resulted in a hybrid methodology that could provide benefits. The Train Low/ Train High model (and the associated Train Low/Race High plan) aims to periodize nutrition in a way that enables athletes to complete certain workouts when carbohydrate availability is low while completing other workouts and all competitions when carbohydrate availability is high. When this plan works, the result is a modest improvement in your ability to oxidize fat during exercise while maintaining the high-quality interval workouts necessary to improve your maximum exercise capacity and your maximum sustainable power output.

There are a lot of ways to reduce carbohydrate availability during exercise, but the two that are most common are starting a workout without replenished carbohydrate stores, and not consuming carbohydrate during prolonged workouts. The first scenario can be achieved by exercising after an overnight fast or training twice in a day without replenishing carbohydrate between workouts. In the second scenario, you are using the first workout to deplete carbohydrate stores and purposely avoiding carbohydrate during the downtime between workouts so you complete the second one with low-carbohydrate availability.

What Happens When You Train Low?

If you do interval workouts with low carbohydrate availability, your power outputs will decline. A number of studies (including Yeo et al. 2008) have reported about an 8 percent decrease in power outputs during high-intensity intervals (5-minute maximal efforts). When it comes to endurance rides, you always slow down as the ride gets longer, but with low carbohydrate availability, you slow down sooner and more substantially. Your perceived exertion will be higher. Essentially, at the end of a 3-hour low-carbohydrate ride, you will feel like—and your muscles will be in a similar condition to—the end of a 5-hour high-carbohydrate ride.

Because of these somewhat logical consequences of training with low carbohydrate availability, the recommended application of the Train Low/

Train High plan would be to conduct your focused interval workouts with high carbohydrate availability and conduct some of your longer endurance rides with low carbohydrate availability. When it comes to competition or fast group rides, high carbohydrate availability is absolutely recommended.

Does It Work?

Yes and no. For instance, Yeo in 2008 found that despite the lower power outputs during high-intensity intervals in a low carbohydrate state, subjects experienced improvement in whole body fat oxidation and resting muscle glycogen storage. But other studies (Akerstrom et al. 2009; De Bock et al. 2008) found that training without consuming carbohydrate during workouts doesn't enhance the adaptations we would normally see from those workouts. This suggests that if you are going to try a Train Low methodology, a lack of carbohydrate replenishment prior to a workout is preferred to restricting carbohydrate feedings during a workout.

The bigger drawback is that while the Train Low philosophy may have a positive impact at the cellular level, its impact on real-world performance is less certain. In short, it improves performance for some athletes and not others, because in the real world you train and compete with your whole body, and your performance is also influenced by your cardiovascular, central nervous, and endocrine systems.

A more recent study by Marquet (2016) shows some interesting promise for real-world performance. In this study, well-trained triathletes were familiarized with a training plan for 3 weeks before being divided into two nutrition periodization groups for the next 3 weeks. The key component of the training program was a high-intensity interval workout in the afternoon and a low-intensity aerobic workout the following morning. Both groups ate the same basic macronutrient composition on a daily basis (6g/kg of carbohydrate, 1.6g/kg of protein, and 1g/kg of fat), but the timing of the nutrients was varied. The "sleep low" group consumed no carbohydrate in the period between the afternoon workout and the end of the following morning's workout, meaning they conducted the easy workout with low carbohydrate availability. They ate and consumed fluids following the afternoon workout, but no carbohydrate. The control group consumed carbohydrate steadily throughout the day and evening.

What Marquet and her colleagues found was that after 3 weeks, athletes in the "sleep low" group improved their 10k running time by 3 percent (about 73 seconds, which is significant!), experienced a reduced fat mass leading to minor overall reduction in body weight, and recorded a 12 percent increase in time-to-exhaustion in a supramaximal cycling test (150 percent of VO_2max, approximately 50–70 second effort). More research is needed, especially with more subjects, but this study shows promise for real-world athletes and time-crunched athletes who could, conceivably, schedule back-to-back workouts in the evening and following morning. This schedule could also work well for commuters.

Is Train Low/Train High Recommended for Time-Crunched Athletes?

Intuitively, athletes think that the fittest riders are the ones who would benefit from new techniques like tweaking carbohydrate availability. Pros who are already close to their maximum potential and are looking for tiny advantages can benefit from Train Low methods. In fact, they were doing it long before it was cool! This is partly because the durations of their events are so long that glycogen depletion is a virtual certainty, and because the nature of professional cycling puts such a premium on low body fat percentages (percentages that are neither sustainable nor necessarily healthy, by the way).

I don't recommend Train Low for high-level amateurs (Cat. I and II in Elites and Masters) on high-volume training plans. It's not because it won't work, but rather because it introduces a lot of risk. These riders already have a very high workload and train 5–6 times a week. There isn't a lot of room for error, and they haven't reached the point where all the fundamental aspects of performance are already optimized (as is the case for the pros). When elite amateurs make mistakes with how and when Train Low methods are used, it often does more harm than good and is harder to recover from.

Train Low/Train High can be beneficial for time-crunched athletes. You typically have 4 workouts per week, consisting of 2–3 interval workouts and a longer weekend endurance ride. There may be some benefit—and no real harm—to completing this longer weekend ride before breakfast (low carbohydrate availability) for a few weeks. Just know you won't feel great, your perceived exertion will be higher, and you should take food with you (remember, low carbohydrate stores seem to be more important than low blood sugar).

You could also try to schedule high-intensity interval workouts in the afternoon and complete low-intensity endurance rides in the morning, as in the Marquet study. The training programs in this book are not designed with that schedule in mind, but if it fits into your personal schedule you may be able to try it.

Compared to elite amateurs on high-volume programs, time-crunched athletes can get away with Train Low because your training load and workout frequency are lower so you can better absorb the additional stress and recover from it without hindering interval performance. I still recommend completing purposeful interval workouts with high carb availability, however. Experiment with one portion of your overall training plan and stick with proven workouts for the rest of it.

The best time for time-crunched athletes to try a Train Low approach is during the weeks between TCTP build cycles. During these 4 to 6 weeks, you should be focusing on endurance rides and reducing high-intensity training stress by reducing the frequency of interval workouts at and above lactate threshold. This can be a good time to consistently follow a Train Low approach to fueling your endurance rides for a few weeks and see how your body responds.

11

FUELING HIGH-INTENSITY WORKOUTS

WHILE THE OVERALL COMPOSITION of your diet and your eating behaviors will determine whether you are consuming enough total energy to support your training and promote optimal recovery, the nutrition decisions you make before, during, and after your high-intensity workouts will directly affect the quality of those training sessions.

For a long time I have started discussions of training nutrition chronologically, looking at pre-workout nutrition first, then during-workout foods, and ending with post-workout nutrition. But when you instead rank these distinct segments of sports nutrition by the impact they have on workout performance, the priority order changes. Through this lens, post-workout nutrition is the most important, because there is a lot more time between workouts than there is between your pre-workout meal or snack and the actual training session.

All of the nutrition and hydration choices you make in the 18–48-hour period between your workouts determine whether you have the carbohydrate stores necessary for a high-quality training session. In contrast, your immediate pre-workout nutrition choices don't do much to change your glycogen stores; they have more impact on how energized you feel. Feeling ready to go is important, but it can't overcome inadequate nutrition choices over the preceding day. So in the following discussion, we're going to start with post-workout refueling first, followed by pre-workout snacks, and then take a look at good choices for supplying exogenous energy during workouts.

STRONGER TOMORROWS: THE KEYS TO POST-WORKOUT NUTRITION

Your nutrition and hydration choices immediately after your rides play important roles in preparing you for successful training sessions in the following days. This is true whether you're on a high-volume, moderate-intensity training program or a high-intensity, low-volume plan, but low-volume trainers have some additional challenges to overcome.

It's likely that you will finish your hard interval workouts having only consumed one bottle of plain water. In my experience, some of you will have chosen an electrolyte drink instead, a few will have consumed a carbohydrate-rich sports drink, and very few will have eaten a gel or any solid food. We can talk about guidelines and recommendations all we want, but the reality is athletes don't consume many calories during high-intensity interval sessions. You can compensate for this somewhat with your pre-workout snack, but after your training session is done, it's important to focus on nutrition and hydration so you can replenish what you've depleted and give your body the nutrients it needs to recover and adapt. Remember, physiological improvements come during recovery, not exercise, so it is important to fuel your recovery properly.

Your body is primed to replenish muscle glycogen stores most rapidly within the first 30 to 60 minutes following exercise, and the sooner the better. This period is known as the "glycogen window," and quite literally there are more gates or "windows" open to allow sugar to enter muscle cells during this time. While this is an important advantage, its importance has been overemphasized for most athletes. If you are training or competing more than once in a single day, it is crucially important to leverage the glycogen window. If you have 24–48 hours between hard workouts, leveraging the glycogen window is not as crucial.

Sodium and Carbs: The Critical Components

Sodium helps replenish sodium lost in sweat, but it also plays an important role in transporting carbohydrate out of the gut and into the bloodstream (part of the reason you rarely see sodium-free sports nutrition products). And, of course, fluid is important for replacing the water that evaporated off your skin to keep you from overheating.

In terms of total amounts, your goal within the first 2 hours after exercising should be to consume 500 to 700 milligrams of sodium and enough water to equal 1.5 times the water weight you lost during the exercise session. In other words, if you lost 2 pounds (32 ounces, or 0.9 kg) during your ride, you should drink 48 ounces of fluid (about 1.4 liters) in the 2 hours after you get back. Within 4 hours after training, you should consume 1.5 grams of carbohydrate per kilogram (g/kg) of body weight. For a 170-pound (77-kilogram) athlete, 1.5 g/kg means 115 g (4 ounces) of carbohydrate.

That can be quite a challenge, especially when you add in the protein and fat calories that come with that carbohydrate, and obviously it becomes even more challenging for heavier athletes. That's why this recommendation is over a 4-hour period. Ideally you should consume the first 50 to 60 grams (1.7 to 2.1 ounces) of that carbohydrate within the first 30 to 60 minutes so you can take advantage of the glycogen window, but the rate of glycogen replenishment doesn't magically go to zero after 60 minutes. Stuffing your face to eat 115 to 135 grams of carbohydrate in an hour isn't fun, nor is it necessary to fully replenish your glycogen stores in time for tomorrow's training session.

Protein and Recovery: More Isn't Better

Protein is critically important to post-workout recovery, but many athletes overemphasize protein and consume much more than they need. This impacts time-crunched athletes because adding more protein than necessary to post-workout nutrition contributes to overfeeding and hinders weight management. A lot of the habits athletes have around protein are rooted in the following myths about the role of protein in recovery.

Myth: Large Amounts of Protein Are Necessary for Recovery

No. Some protein is helpful for recovery, but it is unlikely that you need protein supplementation. The recommended daily allowance (RDA) for protein is 0.8 grams per kilogram of body weight of protein per day. This increases to about 1.2–1.7 g/kg for athletes in a medium- to high-workload training plan (in terms of volume and/or intensity). But consuming more than 2 g/kg of protein doesn't do you any more good in terms of recovery, muscle synthesis, immune function, or energy metabolism. Whether you are a carnivore, omnivore, vegetarian, or vegan, you should be able to consume 1.2–1.7 g/kg of protein daily through your normal meals and snacks. For a 170-pound athlete, it works out to about 4 ounces, or one-quarter pound.

Myth: The Best Time to Consume Protein Is Immediately After Exercise

In terms of timing, you should be careful not to focus too many of your post-workout nutrition choices on protein. Immediately post-workout you want to focus on replenishing carbohydrate, and adding some protein to your food/drink choices may help accelerate the uptake of carbohydrate. So, when should you consume the most protein? Actually, never. It's better to spread your intake throughout the day. You need fuel for building and maintaining muscle tissue, your immune system, and all the other functions of protein throughout the day. And you don't store protein, so unlike fat or carbohydrate you can only use protein from food when you have it on board. In addition, protein is satiating and slows digestion. This is a big part of the reason I'd rather see you spread your protein intake across meals and snacks throughout the day.

Myth: You Need a Recovery Drink After Every Workout

Recovery drinks are great. They conveniently deliver carbohydrate, electrolytes, fluid, and protein, and they are typically consumed immediately after exercise when your body is ready for rapid replenishment. Yet, despite the fact your body is able to replenish glycogen stores most rapidly in this 60–90-minute post-exercise "glycogen window, " you don't necessarily need a recovery drink after every workout.

Replenishment of fluid, electrolytes, carbohydrate, and protein doesn't cease after the first 60–90 minutes post-exercise. It just gradually slows down. If you only trained for 60–90 minutes, glycogen replenishment shouldn't be a big challenge because most likely you didn't empty the tank in the first place. And even if you did, your glycogen stores will be completely replenished in 24 hours just from your normal food intake.

When should you use a recovery drink? If you are training or competing more than once in a single day, a recovery drink after your first session is a good idea. If you are riding back-to-back days of long miles (like following the long-ish Saturday rides in the time-crunched programs when you have another long-ish ride on Sunday), then it's a good idea as well.

A breakpoint I use with some athletes is that a recovery drink may be warranted following rides that accumulate about 1,500–2,000 kilojoules of work (this can vary a bit based on the athlete) or anything more than that. This could be a very hard 90-minute interval session or a 3–4-hour moderate pace ride. The rationale is to base the need for a recovery drink on whether there was sufficient energy expenditure to substantially deplete carbohydrate stores and cause significant training stress.

What a Recovery Drink Should Look Like

Even when a recovery drink makes sense, the most important ingredients are fluid and carbohydrates, followed by electrolytes and protein. Some people get caught up in the exact ratio, whether 2:1 carb/protein is better or worse than

3:1 or 4:1. I think the bigger picture is that they are all better than a protein-heavy drink. Consuming a high-protein recovery drink that contains little to no carbohydrate is not a good idea for recovery. It may supply a nutrient you need for repair and synthesis, but it doesn't supply the nutrient you need for energy replenishment (carbohydrate). The urgency of protein replenishment is not as big as carbohydrate, and you can get the protein you need for repair and synthesis through meals.

Similarly, a drink that contains a lot of protein and a lot of carbohydrate is also not ideal, mostly because it is likely to be very high in calories. Athletes who consume these high-calorie drinks typically overcompensate with total post-workout calories because they follow up the drink with a regular size or over-sized meal.

For a look at what to drink during a workout, see the section "What the Heck Is in My Sports Drink?"

ENERGIZING TODAY: PRE-WORKOUT NUTRITION

Assuming you did a good job replenishing energy stores and fluids in the long hours since your last workout, the role of pre-workout nutrition is pretty simple. You're trying to top off carbohydrate stores and make sure you have adequate blood glucose to continue feeling energized and focused.

You have the stored carbohydrate and fat to power your workouts already; those were supplied by your daily nutrition choices in the hours since your last workout. In contrast, what you eat in the hours before training has more impact on how you feel (energized vs. sluggish), and this has a very real impact on training quality.

If you're getting set to complete a difficult training session—a Power-Interval workout that's going to include 16 to 20 minutes of effort way above your lactate threshold power output—you're going to want to make sure you're energized and alert. There are two components: your pre-workout meal and your pre-workout snack. The differences between the two are how big they are and when they're consumed.

Pre-workout Meal

The most important thing about the last full meal you eat before a training session is that it's out of your stomach and digested before you start training. This is especially important for hard interval workouts, because high-intensity efforts tend to be downright unpleasant on a full stomach. A relatively light meal that's rich in carbohydrate is a good choice, because meals that contain a lot of fat or protein stay in the stomach longer and are digested more slowly. That's a good thing if you're trying to feel full longer, but not good if you're about to go out for a hard workout. Table 11.1 lists examples of good foods to choose before a workout.

When it comes to your pre-workout or pre-race meal, a good rule of thumb is that meal size should get smaller the closer you get to the workout or race. For instance, you can consume 1.5 g of carbohydrate per kilogram of body weight when your final pre-workout meal is 3 hours before your ride, but you want to be closer to 1 g/kg if you're going to train 2 hours after your last significant meal (for a 170-pound athlete, that's about 2.5 ounces).

Just as this isn't the time for a high-fat or high-protein meal, you shouldn't try to fill your daily fiber requirement just before a workout, either. The American Heart Association recommends 25 to 30 grams (0.88–1.0 ounces)

Choosing the Right Pre-workout Food

TABLE 11.1

GOOD FOODS FOR PRE-EXERCISE MEALS	LESS DESIRABLE FOODS FOR PRE-EXERCISE MEALS
High carbohydrate, moderate protein, low fat: pasta, rice, potatoes, sandwiches (roast beef, turkey, peanut butter and jelly), oatmeal, breakfast burrito with eggs and potatoes, pizza (with reduced-fat cheese or less cheese), fruit	High fat and/or protein, low carbohydrate: steak, bacon, sausage, ice cream, chili dogs, cream sauces Low carbohydrate, low calorie: salads (garden, tuna, or chicken), diet soft drinks

of fiber a day to reduce levels of LDL cholesterol (the bad kind) and reduce the risk of heart disease, but fiber also slows digestion, so it's better saved for other meals.

Good choices for your pre-workout meal are pasta, rice, potatoes, sandwiches (roast beef, turkey, peanut butter and jelly), oatmeal with fruit, or a breakfast burrito with eggs and potatoes. Less desirable choices, because they are high in fat and tend to leave athletes feeling sluggish, include fatty meats (steak, bacon, sausage) and dishes that contain a lot of cheese or cream sauces. Other foods that are normally great for you but aren't ideal for pre-workout nutrition are high-fiber, low energy-density choices like a salad.

Pre-workout Snack

There is perhaps nothing more important to the quality of your training sessions than what you eat and drink in the hour immediately prior to getting on your bike. Eat the right things, and you'll feel strong, invigorated, and energized. Eat the wrong things, and you'll feel bloated, sluggish, and nauseated. It's difficult to have a great workout when you feel like you're carrying a bowling ball in your gut.

The key here is to choose foods that will get out of your stomach and into your blood quickly. There are many choices available, and it's important to experiment with various combinations until you find a solution that doesn't come back up halfway through your workout. Your best options, from both the sports nutrition and practical standpoints, are carbohydrate-rich gels and sports drinks. That's not to say you can't have a great workout on a peanut-butter-and-jelly sandwich or a granola bar, but you're more likely to fully digest the carbohydrates in a gel or sports drink and have all that energy available for your muscles.

I've found that using specifically designed sports nutrition products makes it less likely that athletes will experience an upset stomach during a hard workout. These products are simply easier to digest; they get out of the stomach and gut faster than conventional foods. To aid in the digestion and absorption process, make sure you consume at least 8 ounces of fluid (about 0.25 liter) whenever you eat a gel or bar.

Just to show that there is some variability in what works best for individual athletes, my tried-and-true recipe before 2-hour rides is a bit higher in carbohydrate than the standard recommendations. I consume a bottle of sports drink 30 to 60 minutes before training and a gel 10 to 15 minutes before I get on my bike. With a bottle of sports drink and one gel packet, that adds up to about 50 grams (1.75 ounces) of carbohydrate, or 0.65 g of carbohydrate per kilogram (I weigh about 170 pounds, or 77 kilograms). When I get the chance to go out for longer rides, I typically choose foods containing a bit more fat and protein, like a Bonk Breaker energy bar, to help me avoid feeling hungry or having a quick spike in energy early in a long ride.

As you can see in the following list, many other snack combinations provide 50 to 75 grams of carbohydrate and would work in the hour leading up to training, and you can easily bring this down to 30 to 50 grams by consuming smaller portions. Regardless of the option you choose, it's imperative that you consume 16 to 24 ounces of fluid (0.5–0.7 liters) in the hour before training, be it water, fruit juice, or a sports drink.

- 1 cup vanilla yogurt + ½ cup Grape-Nuts cereal + 2 tablespoons raisins
- 1 cup vanilla yogurt + 1 cup fresh fruit
- 1 cup juice + 1 banana
- 1 slice banana-nut bread + 1 cup skim milk
- 1 energy bar + 8 ounces sports drink
- Smoothie: 2 cups skim or soy milk + 1½ cups mango or berries + 2 tablespoons soy protein
- 1½ cups multigrain cereal + 1½ cups skim milk
- 1 bagel + 1 banana + 1 tablespoon nut butter
- 1 cup cottage cheese + 8 whole-wheat crackers + 1 apple

CAFFEINE AND STIMULANTS

Any discussion of pre-workout and during-workout sports nutrition generates questions about using caffeine and other stimulants as ergogenic aids. I'll keep this simple: Caffeine, in amounts normally found in foods, coffee, and tea, is fine and effective. Furthermore, I haven't seen any markedly better stimulant that's not on the World Anti-Doping Agency's list of banned substances or that doesn't come with a federal prison term for possession. In other words, caffeine works.

Caffeine is generally safe in reasonable quantities (200 milligrams or less per dose), and its effects and side effects are well-known and predictable. People keep coming out with new additives and claim all manner of performance enhancements for them, but the truth is, plain old caffeine is hard to beat.

The impact of caffeine on athletic performance is twofold. The more important effect is that it improves motivation, alertness, concentration, and enthusiasm. Considering that the workouts in this program are relatively short and decidedly challenging, adding a little caffeine to your pre-workout snack wouldn't hurt. This is especially true if you find yourself struggling to generate the enthusiasm necessary to start a hard workout after 8 to 10 hours at your day job.

Caffeine's second impact on performance is that it may help your body liberate more fat for use as energy during exercise. This isn't a bad thing, but it's also not going to have a very significant influence on the effectiveness of your workout.

Interestingly, there's some evidence that caffeine may help accelerate glycogen replenishment when it's consumed immediately after a workout. This opens up the possibility of caffeinated recovery drinks but also means you may have a good excuse for your coffee stop after the hard part of your local group ride.

NUTRITION DURING WORKOUTS

Short, high-intensity workouts can have a significant impact on your willingness, ability, and need to consume food and fluids while you're on your bike. In particular, hard workouts inhibit your desire and your opportunities to consume either food or fluids, which is part of the reason that your pre-workout snack is so important. Fortunately, because of the amount of glycogen you can store in your muscles and the fact that you can only process and utilize about 1–1.4 grams of ingested carbohydrate per minute anyway, there is little need to consume any calories during a 1-hour workout.

Before you call or e-mail me to point out the discrepancy between that last sentence and recommendations to eat early and often during rides, let me make an important distinction: If you're planning on having a good ride that lasts more than about 75 minutes, you need to consume carbohydrate within the first 30 minutes on your bike. But if you're going to be done with your hard efforts and either off your bike or into your cool-down within 60 to 75 minutes, you can complete a high-quality training session without consuming a single calorie on the bike. Will your ride be even better if you use a sports drink or a gel during a 1-hour workout? Maybe, but it depends less on the calories themselves and more on what you can tolerate.

Water is the one thing you can't do without during even a 1-hour training session. Depending on the temperature, humidity, and your personal sweat rate, you can lose up to 1.5 liters of fluid (about 50 fluid ounces) in a 1-hour workout. To make matters worse, high-intensity workouts increase core temperature more than low- to moderate-intensity rides, especially if you're

Carb Consumption on Short Rides Versus Long Ones

TABLE
11.2

RIDE LENGTH	CARB INTAKE
75 min. or less	None necessary; drink water
75 min. to 2 hrs.	Electrolyte drink or 1–2 gels
2 to 5 hrs.	Carb and/or electrolyte drinks, water, gels, solid foods
5+ hrs.	Taste, texture, and variety increase in importance

CALORIES IN YOUR POCKET, HYDRATION IN YOUR BOTTLES

What should be in your bottles during workouts: water, or a carbohydrate/electrolyte drink? I am a big fan of sports drinks, but for the vast majority of the rides in a time-crunched program, an energy-dense drink is not necessary. Separating your calories from your hydration is a better strategy. In this scenario, your water bottle serves the purpose of hydration, and the food in your pocket serves the purpose of fueling.

As workload and temperature change, your fluid and calorie needs change independently. When it is hot, you will need more fluid per hour, sometimes twice as much as during cool weather. If the fluid you are carrying contains 35 grams (1.23 ounces) of carbohydrate per 20-ounce serving (0.6 liters), you'll consume 70 grams of carbohydrate per hour if you drink two bottles. That's at the top end of the recommended range of 60 to 90 grams of carbohydrate. Any further calories can overload your gut and lead to gastric distress. Even worse, after the first bottle, you may feel full so you delay drinking and start digging a dehydration hole.

Remember, you can come back from a caloric deficit easily and within minutes by eating. The process of returning to normal hydration status takes much longer, and being dehydrated during that time can have more deleterious effects on your performance.

Separating calories from hydration allows you to adjust your fluid intake in response to temperature without affecting your calorie supply. It also allows you to vary your carbohydrate more easily because it is not tied to what you are drinking. This is important because your food choices can supply a large amount of the sodium you need to replenish. In many cases you can consume the recommended 500 to 700 mg/hour of sodium entirely through food sources while drinking plain water.

riding indoors, and sweat evaporating off your skin is your body's primary cooling system. Sweating out up to 1.5 liters of fluid and failing to drink will absolutely hinder your performance, resulting in lower power outputs for your intervals and a shortened time to exhaustion.

You also lose electrolytes as you sweat (primarily sodium, but also some potassium and traces of other minerals), so you'd ideally consume a sports drink during even short workouts, but again we have to go back to the concept of tolerance. Studies, including one published in 2004 by Dr. Ed Coyle, have shown that as exercise intensity and core temperature increase, athletes gradually lose their drive to drink and eat. Anecdotal evidence not only supports this but also shows that many athletes experience an upset stomach when they consume calories during very hard workouts. At the same time, adding carbohydrate and sodium to the fluid increases an athlete's motivation to drink and increases the amount of fluid you consume every time you lift your bottle to your lips. And the American College of Sports Medicine recommends consuming 500 to 700 milligrams of sodium per hour of aerobic exercise.

I recommend trying to find a compromise that works for you. Many athletes can tolerate electrolyte solutions and lightly flavored carbohydrate/electrolyte sports drinks. Few athletes have any desire to consume energy gels or solid foods. For short workouts, caloric replenishment is not necessary, but the need for electrolytes and fluids means that a sports drink is a good idea for high-intensity workouts as long as it doesn't upset your stomach.

What the Heck Is in My Sports Drink?

A sports drink is essentially water with stuff dissolved in it. Some drinks have lots of different kinds of stuff dissolved in them, most of which just waste space. There is only so much room to dissolve solutes in a drink, and drinks with fewer ingredients can use more of that room for important things such as carbohydrate and sodium. The simplest drinks are the best because they are easiest on the gut and are better at facilitating the transport of sugar and electrolyte across the semipermeable membrane of the intestinal wall.

The concentration of sports drinks is important. When you change the osmolality of the fluid (the total molecular concentration of everything in the drink—carbohydrate, electrolyte, flavoring, additives—per unit volume), it changes how the drink influences the overall mixture in your stomach, and hence how that mixture makes it into the intestine. Sports drinks are formulated to optimize the absorption of carbohydrate, fluid, and electrolyte. If the osmolality of the sports drink is too high because of a bunch of additives, it may contribute to slower gastric emptying. When the osmolality of sports drinks is lower it is more likely to contribute to faster gastric emptying (depending on what else you're eating and drinking), and if it's being consumed on an empty stomach it is formulated to get into the intestine quickly.

If you are designing a sports drink to have a relatively low osmolality but you want it to deliver moderate to high amounts of sodium and/or carbohydrate, you have to eliminate other stuff to make room. That's a big part of the reason we've seen drink manufacturers shift to drinks with shorter ingredient lists.

The ingredients, primarily sugar, sodium, potassium, and flavoring, are in the drink for good reason. Putting electrolytes and flavoring into a fluid makes you want to drink more frequently and consume more fluid each time you drink. There's actually a lot more to the way your sports drink tastes than marketing mumbo jumbo. A lightly flavored drink is preferable to a stronger one because when you consume half a bottle in one long slug, the stronger-tasting drink becomes overwhelming and you stop drinking. A drink that tastes almost watered down when you are at rest will taste just about right when you are exercising. This is why athletes have long diluted commercial sports drinks like original Gatorade, which these days are often flavored to appeal to convenience store customers instead of athletes.

Even taste components and mouth feel are important. A slightly tart drink will encourage you to drink more than an overly sweet one, and citrus flavors also increase the drive to drink. It should be no surprise, then, that almost every drink company has some version of lemon-lime and/or orange in its product line. In addition to the flavor, a sports drink needs to clear the mouth well. When a drink leaves a film in your mouth, as is often the case with overly sweet drinks, it's not only unpleasant, but you're not likely to drink again soon.

Rather than dilute sports drinks, it is better to find a drink with a lighter taste so you can comfortably consume it at full strength. The reason you don't want to dilute heavily flavored commercial sports drinks isn't because doing so lowers the concentration of sugar in the drink, but because it reduces the sodium concentration. Again, this is relative to all the other foods and fluids you are consuming, but if you are consuming a sports drink with the primary goal of staying hydrated—that is, maintaining proper fluid and electrolyte levels—then consuming a watered-down drink provides a lot of fluid and reduced sodium, which over time could contribute to inadequate sodium replenishment in relation to fluid intake.

Ideally, while riding you'll consume enough fluid to replenish at least 80 percent of the water weight you lose by sweating. That's often not a problem during moderate-intensity Tempo rides, but it becomes difficult when you're in the throes of repeated sets of PowerIntervals. That's OK, and the relatively short nature of your workouts should be taken into consideration. The fluids (and electrolytes) you consumed before your workout will help ward off dehydration during short workouts.

The bottom line is that if you consume nothing else during your hard interval workouts, make sure you drink water. Aim for at least one full bottle over the course of an hour, and follow the hydration recommendations in the post-workout nutrition section to make sure you replenish what you've lost.

Fueling Early-Morning Workouts

Early morning is a great time for busy professionals to squeeze in a workout. You can be done with your workout and showered before your kids wake up or your phone starts buzzing. A lot of people prefer to start their day with a workout because it's their time for themselves and allows them to begin the day with a positive accomplishment.

Fueling early-morning interval workouts is a challenge, because you haven't eaten for 8 to 10 hours and you burned through about 80 percent of your liver glycogen overnight. All the same, you don't have time to eat and wait around for an hour or more before getting on your bike. So, what can you do to ensure you have a great morning workout?

Keep it simple and small: Your muscles are full of glycogen and ready to go; it's your blood sugar that's low because your liver glycogen stores are mostly depleted. Low blood sugar means less fuel for your brain, and a hungry brain has trouble staying focused on completing intense intervals at high power outputs. You just need something light that delivers simple and complex carbohydrates, and maybe a little protein to make it more satiating. A sports drink or a gel would work, as would any of the aforementioned pre-workout snacks. If you normally consume caffeine, a shot of espresso or a small cup of coffee isn't a bad idea, but make sure you also consume about 16 ounces (about 0.5 liter) of plain water or fruit juice.

Eat first: It always takes a little time to get dressed and set up for your ride, so eat before you start that process. This means eating as soon as you get out of bed, and then going about the business of getting ready to train.

Get started: Early-morning workout time disappears fast, so get started even if it means doing a slightly longer warm-up spin to let your food settle. If you find you really need a little more time to digest your snack before you work out, be careful not to get too engaged in something like cruising the news or checking your e-mail.

Fueling Your Longer Rides

During longer workouts, events, and races, your nutrition requirements are somewhat different. When you're going to be on the bike for more than 75 minutes, it's important to start consuming carbohydrates, electrolytes, and fluid early on and continue to do so all the way through the end of the ride. The standard guidelines for carbohydrate consumption during endurance exercise call for 30 to 60 grams (1 to 2 ounces) of carbohydrate per hour, more toward the high end of the range as intensity increases.

From watching athletes train for more than 20 years, I can tell you that 50 to 60 grams of carbohydrate in an hour is good for racing and hard group rides, but riders on moderate-intensity group rides and centuries tend to gravitate more toward 35 to 40 grams (1.25 to 1.4 ounces) per hour. And if you're wondering if body weight has an impact on the guidelines, the answer is yes and no. The 30- to 60-gram range is pretty large, and both small and large riders tend to fit within it, but smaller riders often do well at the lower end and larger riders sometimes need to be at the higher end. That said, a smaller rider who is working hard may need to consume 50 grams of carbohydrate an hour while a bigger rider who is just cruising along may only need 30 to 40 grams.

Another way of gauging calorie consumption during longer rides is as a percentage of your hourly workload in kilojoules. Remember that you start your rides with about 1,600 calories of stored carbohydrate, and you can make that stored energy last longer by adding exogenous carbohydrate in the form of a sports drink, energy bar, or gel while you're riding. But when you see 600 kilojoules on your handlebar display after the first hour, don't make the mistake of thinking you should be consuming anywhere near that number of calories. Instead, you want to consume 20 to 30 percent of your hourly caloric expenditure, which in this case would be 120 to 180 calories or 30 to 45 grams

JASON KOOP'S SUPERSECRET RICE BALLS

One of the greatest truths about sports nutrition is that even the best foods are useless if they stay in your pocket. You have to put those calories, electrolytes, and fluids into your body for them to do you any good. That means you have to like how they taste, how they smell, how they feel in your mouth, and how easy they are to unwrap and get down your throat. This is part of the reason homemade, portable sports nutrition foods have exploded in popularity over the past few years.

CTS coach Jason Koop is primarily an ultrarunner, as well as being coaching director for CTS and the author of *Training Essentials for Ultrarunning*. When he was a novice endurance athlete, he loved Krispy Kreme doughnuts, and one of his early experiments in sports nutrition was to cram three or four doughnuts into a sandwich bag and squeeze them out of a torn corner, like you would with a carbohydrate gel. I vividly remember watching him extrude doughnuts from a plastic bag during a century ride in Colorado when he was a young coach, and I have to tell you it was a little hard to ride next to him.

Thankfully, his tastes have improved since then, and he developed two variations of a rice ball that both meet the during-workout and during-competition nutrition guidelines in this chapter and have the taste, texture, and convenience characteristics that make them a go-to favorite.

BACON AND EGG RICE BALLS

Makes about 12 rice balls

2 eggs

2 strips bacon

1½ cups (290 grams) uncooked basmati rice

2 oz. (60 grams) grated Parmesan cheese

Salt to taste

1. Cook the rice.

2. Scramble and cook the eggs.

3. Cook the bacon. Drain excess fat and chop.

4. Combine rice, eggs, bacon, cheese, and salt in a large mixing bowl.

5. Scoop into 12 sandwich bags and tie the end off.

Nutrition (per ball)
Calories: 133
Carbohydrate: 18 g
Protein: 4 g
Fat: 5 g
Sodium: 354 mg

SWEET AND SALTY RICE BALLS (VEGETARIAN)

Makes about 12 rice balls

2 eggs

1½ cups (290 grams) uncooked basmati rice

2 T (30 ml) honey

1 T (15 ml) soy sauce

1. Cook the rice.

2. Scramble and cook the eggs.

3. Combine rice, eggs, honey, and soy sauce in a large mixing bowl.

4. Scoop into 12 sandwich bags and tie the end off.

Nutrition (per ball)
Calories: 115
Carbohydrate: 20 g
Protein: 2 g
Fat: 3 g
Sodium: 327 mg

of carbohydrate (1 to 1.6 ounces). And 600 kilojoules an hour is a good ball-park figure for most amateur cyclists. During a hard interval workout you might get up to 800 kj/hr, and at a moderate cruising pace with a group you might be down at 450 to 500 kj/hr.

What do numbers like 35 to 50 grams of carbohydrate per hour mean in terms of items you can hold in your hand? Most energy gels contain about 25 grams of carbohydrate per packet. There is more variation in the amount of carbohydrate found in sports drinks per serving. Bonk Breaker Real Hydration, for example, is an electrolyte-focused hydration drink that contains 8 grams of carbohydrate in a serving. If you use other brands, you may consume anywhere from 20–25 grams of carbohydrate in a serving. Most energy bars targeted at endurance athletes contain 30 to 45 grams of carbohy-drate per bar (or per serving). Throughout your training, it's best to diversify your sports nutrition, in terms of type and texture, so you can fuel yourself properly as product availability and your taste preferences change.

Here's a tip for everyone who prefers to use energy gels or bars: You have to drink about 8 ounces of water (about 0.25 liter) with the gel for it to work properly. You're consuming a concentrated, viscous source of carbohydrate, and a few slugs of water will help your body break it down, get it out of the stomach, and absorb it from the gut more quickly. A gel plus water means you'll get to use more of the carbohydrate you just consumed. If you just down the gel and skip the water, you'll absorb most of the carbohydrate, but you'll absorb it more slowly.

In terms of hydration on longer rides, you still want to consume enough fluid to replace at least 80 percent of the fluid you're losing from sweat. The bare minimum is one standard bottle (standard bottles are typically 20 ounces or 500 milliliters, depending on where they are made) per hour, but that will only be adequate for low-intensity rides on cool days. In warmer conditions, or for any moderate- to high-intensity ride, shoot for two bottles an hour. And if it's a particularly hot day, you may need to add a third bottle.

SAVING YOURSELF

Every cyclist has felt it: a sudden emptiness in your gut, a twitch in a calf or hamstring muscle, or a momentary bout of light-headedness. You didn't eat enough or drink enough, and now you're about to bonk, cramp, or both. Your body is telling you it needs food and/or fluids right now, and if you refuse to listen, your body will begin to shut down. You screwed up and you know it, but it's still possible to save yourself and continue to have a good ride or race.

Time is of the essence, and desperate times call for—or at least excuse— desperate measures. If you're bonking, you need carbohydrate fast. That means simple sugars and a lot of them. Down two energy gels right away (with at least half a bottle of water), or try to consume a full bottle of carbohydrate-rich sports drink.

If you're out of sports drink or you've already eaten all the food in your pockets, it's time to hit the candy aisle of the convenience store. Everyone has favorite emergency foods; some go for chocolate chip cookies and Mountain Dew while others go for Little Debbie Oatmeal Cream cookies and Coke. My personal favorites are a Snickers bar and a Lipton Iced Tea (sugar and caffeine equal to a Coke but no carbonation). Obviously, these options are not the preferred choices for sports nutrition—they almost always put too much sugar into your belly—but they'll do the trick in a pinch. You'll get a boost from the sodium, sugar, and caffeine, and buy yourself enough time to get back on track with your nutrition.

If you're starting to cramp you need to look for electrolytes, primarily sodium and potassium. Not all cramps are caused by a lack of electrolytes, but it's very difficult to pinpoint exactly what's causing the situation in your calf while it's happening, and there's a chance that consuming electrolytes will help solve the problem. If consuming electrolytes works, you get to keep going.   >

If it doesn't, you'll still have to deal with the cramp, but at least you'll have more electrolytes onboard.

In other words, as soon as you feel a pre-cramp twinge in your calf, hamstring, or quadriceps, try to immediately consume 200 to 400 milligrams of electrolytes. Depending on the products available, this can mean one or two energy gels and/or a full bottle of sports drink. Often this will mean consuming more carbohydrate than you ideally want at one time, but right now the cramp is going to harm your performance a lot more than over-consuming carbohydrate will.

Another theory says that cramping is due to muscle fatigue, and neither food nor electrolytes will help if that's the case. Still, a shot of electrolytes is worth a try.

The newest theory on cramp prevention and alleviation centers on the nervous system. The idea is that cramps are caused by nervous system pathways that get "stuck," refusing to relax muscles once they have contracted. The solution, as the theory goes, is disruption. Strong tastes that are shockingly bitter, spicy, or salty may disrupt the nervous system enough to "reset" the system. This is part of the appeal of pickle juice or mustard. They are both high in sodium, but they are also very strong and somewhat shocking flavors in the middle of an endurance event. The science on nervous system disruption is new and ongoing, but it's potentially promising. In the meantime, slowing down and loading up on electrolytes is a good option that's likely to help and unlikely to make the cramping worse.

Even after more than 30 years as a cyclist, I had to save myself the second time I rode the Leadville 100. It was hot that year, and I made some nutritional mistakes in the first 2 hours of the race because I was too focused on staying with a fast group of riders. About halfway up the 10-mile climb to the turnaround at the Columbine Mine, I felt my right calf twitch. Crap. I had more than 5 hours left to ride, and if I started cramping that far out, it was likely I wouldn't make it to the finish. Over the next 10 minutes I pounded three gels and consumed a full bottle of sports drink, way more carbohydrate and sodium than I, or any sports dietitian, would recommend. But the reasons we don't recommend such rapid consumption are that absorption rates slow down and there's a significant risk you'll end up with an upset stomach.

In my opinion, when the building is on fire you dump as much water on it as you need to put the fire out, and you worry about the possibility of water damage later. I needed sodium, and if that meant consuming too much carbohydrate to get it, then so be it. If you cramp or bonk it's all over, so if you screwed up and put yourself in a bad nutritional position, eat and drink a lot in an attempt to bring yourself back from the brink. You might have to deal with an upset stomach later (fortunately, I didn't), but the alternative is cramping or bonking right then and there. In other words, you're avoiding an immediate certainty in exchange for a future possibility.

If you do end up with an upset stomach, there are three things you need to do: slow down, sip plain water, and cool off. Most instances of gastric distress during exercise are caused by reduced gut motility. When you overheat, blood is directed to the skin and working muscles, leaving less blood flow for the gut. When digestion slows, food stays in the gut longer than normal, and that can lead to the production of gas, which leads to bloating and nausea. Slowing down reduces heat stress by reducing the amount of heat being produced by working muscles. This, along with proactively cooling off by dousing yourself with water, can reduce skin and core temperature and assist in redistributing blood flow so gut motility increases again. Sipping water, not guzzling it, can also help to get the gut moving again.

Although my overall recommendation is to separate your hydration from your calories, carbohydrate-rich sports drinks can be convenient and useful during longer rides. Some athletes like to start out with a bottle of sports drink and refill with water after that is consumed. Others like to carry a single-serve sleeve of drink mix for later in the ride when the taste and sodium are helpful for increasing your drive to drink, and the drink is an easy way to get fluid, electrolytes, and carbohydrates all in one place.

FOCUSED FUELING: WHERE DIET AND EXERCISE COLLIDE

In Chapter 10 I talked extensively about eating behaviors, including caloric overcompensation. Athletes tend to overestimate the energy cost of a workout and as a result consume too many calories ahead of time in anticipation, gorge on huge meals after training, reward themselves with poor nutrition choices after training, or some combination of the three. The vast majority of the workouts in the Time-Crunched Training Program are 90 minutes or shorter, and even though many are high-intensity workouts, you can be optimally fueled by focusing primarily on good nutrition habits during your rides and positive eating behaviors and nutrition choices in the hour before and the hour after training.

For many athletes, this may mean consuming more sports nutrition products than you do right now. And from both a weight-management and a performance perspective, especially for workouts lasting 2 hours or less, it's better to consume calories you specifically want to use for training as close as possible to the times when you will need them.

A small snack (25 to 35 grams of carbohydrate, or about 1 ounce) in the hour before a 60-minute workout staves off hunger and keeps you alert and focused, while the carbohydrate you have stored in your muscles takes care of the actual fuel for training. For workouts that are 90 minutes to 2 hours, a 100-calorie energy gel eaten during your workout will enhance the quality of the efforts you perform as little as 10 minutes after that. In these cases, your pre-workout snack and the calories you ingest during exercise have a direct and acute impact on the quality of your training session.

When you focus on fueling immediately before and during your workouts, you can avoid consuming more calories than you need. In thousands of dietary analyses, one pattern that emerges is that many athletes consume more food than necessary prior to relatively short workouts. They increase the size of their meals and the frequency of snacks in anticipation of a workout, but the total caloric increase over the course of a day can easily be out of proportion to the actual demands of the day's exercise session.

Focused fueling helps eliminate overeating for time-crunched athletes by reinforcing the notion that you don't need to change your baseline eating habits; just add training-specific calories in the hour before training and fuel up early during your longer workouts with high-carbohydrate gels and sports drinks. Because gels are typically only about 100 calories, it's difficult to gorge yourself on them, and you'll be in better shape than if you had downed a 600-calorie treat at a coffee shop.

Following a high-intensity training session, base your decision on whether you need a recovery drink on the energy expenditure of the workout. As I mentioned in the section on post-workout nutrition, a recovery drink may be warranted following rides that accumulate about or more than 1,500–2,000 kilojoules of work. This could be a very hard interval session or a longer ride at a more moderate pace. In any case, the rationale is to base the need for a recovery drink on whether there was sufficient energy expenditure to substantially deplete carbohydrate stores and cause significant training stress.

In my experience, the best way for time-crunched athletes to manage caloric intake, make great training progress, and lose some weight at the same time is to eat as you normally do during most of the day and let your pre-, during-, and post-workout sports nutrition habits balance a significant portion of the calories you burn during training.

12

THE TIME-CRUNCHED KITCHEN

THERE'S A CONSTANT PUSH-AND-PULL in our busy lives between trying to find efficiencies so we can squeeze more activities into the day and trying to slow down, be more mindful, and be more engaged in the activities we find valuable. The premise of this book is that being an athlete is valuable to your overall well-being, and therefore it is worth the effort to find ways to fit training into your schedule.

Your food choices play an important role in the success of your training and weight management, but if you're struggling to find 60–90 minutes to ride during 2–3 weekdays, then chances are good that you don't have hours to while away in the grocery store and in your kitchen. Athletes perform best by eating great fuel, but after years of working with time-crunched athletes it has become abundantly clear to me that they need help finding ways to save time shopping and preparing their meals.

I love good food and appreciate the skill required to make great food. That skill, by the way, is not something I possess. I would say I'm a reasonably good cook when I have enough time in the kitchen to pull something together, but I know that to truly enjoy great food I need to visit the homes and restaurants of friends like chefs Michael Chiarello and Matthew Accarrino. Both have contributed greatly to my understanding of how flavors and ingredients can make foods with low energy-density taste richer and more satisfying.

Professional chefs are also masters of efficiency. So much work goes into preparing hundreds of dishes a night that any way to save time is extremely valuable. You can benefit from many of these time-saving techniques, too, because the goal is to reduce the time it takes to shop for and prepare your food while still maximizing the nutritional quality of your meals and the level of enjoyment you get from eating them.

SHOPPING TIPS

Jim Rutberg loves the grocery store. His wife, Leslie, knows this all too well because a "quick trip to the store" is rarely quick when he's the one doing it. Having written extensively about sports nutrition, Jim tends to wander up and down the aisles in search of new inspiration for athlete-oriented meals and snacks. In recent years, however, he has had to change his shopping habits considerably. With two young boys at home and all of the extracurricular activities and after-school sports that come with them, he has no time to linger at the store anymore. A lot of time-crunched athletes face similar constraints, and unlike Jim, many of us don't particularly enjoy grocery shopping all that much. So, let's take a look at how you can get in and out of the grocery store faster while taking home the right ingredients to fuel your workouts (and keep the family happy).

The Basics

Let's start with a few basic pieces of advice. Key among them is to have a plan and a list. Grocery stores are designed to be inconvenient, because keeping shoppers in the store longer increases the amount of food that goes into the cart. For years I have envisioned a device, similar to the pricing gun couples use in home furnishings stores to build a wedding registry list, that would enable grocery store shoppers to scan items as they go into the cart. Such a device would make it easier for shoppers to manage their budget, since it could keep a running tab of the total grocery bill. Loading a shopping list into the device, or pulling up a list from a previous shopping trip, would enable the device to plot the quickest route through the store, too. As of 2017, the only store apps I know of that handle in-store product mapping are provided by Target, Walmart, and Lowes home improvement stores nationwide, and Meijer stores in the Midwest. I'm sure Point Inside, the software company behind the apps for Target, Lowes, and Meijer, hopes it will catch on more widely, and so do I.

Meanwhile, the best two ways to get through the store without loading up on stuff you didn't intend to buy are, first, to frequent the same store so that you learn the layout and find the items you want quickly, and, second, to start with a list so you stay focused on getting the items you need without being distracted by "ooh, that looks good" motivations.

The other big piece of basic but sage advice is to never go to the grocery store when you are hungry. Being hungry affects not only our buying habits but also our food choices. In a 2015 study at the Carlson School of Management, participants were divided into a hungry group and a fed group. Both groups were asked to request as many binder clips—a non-food item— as they wanted. The hungry group "purchased" 64 percent more binder clips than the fed group. Being hungry, the researchers theorized, focuses a person's attention on acquisition (Xu et al. 2015).

What do binder clips have to do with grocery shopping? If you are hungry you may want food, but that desire also affects your drive to acquire both food and non-food items. In another study more specific to the impact of hunger on grocery purchases, Aner Tal and colleagues found that a 5-hour fast prior to food shopping led people to choose higher-calorie items (Tal et al. 2015). In their study, both fed and fasted groups purchased the same total number of items, so hunger didn't increase the amount of food purchased.

It did, however, change the foods shoppers were drawn to. This can have significant implications for athletes who are trying to focus their nutrition strategy on foods that have high nutrient density but lower energy density.

Organize Your List by Store Layout, Not Food Categories

A lot of people write their shopping lists based on the traditional food pyramid. As a result, the list is divided by produce, dairy, proteins (meat, fish, poultry), and grains (bread, pasta, rice). The problem is, grocery stores aren't organized that way, and as a result you end up zig-zagging your way through the store and backtracking through the aisles. Instead, do most of your shopping in the same store and learn the layout. Then organize your list according to the layout of the store.

Take the Smaller Cart

Just as using larger plates means you will put more food on them, using giant shopping carts will increase the amount of food you purchase. Even with a shopping list, one of the evaluations we all make while grocery shopping is, "Is this enough?" A larger cart makes it seem like you are not buying very much, which entices you to add more items.

If it's a quick trip for a few items, a basket is an even better choice. When you have to physically carry your items while you're shopping, you will think twice before adding extra weight and lingering in the store.

Order Nonperishable Items Online

Technology is changing the way we shop for everything, including groceries. There are a number of ways to shop for groceries online, either directly from your local grocery store or through larger services like Amazon. There are typically some delivery fees, but as with other services you have to evaluate the value of your time. Adding a few dollars to the grocery bill to save yourself significant time might be worthwhile.

A lot of shoppers, myself included, like to select produce and fresh proteins (meat, fish, poultry) personally, and this is where online grocery shopping has its biggest limitation. You are trusting someone else to select your fresh food, and if you don't like what shows up on your doorstep there's not much you can do about it. As a result, the best items to order online are the ones where there is no discernable difference between the choices on the shelf or refrigerator case. Nonperishable items like canned and bottled goods, dry goods, and cleaning supplies certainly fit this criteria. So do packaged perishable items like milk, cheese, and eggs (unless you're one of those people who searches the shelf for the latest possible expiration date on a milk carton). Online ordering won't prevent you from having to go to the grocery store, but it can significantly shorten your grocery store trips.

Go Early or Late

To get in and out of the grocery store faster, go when there are fewer people shopping. This is one of the tips that has helped Jim the most. With an 8- and 10-year-old at home, bedtime is about 7:30 p.m. Going shopping on the way home from work at 5-ish meant being at the grocery store with a lot of other people on their way home from work, and seriously cut into the already limited time he could spend with his kids before their bedtime. He was also hungry on his way home from work, and that influenced his buying habits. So he changed his routine. He now goes home after work and has dinner with his family, helps with homework and getting the boys to bed, and then heads out to the grocery store around 8 p.m. Not only is the store far less crowded, but it's the end of the day, so there's added incentive not to dawdle.

Don't Fear Frozen Foods

There's a lot of junk in the frozen food section of the grocery store, but for the time-crunched athlete it can also be a gold mine. Flash-freezing techniques have enabled food producers to vastly improve the quality of frozen fruits, vegetables, and even fish. The key is to purchase frozen foods that are as close to their natural state as possible. This means flash-frozen berries without added sugar or syrup, and frozen vegetables without added sauce. One product that benefits from a bit of processing is frozen shrimp, because you can get them with the heads and tails already removed, and sometimes already peeled.

Keep in mind that just because something is frozen, that doesn't mean it will keep forever. When fruits and vegetables spend too much time in your freezer and become encrusted with ice, that extra moisture becomes problematic when you thaw the food and end up with mushy, broken-down glop. Similarly, when you freeze fruits or vegetables yourself, the faster you can get the food to freeze, the better. For something like berries, that means spreading them out on a tray and putting them in the freezer, because they will freeze more quickly individually. Once frozen, gather them into a sealed container. When fruit freezes slowly, larger ice crystals form and that destroys the cell walls in the fruit; when you thaw it you get mush.

FOOD STORAGE TIPS

Time-crunched athletes often try making fewer, larger grocery store runs with the goal of cutting down trips to the store and having more of the foods you need at arm's reach in your own kitchen. The problem is, fresh whole foods go bad if you don't eat them quickly enough.

The best example of this is the "farm basket." The service goes by different names in different places, but basically it's a farm share where you get a delivery box full of fresh, awesome, locally grown, seasonal fruits and vegetables straight from the farm. I love the concept, but holy moly that's a lot of turnips! The biggest challenge with farm shares is often what to do with all that produce. If you don't eat it fast enough it goes bad, and even if it has a longer shelf life, more produce is coming next week so you better eat up.

Many farm shares today are starting to realize there needs to be a way to adjust the quantities and selections in those produce boxes. And many consumers have learned the best way to manage the volume is to "share the share" within a group of friends.

Nevertheless, the issue of food waste is a big one, not only economically but also environmentally and morally. I know I left it up to you to determine where you wanted to sit on the ethical and environmental spectrum of food politics, but when it comes to food waste, I think we can all agree that throwing out up to 30 percent of all the food we produce is bad all around. In the spirit of thinking globally and acting locally, you can save yourself some money and make the best use of those groceries with the following food storage tips:

Protect your potatoes: You probably already know that potatoes like a cool, dry environment, but to keep them from sprouting you can throw an apple in with them. The ethylene gas given off the apple does the trick. On the other hand, two foods you don't store together are potatoes and onions. They both like it cool and dry, but when they are stored together the onions accelerate sprouting in the potatoes.

Not everything goes in the fridge! Some fruits and vegetables will last longer if you keep them on your counter. Stone fruit (peaches, plums, nectarines) are one example of this. Keep them on the counter at room temperature, stem side down. Personally, I love peaches and plums in the summer when they are cold, so I'll often plan ahead and put the ripe one I plan on eating in the fridge as I leave for a ride. When I get back it's perfect!

Other fruits and vegetables that fare better on the counter are melons, tomatoes, avocados, bananas, kiwi fruit, mangos, papayas, and pineapples. Once cut up, these fruits should be refrigerated, as with melons and pineapples where you may not finish the entire fruit within one sitting.

SAVE THE AVOCADOS!

Avocados are a great food for endurance athletes. They are a good source of fat and fiber and contain some protein. You can mash them up into guacamole, or chunk them on top of eggs, a burrito, or a ton of other dishes. If you're not into eating animal products, avocado often makes a great replacement for butter or mayonnaise.

Avocados can be expensive, and once cut, the exposed surface of an avocado turns brown within a few hours. This is the same type of oxidation that happens with apples and other fruit once exposed to the air. Here are some of the ways you can preserve your avocados:

Keep the pit in it: Store the unused portion of avocado with the pit still inside. The exposed surface of the fruit may still get waxy or brown, but the rest of the avocado beneath stays green and ready to eat.

Store it with cut onions: The same chemicals that make you cry when you chop onions can protect your avocado from oxidizing. Place the unused portion of avocado in an airtight container with a few cuts of onion. You can also cover the top of leftover guacamole with chopped onions to keep the guacamole from oxidizing.

Add a squeeze of lemon or lime: The acid in citrus can keep many fruits from oxidizing, including avocados. This trick will keep cut apples from turning brown, too.

Create a seal: It is exposure to air that browns the avocado, so creating a seal that keeps oxygen out can help preserve them. Tightly wrapping the unused portion in plastic wrap can work, and some people brush the exposed surface of the avocado with olive oil to seal it. If you have a bowl of leftover guacamole, don't just cover the top of the container; press the plastic wrap right onto the surface of the guacamole to seal it off.

Keeping Butter and Eggs

When in doubt, put butter and eggs in the fridge. However, butter can be safely left on the counter as long as you'll use it within a few days. Its high fat content and low water content means it resists microbial growth quite well. Salted butter stays fresh longer on the counter than unsalted, because the salt further increases resistance to bacterial growth. Why bother keeping butter on the counter? It spreads a lot more easily, but that's really the only benefit.

As for eggs, in the United States they should stay refrigerated. Why, especially when they are not refrigerated in other parts of the world? Well, the reason has to do with the way eggs are produced and sold in this country. When an egg comes out of a hen, there is a very thin coating on the outside of the shell that protects the shell from being porous. That keeps bacteria out. But in the United States we like gleaming white eggs, so egg producers wash them, and that removes this protective coating. To keep bacteria growth at bay, the eggs are then refrigerated all the way through the supply chain to the grocery store and your home. If you leave them out and they warm up, they can sweat, and that can increase the chances that bacteria will get into the egg.

Keep in mind, however, that egg-laying hens in the United States are not vaccinated against salmonella, so washed shell or not, raw or undercooked eggs can still contain salmonella if the hen carried the bacteria. The upside to refrigerated eggs is that they have a much longer shelf life.

Keeping Fruits and Vegetables Fresher Longer

Wilted and limp vegetables are such a sad sight. Obviously, the best way to avoid this is to eat them soon after you get them home. But what about storing them? You know those drawers in your fridge? Many people just use them to separate fruits and vegetables for convenience, but if you are more strategic about it you can keep food fresh longer. The drawers should have small window openings that can be opened or shut depending on how much humidity you want to have in the drawer. Closing the vents increases the humidity; opening them decreases it.

Green leafy vegetables like to be in a more humid environment, but not directly wet, so closing the vent works well for them. Pears and apples, on the other hand, give off ethylene gas as they ripen, and if that gas is trapped inside a high-humidity drawer with the vents closed, that gas will accelerate the ripening of other fruits and vegetables nearby.

The following should be kept in the high-humidity drawer (vent closed): green, leafy vegetables like lettuce, kale, and spinach; broccoli, cauliflower, cucumbers, eggplant, green beans, fresh herbs (cilantro, parsley), peas, peppers, and cabbage. These are all vulnerable to moisture loss, so they do well in higher humidity.

The low-humidity drawer is better for fruits and vegetables that either produce a lot of ethylene gas or are not susceptible to water loss. This group includes apples, pears, kiwis, mangoes, papayas, and avocados (if you refrigerate them at all).

What about berries? Number one, berries are vulnerable to ethylene gas, so you don't want to put them in the low-humidity drawer with the apples and pears. At the same time, moisture is the enemy of your berries, because it accelerates the growth of mold. The best option is to eat berries within a few days of purchasing them because no storage method beyond freezing them makes them last very long.

If you want to give fresh berries a bit of a longer shelf life, though, you first need to get the mold spores off them. Two methods for doing this are dunking berries in a vinegar-and-water solution (1 cup vinegar to 3 cups water) or in a hot-water solution (125–140 degrees, not boiling!) to kill the mold spores. If using the vinegar method, rinse the berries afterward. Following either method, dry the berries and place them in a fresh, sealed container lined with a paper towel.

SAVING TIME IN THE KITCHEN

It is easy to say that you will prepare fresh, home-cooked meals for breakfast, lunch, and dinner. But many times, athletes get home from a long day at work, and possibly a training session after work, and they are tired. At that moment, the idea of getting fresh ingredients out of the fridge and spending time preparing a meal presents a challenge, and often that leads us to convenience foods or even fast food. In order to actually eat the way you intend to, you have to lower the barriers to preparing meals.

Let the Grocery Store Do the Work

Time is money, so while it may be a little more expensive to purchase the pre-cut melon or pineapple or sliced/diced vegetables, if that increases the likelihood you'll actually eat those foods then it is worth the expense. As I mentioned earlier, up to 30 percent of all food purchased goes to waste. Some of that is due to buying more food than we will realistically consume before it goes bad, but it can also be due to the time required to prepare those foods. This may sound insane—it really only takes a few minutes to slice up a pineapple—but take a critical look at your own behaviors. Have you purchased food with the intent of cooking it but been too busy to do so and ended up throwing it out? If you have, then the cost savings of purchasing the food uncut is meaningless because in the end you wasted that money anyway.

Beyond the money or the reduction in food waste, the important thing from a nutritional standpoint is that lowering the barrier to preparing your own meal with vegetables and lean proteins means you will increase the nutritional quality of your diet. Some people avoid pre-cut vegetables because it makes them feel lazy, like they can't even bother to cut up vegetables. You have to get over that. Saving time isn't about avoiding tasks you could physically do, it's about creating time for things you want to do.

Stock Up on These Sauces and Starters

There will always be someone out there who swears by making everything from scratch, and more power to them. But for the rest of us, there are some prepared foods that save time and are realistically no better or worse for you compared to making it yourself. Here is a good starter list:

Broth: Whether it's beef, chicken, or vegetable, broth is a good item to have on hand. Cooking rice in broth adds flavor and richness to plain rice.

Coconut milk: Great for curries, but can also add richness to smoothies, oatmeal, soups, and sautés.

Bottled tomato sauce (e.g., marinara): Because Chef Chiarello's specialty is Italian cooking he might have a heart attack when he reads this, but there is nothing wrong with bottled tomato sauce.

Green chile and your favorite salsa: You could make them yourself, but why? Just check the ingredients, because some brands add sugar to salsa, and there's no reason for that.

The Best Canned Foods to Have on Hand

If you associate canned food with mushy waterlogged vegetables and sickeningly sweet fruit packaged in syrup, it's time to revisit canned fruits, vegetables, and lean proteins. Or at least some of them. Here are the best choices from the canned food aisle:

Beans: Choose from black, red, pinto, garbanzo, kidney, or whatever you fancy. You can't really go wrong with a can of beans. Just drain, rinse, and put to use in a variety of recipes to add some valuable plant-based protein.

Green chile: Maybe it's because I've been living just north of the prime green-chile-growing areas of Colorado and New Mexico, but those little cans of diced green chile peppers are a pantry essential.

Diced tomatoes: There's nothing else in the can, and it saves you the time and mess of doing it yourself.

Tuna: Just make sure it's packed in water instead of oil.

LET'S TALK BACON

It must be a good time to be hog farmer, because the popularity of bacon seems to be rising every month. Bacon is everywhere and in everything! If you recall, however, it was one of the fatty meats I recommended avoiding in Chapter 10, along with ham, sausage, and fatty cuts of beef. I'm sorry to break it to you, but there is no essential nutrient in bacon that humans need and can't get from a leaner protein source.

Here's the thing about bacon, though: It tastes really good. In this case, remember that a little goes a long way, which means the flavor of bacon is so strong that adding a small amount to your food will influence the flavor quite a lot without overdoing it in calories.

Bacon's savory and salty richness is something that can make a meal more satisfying, so it doesn't make sense to call for an all-out prohibition. If you like bacon, enjoy it but consume it sparingly. Good as it may taste, it really has absolutely no redeeming qualities you can't get from a better protein source.

Fruit: While I personally prefer frozen fruit to canned fruit, and fresh fruit above all, canned peaches, pears, and other fruits can be convenient when they are out of season. Choose varieties packed in their own juice with no sugar added.

Pumpkin: Look for pureed pumpkin, not pumpkin pie filling. Pureed pumpkin can be used in a variety of soups and in place of oil in baking.

TIME-CRUNCHED ATHLETE RECIPES FROM CHEF MICHAEL CHIARELLO

The restaurant business is tough, and the chefs and restaurateurs at the top of the industry combine their culinary expertise with the drive and endurance of a professional athlete and the business acumen of a Silicon Valley titan. Chef

Michael Chiarello has been on the top of his game for a long time, and his passion for cycling has helped him stay there.

Michael's rise to the top of the culinary world started in his family's kitchen. He was brought up on traditional family recipes and given a strong respect for high-quality ingredients straight from the farmer and butcher. A graduate of the Culinary Institute of America in 1982, he was awarded Chef of the Year by *Food and Wine Magazine* just three years later.

As Michael opened a series of acclaimed restaurants, he also ventured into media, writing multiple cookbooks and creating cooking shows for PBS and Food Network, including the Emmy–award winning show *Easy Entertaining*. He became even more widely recognized when he was a finalist in the first season of Bravo TV's *Top Chef Masters* competition show, and he has appeared as a judge on *Top Chef* and subsequent seasons of *Top Chef Masters*. He has also appeared on *The Next Iron Chef* and is a frequent guest on daytime talk shows and cooking shows.

The center of Michael Chiarello's restaurant and winery empire is Yountville, in California's Napa Valley. Not only are the weather and terrain perfect for creating world-class wine and supporting farms that supply his restaurants with essential ingredients, but the Napa Valley is also a perfect place for cycling. Not far from the crowded streets of San Francisco, the hills and quiet roads of Napa Valley provide a grand destination for Bay Area cyclists. On weekends, the parking lot at Bottega, Chiarello's flagship restaurant in Yountville, is filled with cyclists as well as diners.

Cycling has long been Chiarello's pressure valve, a way to step away from the constant multitasking that characterizes working in and running top-tier restaurants. The bike provides rare time to himself and with his own thoughts. As with many athletes, riding isn't always about clearing the mind and focusing only on the ride itself. It can also be about finding time to focus on big decisions or work out creative ideas without the distraction of other people around. Exercise is a proven stress reliever, but it is also great for unleashing a person's productivity and creativity.

About the Recipes

As you might guess from his last name, Michael specializes in Italian cuisine, and many of the recipes presented here reflect those themes. Rather than heavy lasagnas and cream sauces, Chef Chiarello focuses on lighter fare that is still hearty and extremely tasty. The caponata, for instance, is a hearty roasted vegetable dish that is perfect for dinner and leftovers for lunch. The piadine— there are two variations—makes a great post-ride lunch. Michael's famous omelet technique is also included; fill your omelet with the vegetables of your choice. There are also snacks and the chef's signature "NapaStyle Fitness Bar," a crowd favorite.

In keeping with the ideas presented in Chapter 10, I am purposely not including a nutritional breakdown for the recipes in this section. After years of trying to strictly control the caloric intake and macronutrient percentages of athletes' nutrition plans, the overwhelming reality is that fresh ingredients and positive eating behaviors matter more than the precise number of carbohydrate or fat grams you consume. Time and again, time-crunched athletes we work with demonstrate that they have gotten the message about staying away from junk food, processed food, and empty calories. I have faith that you understand the value of consuming fresh, whole foods, and these recipes are based entirely on that premise.

The recipes in this section do not constitute a meal plan. They are not intended to be your only meals and snacks while you are following one of the training plans described in Part 2. Instead they represent a selection of easy-to-prepare meals and snacks that will complement your athletic lifestyle, created by an award-winning chef who shares your passion for performance and endurance sports.

CHIARELLO'S CLASSIC OMELET TECHNIQUE

An omelet is a wonderful foundation for a great breakfast, especially when you fill or top it with fresh vegetables. This preparation technique produces an evenly cooked product and does away with omelets that are overcooked and tough on the outside and runny on the inside.

MAKES ONE OMELET

3 large eggs
½ teaspoon salt (2.5 grams)
¼ teaspoon freshly ground black pepper (0.45 grams)
1 teaspoon unsalted butter (5 grams)
Melted butter, optional

1. Break the eggs into a bowl and season with salt and pepper; lightly beat with a fork.

2. Heat a 10-inch (25cm) nonstick sauté pan with 1 teaspoon unsalted butter. When butter begins to crackle pour in beaten eggs and cook for 10 seconds, just so the eggs begin to set on the bottom. Immediately scrape the sides toward the middle using a silicone spatula or pancake turner. Stir almost continuously, until the omelet is cooked to your liking. Allow 2 minutes for a well-cooked omelet.

3. While tilting the pan, flip one-half of the omelet over toward the middle. Add the filling of your choice and continue rolling the omelet over itself. Roll the omelet onto a serving plate. Make a slit with a paring knife to expose some of the filling, if desired.

Chef's Note: In addition to fresh vegetables and a variety of cheeses, the Salami Bits and Caponata included in this section make great fillings for omelets.

STRAWBERRY PANCAKES

These pancakes are the start of a great day on the bike. Mix batches of the dry ingredients in this recipe together ahead of time and store them to make your morning routine quicker. These are rich in carbohydrate, so you may want to round out your breakfast with yogurt or an egg to provide more protein and fat.

SERVES 2

1 large egg, at room temperature

1¼ cups all-purpose flour (150 grams)

1 teaspoon sugar (4 grams)

1 teaspoon baking powder (5 grams)

½ teaspoon salt (2.5 grams)

1¼ cups buttermilk (300 grams)

2 tablespoons melted butter (28 grams)

Stovetop Strawberry Preserves (recipe follows)

1. In a medium bowl, beat the egg. Add buttermilk and whisk together.

2. Mix together dry ingredients. (For a smoother batter and fluffier pancakes, use a sifter to combine the dry ingredients.)

3. Add the dry ingredients to the egg-buttermilk mixture and stir well, until batter is smooth.

4. Heat the griddle. To test, sprinkle with drops of water. If bubbles "skitter around," heat is just right.

5. Brush the griddle with the melted butter.

6. Slowly pour batter onto griddle to desired pancake size. Keep an eye on how the pancakes settle so as to determine where to make the next one (so they do not touch).

7. When pancakes are puffed and full of bubbles, flip and cook the other side.

8. Keep cooked pancakes hot by placing them between folds of a warm towel in warm oven. (Don't stack them!)

9. Serve hot, smothered with Stovetop Strawberry Preserves.

STOVETOP STRAWBERRY PRESERVES

The great thing about this recipe is that you will end up with 3–4 cups (720–960 milliliters) of preserves (or you can cut it down pretty easily). Why make your own preserves when plenty are available at the grocery store? Flavor. The addition of fresh lemon juice, black pepper, and rosemary give this recipe a unique flavor that is well worth the minimal effort. Experiment with other seasonal fruits as well!

MAKES 3–4 CUPS

4 pints fresh strawberries, washed, cored, and quartered
 (about 64 medium strawberries)
½ cup sugar (100 grams)
Pinch of salt and black pepper
2 lemons, juiced
1 teaspoon chopped fresh rosemary leaves (0.70 grams)

1. In a skillet with high sides, add all ingredients and stir to combine.

2. Bring to a boil and then lower heat to a simmer. Cook until thick and spoonable, about 30 minutes, stirring occasionally.

3. Transfer preserves to a bowl and let cool until warm or room temperature. Serve with toasted bread, baked goods, or on pancakes.

4. Refrigerate unused portion.

FRESH FRUIT SMOOTHIE

The world is not lacking for smoothie recipes, but Chef Chiarello's is one of my favorites. It is light but packed with flavor and energy. Personally, I cut the recipe in half to make a single 12-ounce smoothie (350 milliliters). The addition of lemon juice adds some tartness, and if you like coconut milk it's a great substitution for the soy milk.

MAKES 24–28 OUNCES/700–830 MILLILITERS

½ cup soy milk or other milk (125 milliliters)

½ cup white grape juice (125 milliliters)

1 cup strawberries, stemmed (225 milliliters)

½ cup pineapple chunks (120 milliliters)

Small handful fresh seedless grapes

½ lemon, juiced (for tartness if desired)

Pinch salt

1. Place all ingredients in a blender and blend until smooth.

2. If you'd like an iced smoothie, blend ingredients first and then add ice and blend to desired consistency.

GRILLED AVOCADO, TOMATO, AND RED ONION SALAD

As written, this recipe serves four people, so feel free to cut it down if you're only making enough for 1 or 2 people, as it is best served immediately. One thing I like about this dish—aside from the fact it tastes amazing—is that it is rich and filling, yet small, quick to prepare, and incredibly fresh.

SERVES 4

10 tomatoes, quartered
4 avocados, pitted, halved, and peeled
1 red onion, sliced
½ lemon, juiced
Extra-virgin olive oil, for drizzling
1 cup prepared basil pesto (240 milliliters)
½ cup pine nuts (120 milliliters/70 grams)
Grated Parmigiano-Reggiano cheese, to taste

1. Preheat a gas or charcoal grill over medium heat.

2. Arrange quartered tomatoes on a serving tray, and set aside.

3. Place avocado halves in a bowl and drizzle with olive oil. In another bowl, combine the red onion slices with the lemon juice and a drizzle of olive oil.

4. Grill the avocado halves cut side down for about 30 to 45 seconds, keeping grill open (do not cover).

5. Remove avocados from grill and place them on top of the tomatoes with empty pit holes facing up. Fill the pit holes with the onion mixture, then top with pesto.

6. Sprinkle pine nuts and cheese on top.

SPAGHETTI SQUASH WITH MARINARA

This recipe is definitely big enough to feed a family, with leftovers. And while it takes 30–40 minutes to roast the squash, this is not a recipe that takes a lot of tending. Stick it in the oven, set a timer, and you can go get a little work done, help the kids with homework, or spend some quality time with your partner.

SERVES 6

2 whole spaghetti squash

Extra-virgin olive oil

Sea salt and freshly ground black pepper

4 cups prepared (jarred) marinara sauce (960 milliliters)

1. Preheat the oven to 450°F (230°C). Line a baking tray with aluminum foil.

2. Cut each squash in half lengthwise and scrape out the seeds. Brush flesh side of each squash with olive oil, and season with salt and pepper.

3. Place squash halves flesh-side down and roast 30 to 40 minutes, until you can easily insert a knife into the flesh. Remove from the oven and let rest until cool enough to handle.

4. Heat the marinara sauce in a large sauté pan.

5. When squash is cool enough to handle, use a large kitchen spoon to scrape the strands of squash from the inside of the skin.

6. Add the squash strands to the pan and toss with the marinara sauce. No additional cooking is necessary. Serve and enjoy.

PIADINI WITH CAESAR SALAD AND ROASTED GARLIC PASTE

While this recipe makes 4 piadini (small pizzas), the yield for the Garlic Paste recipe will be more than you need. It keeps in the refrigerator quite well. And once you have some garlic paste made, this is an easy and quick dish to make on the grill.

MAKES 4

1 pound pre-made pizza dough (450 grams)

12 cups loosely packed torn romaine lettuce (about 2 heads)

Your favorite Caesar salad dressing, to taste

Olive oil

4–6 tablespoons Roasted Garlic Paste (60–90 milliliters); recipe follows

1 tablespoon finely chopped fresh thyme leaves (0.8 grams)

6 tablespoons freshly grated Parmigiano-Reggiano (30 grams)

1. Preheat a gas or charcoal grill to high.

2. Put the lettuce in a bowl. Pour desired amount of Caesar dressing over and toss well.

3. Divide the dough into 4 equal balls. On a floured board, stretch and roll the dough into thin discs with a rolling pin. The dough may also be stretched by hand, but rolling will give you a thinner crust.

4. Coat the flattened dough discs with olive oil and place, oiled side down, on the hot grill. (Alternatively, you can grill the dough indoors on a cast-iron stovetop grill pan that has been preheated over medium-high.)

5. When you start to see bubbles on the surface of the dough, turn it over and grill until it is slightly browned on the bottom. Brush each piadini with a generous tablespoon of the garlic paste and sprinkle with the thyme. Remove from the grill with tongs and top with the Caesar salad. Sprinkle cheese on top, fold in half, and eat.

ROASTED GARLIC PASTE

YIELDS ABOUT ½ CUP (120 MILLILITERS)

2 whole garlic heads

¼ cup pure olive oil (55 grams/60 milliliters)

Sea salt and freshly ground pepper

1. Preheat the oven to 375°F (190°C).

2. Peel the outermost layers of skin off the heads of garlic. Cut off the top one-third of each head to open the cloves. Put the heads, cut side up, in a small baking dish and pour the olive oil over them. Season with salt and pepper.

3. Cover dish tightly with foil, place in the oven, and roast until cloves are softened, about 45 minutes. Uncover the dish and continue to roast until the cloves begin to pop out of their skins and brown, about 15 minutes. Let cool.

4. When cool enough to handle easily, squeeze the roasted garlic into a small bowl. Press against the skins very well to get out all the sweet roasted garlic you can. Add the oil from the baking dish and mix well with a fork, forming a paste. Store leftover paste tightly covered in the refrigerator.

PIADINI WITH APPLES, HONEY, AND BLUE CHEESE

The frisee lettuce (also called curly endive) is the key to this dish because of its frizzy and crunchy texture and somewhat bitter flavor.

MAKES 4

1 pound pre-made pizza dough (450 grams)

2 to 3 heads frisee lettuce

2 apples (Granny Smith for tartness, and/or Pink Lady for sweetness),
   cored and sliced

Olive oil

1 lemon, juiced

5 tablespoons honey (110 grams)

Salt and pepper

4 ounces blue cheese (110 grams)

1. Preheat a gas or charcoal grill to high.

2. Wash, dry, and roughly tear the frisee into a salad bowl. Then add the sliced apples. Drizzle with olive oil, lemon juice, and 1 tablespoon (22 grams) of the honey; add salt and pepper. Toss lightly, then set aside.

3. Divide the pizza dough into 4 sections. On a floured board, stretch and roll each piece into a thin disk with a rolling pin. The dough may also be stretched by hand, but rolling will give you a thinner crust.

4. Coat top of each flattened dough disc with olive oil and place, oiled side down, onto the hot grill. (Alternatively, you can grill the dough indoors on a cast-iron stovetop grill pan. Set the burners to medium-high and make sure to preheat the pan.) When you see bubbles on the surface, flip and grill the second side. The first side of each piadini should be slightly browned.

5. Put 1 tablespoon (22 grams) of honey and 1 blob of blue cheese, to taste, on the top of each piadini. Close the grill and wait for the cheese to melt. When it is nice and gooey, place the piadini on a platter and top with the cool salad and apples.

6. Fold the grilled bread over the toppings and enjoy.

GRILLED CORN SALSA

There is nothing like fresh corn on the cob in the height of the summer, and this salsa will put anything in a jar to shame! This recipe makes a big batch, so you can share. You can eat it with tortilla chips, but it is even better on soft tacos or as a topping for grilled fish.

SERVES 10

10 large ears corn, husked

$\frac{1}{3}$ cup extra-virgin olive oil (80 milliliters), plus more for brushing

Salt and freshly ground pepper

8 vine-ripened tomatoes, about 1 pound/450 grams total

1 cup finely diced red onion (240 milliliters)

4 tablespoons red wine vinegar (60 milliliters), or more to taste

$\frac{1}{2}$ cup julienned fresh basil leaves (12 grams)

1. Brush the corn liberally with olive oil and season with salt and pepper. Grill, turning every few minutes, until light gold all over and cooked, about 12 minutes. Let cool and cut off the kernels. Discard the cobs. Place kernels in a large mixing bowl.

2. Core the tomatoes and cut a small X on the bottom of each. Brush with olive oil, season with salt and pepper, and place on the grill, X side down, away from direct heat. Cover the grill and cook until the tomatoes begin to soften but are not cooked all the way through (or they will melt through the grate!), about 15 minutes. Set aside until cool enough to handle, then peel. Cut the tomatoes in half crosswise and squeeze out the juice and the seeds through a sieve into a bowl. Reserve the juices and chop the flesh.

3. Put the onions in a nonreactive (stainless-steel, ceramic, glass, or metal cookware with enamel coating) medium bowl and toss with 2 tablespoons/30 milliliters of the vinegar. Let marinate until the onions turn pink, about 10 minutes.

4. Add the chopped tomatoes, reserved tomato juice, onions, basil, and $\frac{1}{3}$ cup olive oil (80 milliliters) to the corn. Toss well. Taste for seasoning and adjust with salt, pepper, and remaining 2 tablespoons of vinegar. The salsa is best eaten the same day but will keep, covered and refrigerated, a day or so.

CAPONATA "AGRODOLCE"

Caponata is a Sicilian dish based on eggplant (aubergine). This recipe is a little more advanced and takes some time, but it's worth the effort, not just because of the flavor but especially because it yields a big bowl of caponata that can be kept in the fridge or divided into portions and frozen. The high-lights of the dish are the eggplant, squash, zucchini, and the sweet-and-sour ("agrodolce") sauce.

SERVES 6

6 ribs celery, cut into ¼-inch slices (6 millimeters)

3 medium eggplant, diced into ¼-inch pieces (6 millimeters)

3 small yellow squash, quartered and cut into ¼-inch pieces (6 millimeters)

3 small zucchini, quartered and cut into ¼-inch pieces (6 millimeters)

Olive oil (for roasting the vegetables)

2 tablespoons chopped fresh oregano (6 grams)

2 tablespoons chopped fresh parsley (4 grams)

3 cloves garlic, thinly sliced or crushed

2 onions, chopped into ¼-inch pieces (6 millimeters)

2 tablespoons sugar (25 grams)

1 ½ cups red wine vinegar (360 milliliters)

1 cup prepared roasted red peppers, thinly sliced (240 milliliters)

1 cup pitted and chopped Kalamata olives (240 milliliters)

1 cup capers (240 milliliters)

2 cups prepared (jarred) marinara sauce
   (480 milliliters)

Salt and freshly ground pepper, to taste

1. Heat oven to 450°F (230°C) and place baking pans in oven to preheat. Place cut vegetables in separate bowls and coat lightly with olive oil. Pan roast all of the vegetables (eggplant, squash, zucchini, celery) separately in very hot pans. Spread cooked vegetables on a tray lined with paper towels to drain and cool slightly.

2. In a large sauce pan, sauté the onion and garlic in olive oil until softened. Place in a large bowl with the roasted vegetables, and mix gently.

3. Combine the chopped oregano and parsley in a small bowl.

4. To make the agrodolce, combine vinegar and sugar in a small sauce pan and cook over medium heat to reduce by half. It should have the consistency of a light syrup.

5. While vegetables are still warm, add the roasted peppers, olives, and capers.

6. Pour the agrodolce sauce over the vegetable mixture and toss.

7. Add the prepared marinara sauce and finally the oregano and parsley; stir gently. Add salt and pepper to taste.

NAPASTYLE FITNESS BARS

This recipe, while incredibly tasty, illustrates why most people buy pre-made bars like the Bonk Breakers we provide at CTS camps. It takes a lot of ingredients to get the consistency and taste of a during-workout bar just right. These bars, though, are worth the effort. I particularly like them during Endurance Blocks (see Chapter 14), multi-day cycling events, and endurance mountain bike events. The longer you're on the bike, the more you'll crave something different, and these bars fit the bill perfectly.

MAKES ABOUT 18 BARS

1 cup quick-cooking oats (240 grams)

½ cup sliced almonds (240 milliliters)

½ cup dark raisins (240 milliliters)

½ cup golden raisins (240 milliliters)

½ cup dried apricots (240 milliliters)

⅓ cup unsalted butter, room temperature (75 grams)

½ cup packed brown sugar (100 grams)

¼ cup golden molasses (60 milliliters)

1 egg

1 cup unbleached all-purpose flour (120 grams)

¼ cup whole-wheat flour (30 grams)

½ cup nonfat dry milk (65 grams)

¼ cup toasted wheat germ (60 milliliters)

1½ teaspoons baking powder (7.5 grams)

½ teaspoon baking soda (3 grams)

½ teaspoon vanilla extract (2.5 milliliters)

Pinch sea salt

½ cup milk (preferably 2 percent) (120 milliliters)

1 tablespoon unsalted butter (14 grams) for baking pan

1. Preheat oven to 300°F (150°C).

2. Place oats and sliced almonds on a baking sheet. Toast in oven for 10 minutes and then set aside.

3. Place dark and golden raisins, apricots, and the toasted oats and almonds in a food processor and pulse until coarsely chopped. Set mixture aside.

4. Increase oven temperature to 325°F (160°C).

5. In the bowl of a heavy-duty mixer fitted with a paddle, beat ⅓ cup unsalted butter, brown sugar, molasses, and the egg until light and fluffy.

6. In a large bowl, combine the unbleached all-purpose flour, whole-wheat flour, nonfat dry milk, toasted wheat germ, baking powder, baking soda, vanilla, and a pinch of salt. Add oats-and-fruit mixture, butter mixture, and milk, and mix thoroughly.

7. Butter a 13 × 9 × 2-inch baking pan (30 × 22 × 5cm). Pour in the batter and spread evenly. Bake for about 30 minutes, until set. Cool in the pan.

8. Cut into bars. To store, wrap bars individually in plastic wrap. Freezes well.

NAPASTYLE TOASTED SPICE RUB ALMONDS

Almonds are a great snack for athletes, but after a while you're going to need something more than raw or roasted almonds. This recipe gives your almonds a nice kick. Toasting freshens spices, releases their oils, and makes them more fragrant, as well as adding a new dimension of flavor. You will have more spice rub than you'll need for this recipe alone. It keeps well, though, so store it in a glass jar in a cool, dry place, or freeze. Chef Chiarello advises that you taste your chili powder and, if it's too spicy and hot, cut back the amount. California chiles are almost sweet, not hot.

MAKES 1 POUND

1 pound raw almonds, preferably unsalted (450 grams)

2 tablespoons unsalted butter (28 grams)

2 teaspoons sea salt (10 grams)

3 tablespoons Toasted Spice Rub (45 milliliters); recipe follows

1. Preheat oven to 350°F (175°C).

2. Blanch the almonds in boiling water, rinse with cold water, and blot dry. Pinching the almonds with your fingers should peel the skins off.

3. Melt butter in a large ovenproof skillet over moderate heat and let bubble until it turns light brown and smells nutty. Add the almonds and salt and cook, stirring occasionally, over moderate heat until the almonds begin to color, about 5 minutes.

4. Add spice mix, toss to mix, and coat thoroughly.

5. Transfer the skillet to the oven and bake until the almonds are medium-brown, about 15 minutes. Remove from the oven, taste for flavor, add more spice mix or salt, if necessary.

6. Return to the oven for 5 more minutes. Transfer the nuts to a sheet pan; they will crisp as they cool.

7. Store the cooled almonds in an airtight container at room temperature.

TOASTED SPICE RUB

COATS 4 POUNDS OF ALMONDS

¼ cup fennel seeds (23 grams)

1 tablespoon coriander seeds (1.8 grams)

1 tablespoon black peppercorns (14 milliliters)

1½ teaspoons red pepper flakes (2.7 grams)

¼ cup (1 ounce) pure California chili powder (28 grams)

2 tablespoons kosher salt (36 grams)

2 tablespoons ground cinnamon (5 grams)

1. Toast the fennel seeds, coriander seeds, and peppercorns in a small, heavy pan over medium heat. When the fennel turns light brown, you're ready for the next step.

2. You're going to want to work quickly on this step. Turn on the exhaust fan, add the red pepper flakes, and toss thoroughly while under the fan. Immediately transfer the spice mixture to a plate to cool slightly.

3. Put chili powder, salt, and cinnamon in a blender. Add the spice mix and blend until the spices are evenly ground.

4. Pour into a bowl. The spice mix is now ready to be used in the preparation of the almonds.

NAPA ROAD MIX

It's time to raid the bulk bins at the grocery store! This mix is perfect for a long road trip to a cycling event, a hike, or as something different during a long road or mountain bike ride.

SERVES 3

¼ cup dried pears, cut lengthwise in halves or thirds (60 milliliters)

¼ cup dried nectarines, cut into quarters (60 milliliters)

¼ cup dried Calimyrna figs, cut into halves (60 milliliters)

¼ cup dried cherries (60 milliliters)

¼ cup Medjool dates, pitted and cut in half lengthwise (60 milliliters)

¼ cup hazelnuts, toasted and peeled (60 milliliters)

¼ cup almonds, toasted (60 milliliters)

⅓ cup pumpkin seeds, toasted (80 milliliters)

½ cup sesame "fries" or sticks (120 milliliters)

½ cup sesame "bits" or crackers (120 milliliters)

1. In a bowl mix together the first 8 ingredients. Carefully blend in the sesame "fries" and "bits" so they don't get crushed. Transfer the mixture to zip-lock bags or other storage container.

SALAMI BITS

I noted earlier that a little bacon goes a long way because it has such a strong flavor. Chef Chiarello recommends salami to put an Italian twist on the idea of using a small amount of a bold flavor to enhance a dish. These salami bits are a great addition to omelets, salads, and sandwiches.

MAKES 1 POUND

1 pound salami, very finely minced or ground with the medium blade
  of a meat grinder (450 grams)
2 tablespoons olive oil (30 milliliters)

1. Heat a large sauté pan over medium-high heat. Place salami in heated pan. Drizzle with olive oil, and cook while stirring. The salami will give off steam in about 5 minutes while it releases its moisture.

2. Listen and watch the pan. When the hiss of steam turns to a sizzle, turn the heat down to medium and cook, stirring occasionally, until the salami bits are crisp.

3. Using a slotted spoon, transfer the bits to several thicknesses of paper towel to drain. The bits will crisp even more as they cool.

4. Use immediately or package and freeze. If frozen, warm them in a skillet or toaster oven so they stay crisp to serve.

BAKED PLANTAIN ROUNDS

While the recipe calls for 4 green plantains, you can easily adjust to any amount. Though they may look like green bananas, green plantains are starchy rather than sweet. As a result, this recipe yields a more savory chip. Because plantains do not have a strong flavor on their own, you have the opportunity to add various additional spices to add some heat or other flavors.

SERVES 4

4 green plantains

Olive oil (enough to lightly coat plantain slices)

Salt and freshly ground pepper

1. Preheat oven to 400°F (200°C).

2. Remove plantain peel with a knife. Thinly slice using a mandoline or a sharp knife.

3. In a bowl, toss plantain slices with olive oil, salt, pepper, and any additional spices you choose. Spread in a single layer on a cookie sheet.

4. Bake for 15 to 17 minutes, until golden brown, turning slices after about 8 minutes. Watch closely after turning; they can burn quickly.

5. Remove from oven and serve. Chips are best eaten immediately, but they'll keep for about a day.

BONUS RECIPES FROM MATT ACCARRINO

Michelin star chef Matthew Accarrino was a cyclist before he was a chef. As a teenager, Matthew raced as a junior until his right femur shattered due to a benign tumor that had been growing there undetected. Recovery took two years, during which he watched a lot of cooking shows on television, particularly those featuring chefs Emeril Lagasse, Julia Child, and Jacques Pépin. They were his first teachers, and later, as he made his way into the profession, he went to work for Lagasse. Fast-forward to the present day and you'll find Accarrino in San Francisco presiding over his own restaurant, SPQR, named after the initials for the city of Rome. For four consecutive years (2013–2016), he has been nominated by the James Beard Foundation for Best Chef: West, and SPQR has been annually recognized with a Michelin star.

Chef Accarrino returned to cycling several years ago and has since participated in several CTS camps and Endurance Bucket List events, including the Amgen Tour of California Race Experience and USA Pro Challenge Race Experience. During these events, our athletes rode every stage of the races a few hours before the pro peloton. Matthew also built relationships with professional teams and events, and he's applied his knowledge and experience of cooking and cycling to help improve the culinary options available to professional cyclists. When he traveled to races and training camps with the Holowesko-Citadel Professional Cycling Team, he helped transform meal times from a basic necessity to a thoroughly enjoyable and satisfying experience. When athletes are tired in the middle of big blocks of racing or training, better meals have a substantial positive effect on a rider's personal outlook and the team's overall morale.

Matthew was gracious enough to contribute a few recipes to this book. The rice pudding recipe comes straight from his experience at the Holowesko-Citadel team, and the sweet potato and beet pesto recipes are easy-to-prepare dishes that pack big punches nutritionally.

RED BEET PESTO

Some athletes consume beet juice products for the potential increase in blood levels of nitric oxide, which may in turn improve endurance performance. While you won't consume enough beets from this recipe to see an ergogenic effect, it certainly won't hurt your performance. Beets are in season late in the summer and into the fall; the deep red-pink color of this pesto makes it a startling addition to a Halloween party!

SERVES 4

3-4 medium roasted red beets, peeled and cut into 1-inch pieces
   (25 millimeters)

1 teaspoon red wine vinegar (5 milliliters)

⅓–½ cup olive oil, divided use (70–120 milliliters)

1¼ teaspoons salt (7.5 grams)

Freshly ground pepper, to taste

1 garlic clove, crushed (mellow roasted garlic works well here)

½ cup slivered almonds, toasted (120 milliliters)

1 tablespoon parsley leaves, optional (3.8 grams)

¼ cup grated Parmigiano-Reggiano or pecorino cheese (20 grams)

To roast the beets

1. Create a foil packet (pull a length of foil and fold over in half, seal the edges by folding together in ¼-inch [6mm] folds). You should have a pocket with an opening on one side.

2. Place washed beets in a bowl. Sprinkle with a tablespoon of olive oil and season with salt and pepper. Add a teaspoon of red wine vinegar and transfer beets and juices to the foil packet. Seal and transfer to a baking tray. Transfer to a 350°F (175°C) oven and roast for 35 to 50 minutes. The beets are done when a skewer or paring knife inserted in the beets comes out easily. Let cool in the packet.

To make the pesto

1. Place the roasted beets, garlic, almonds, and remaining olive oil in a food processor. Pulse to chop finely. If you are using parsley, pulse it in now until finely cut.

2. Add the cheese and pulse. Taste and adjust seasoning with salt or a few drops of red wine vinegar if desired.

SWEET POTATO AND QUINOA SKILLET CAKES

I like making this recipe as one or two big skillet cakes, rather than a larger number of palm-sized cakes. It's easy and once you're done you just slice it like a pie or pizza. You can really be creative with how you spice these cakes and make them more sweet or savory depending on your preference.

SERVES 2

2–3 medium-to-large sweet potatoes (peeled and grated, enough for
    3–4 cups/720–960 milliliters)

½ cup cooked quinoa (120 milliliters)

½ cup cooked or canned garbanzo beans, mashed (120 milliliters)

1½–2 tablespoons olive oil (20–30 milliliters)

1–2 teaspoons salt (5–10 grams)

2 green onions, finely cut

½ teaspoon garlic powder (1.5 grams)

2 tablespoons wheat flour; rice flour or gluten free mix can be used (16 grams)

Spice blend, za'atar, salt and pepper to taste

1–2 eggs

1. Peel and grate raw sweet potatoes. Using a kitchen towel, wring out the shredded potato to remove some of the excess moisture.

2. Toss the shredded sweet potato, cooked quinoa, and mashed garbanzo beans with olive oil and salt.

3. Add the green onions, garlic powder, flour, and desired spice blend, and eggs. Mix well.

4. In a preheated large skillet over medium heat, add a film of olive oil or spray generously with nonstick spray. Place enough of the mixture to form a cake that is ½ inch (1cm) thick and covers the bottom of the skillet. This recipe will likely take 2 batches; alternately you may make several smaller cakes.

5. Cook until golden on one side and then gently flip. If you are uncomfortable flipping a large cake, slide the cake from the pan to a plate golden side down. Invert the pan over the cake on the plate and turn over to flip the cake back into the pan on the side that needs to be cooked. Finish cooking the cake until golden on the second side and cooked through.

6. Transfer to a board and cut into serving pieces.

7. Serve alongside roasted vegetables, meat, or fish, with sprinkled soy sauce, hot sauce, or your favorite condiment.

GREEN SALAD WITH ROASTED SWEET POTATOES

This recipe illustrates Matthew's belief that you can pack a lot of flavor into a dish without adding a ton of extra calories. There are strong flavors in this dish, from the vinegar to the arugula, toasted nuts, and your favorite spice blend.

SERVES 2 TO 4

2–3 medium-to-large sweet potatoes

1 small-to-medium red onion

1½–2 tablespoons olive oil (20–30 milliliters)

Salt, to taste (probably about 1–2 teaspoons) (5–10 grams)

1 green onion, finely cut on the diagonal

1½ cups greens; baby arugula or spinach are great options (360 milliliters)

2 tablespoons toasted nuts (Matthew recommends pistachios, walnuts, pecans, or almonds) (30 milliliters)

3 tablespoons crumbled feta cheese (45 milliliters)

Spice blend of your choice (dukkah or za'atar are great options)

1 tablespoon honey (15 milliliters)

2 tablespoons balsamic vinegar (30 milliliters)

1. Preheat oven to 375°F (190°C).

2. Peel sweet potatoes and cut into medium pieces. Peel red onion and cut into wedges.

3. Toss the potatoes and onions with olive oil and salt. Place on a foil-lined baking tray and roast until softened and caramelized, about 35–45 minutes. Let cool slightly.

4. Transfer to a serving platter and top with green onion, greens, nuts, and feta. Finish with a generous sprinkle of the spice and a pinch of sea salt.

5. Combine honey and vinegar, drizzle over top of the salad, and serve.

EASY RICE "PUDDING"

Here's what Matthew says about this recipe: "As an avid cyclist and amateur racer, I found the opportunity to work closely with a pro cycling team very interesting. This recipe was developed after time spent cooking for the Holowesko-Citadel professional cycling team. The first time I cooked for them, the team's guidelines said to always make sure there was plenty of plain rice at every meal. But the guys liked the other food so much they never seemed to eat the rice. I hate to waste food, so I needed to figure out a better way to serve the rice. How about dessert? This is a great option for that; it feels rich but skips the refined sugar, cream, and eggs in favor of a lighter version. Great warm or chilled, eat it for breakfast, recovery, or dessert. It keeps for a few days in the refrigerator, and you can make it with leftover rice as well. Just heat the rice first, and then add the other ingredients."

SERVES 2

1 cup jasmine or basmati rice (240 milliliters)

2¼ cups water (540 milliliters)

1 teaspoon salt (5 grams)

2 teaspoons vanilla extract (10 milliliters)

2–3 ounces maple syrup, agave, or honey (60–90 milliliters)

1¾–2 cups almond or soy milk, unsweetened or lightly sweetened
(420–480 milliliters)

1–1½ teaspoons ground cinnamon (2.5–4 grams)

1. Briefly rinse the rice and drain. Transfer to a rice cooker and follow manufacturers' instructions, or put it into a saucepan with lid. Add the water and salt and bring to a boil. Reduce to a simmer.

2. Cook rice for 14–18 minutes and turn off heat. Allow to rest for 10 minutes.

3. Stir in the remaining ingredients. Serve warm or chilled with fruit on top and/or granola for crunch.

13

HYDRATION AND HEAT-STRESS MANAGEMENT

USING THE CONCEPTS AND TRAINING PROGRAMS in this book, time-crunched athletes can achieve high-performance fitness and compete against athletes who spend a lot more time on their bikes. However, as explained in Chapter 3 and as we will reiterate in Chapter 15 (Making the Most of Your Fitness), low-volume high-intensity training plans don't provide the same depth of fitness that high-volume athletes achieve. As a result, optimizing your on-the-bike and off-the-bike habits is part of being a successful time-crunched athlete. Hydration and heat-stress management are important for all athletes and are two areas where time-crunched athletes can gain a competitive advantage.

THE ESSENTIAL ROLES OF FLUIDS

When it comes to sports nutrition for athletes, fluids are even more important than calories. During exercise, macronutrients have one essential job: to provide energy to working muscles. Water, in contrast, plays a wide variety of roles, and each of them is mission-critical.

Core Temperature Regulation

Regulating your core temperature is water's most obvious role during exercise. As you exercise, some of the energy you burn produces the work that moves you forward, but unfortunately even more energy is wasted as heat. This is the price we pay for our overall lack of efficiency. For cyclists, only about 20–25 percent of the energy we burn actually creates mechanical work. The problem is that the human body operates properly only within a narrow temperature range, from 95 to 104°F (35 to 40°C). A lot of the heat generated from exercise has to be dissipated in order to maintain core temperature within the optimal range.

Sweat is the body's primary cooling mechanism, with evaporative cooling carrying heat away from the body. As your core temperature rises, sweat glands all over your body start producing more sweat by drawing fluid from the space around them and secreting it onto the surface of the skin. That fluid gets replaced by fluid from your blood plasma, making your blood volume a major reservoir of potential sweat.

As we'll cover in more detail later in this chapter, the amount of fluid an athlete needs to consume depends largely on sweat rate, which can vary greatly depending on exercise intensity, air temperature, wind conditions, and humidity.

Gut Motility and Digestion

Without enough fluid, you cannot digest food, which means your nutrition strategy is entirely dependent on your hydration status. After food gets broken down in the stomach and travels to the small intestine, the nutrients, fluid, and everything else you want from that food have to be transported through the selective semipermeable membrane that makes up the wall of your intestine. To get carbohydrate from the intestine into the blood, you need to have enough water in the intestine to facilitate the transport. If you don't, the food sits there until enough water becomes available, either because you drink more or because it is pulled from your body into your intestine.

This latter mechanism isn't ideal in any circumstance, but it is not a big problem when you are at rest and well hydrated. When you are exercising and pumping sweat onto your skin to cool off, however, your body prioritizes thermoregulation over digestion, and digestion slows dramatically. This is often the tipping point for gastrointestinal distress because once gut motility drops, it can take a long time for it to return to normal, and food that sits in the gut generates gas, leading to pressure, bloating, and a cascade of gastrointestinal issues you want to avoid.

Blood Volume

You have about 9.5 to 11.6 pints (4.5 to 5.5 liters) of blood in your body, and it never stops moving. Athletes and coaches focus on the blood's role in delivering oxygen to working muscles, but blood also delivers nutrients to your cells and takes away the waste they produce. It carries heat away from the core to the extremities and skin in order to maintain a healthy body temperature. And blood plasma provides the fluid that ends up being excreted as sweat. One of the key responses to training and acclimatization to heat and/or altitude is an increase in blood plasma volume. It's your body's way of filling the reservoir to be prepared for the anticipated activity and environment.

When you run low on fluids and plasma volume drops, your body starts prioritizing how to use what's left. In cold temperatures, athletes with a better hydration status stay warmer longer. Dehydration hastens the onset of hypothermia. When it's hot outside and your plasma volume gets a little low, your resting and exercise heart rates increase. Your heart has to pump faster to deliver the same amount of oxygen using less fluid. When plasma volume gets even lower, your body prioritizes sweating over digestion. If the situation gets dire, it prioritizes oxygen delivery over sweating, and you end up with heatstroke.

Waste Removal

Removal of metabolic waste products is another crucial role for fluids. The kidneys filter waste products out of your blood and excrete them in urine. With mild dehydration, your urine production diminishes, and the color of your urine starts to darken. More severe dehydration can damage your kidneys and alter the pH of your blood.

WHY HYDRATION STATUS MATTERS FOR TIME-CRUNCHED ATHLETES

Hydration status gets a lot more attention for athletes on high-volume training plans, and particularly for marathon and ultramarathon runners. With greater time spent exercising, these athletes spend more time sweating, and the need to replenish lost fluids becomes more obvious. The unique challenge that time-crunched athletes face is that individual workouts are often too short to experience a significant hydration-related decline in performance *during* the workout itself. In other words, time-crunched athletes often reach the end of the workout before they can see obvious signs that dehydration is causing a loss in power or motivation to continue.

You could see this as a positive, in that the workouts are over before dehydration hurts performance, but the problem is that many time-crunched athletes fail to properly rehydrate following workouts because they are not getting feedback telling them they need to. Thus begins a slow and gradual decline into chronic dehydration that negatively affects all workouts, robbing athletes of the opportunity for higher power outputs and higher-quality training sessions.

Simply weighing yourself before and after your training sessions is a good place to start monitoring your fluid intake, but doing so only tells you whether you adequately replenished the fluids lost since the beginning of the workout. This method says nothing about your hydration status at the beginning of the workout, yet that is arguably more important than the amount of fluid you lose during a relatively short workout.

Day-to-Day Hydration Status

Fluid and electrolyte replenishment during exercise is heavily dependent on sweat rate and temperature. Fluid loss can range from 500 ml/hour to more than 2 L/hour, and electrolyte loss is greatly influenced by the composition of your sweat. Recommendations for fluid and sodium intake directly before, during, and after exercise are discussed in Chapter 11. But hydration status is never static, so let's examine recommendations that will help you stay well hydrated on a day-to-day basis.

Dehydration is often evaluated based on body weight. But many athletes don't realize they start their day or their workout already dehydrated. A 2 percent loss of body weight during your workout may not be truly 2 percent dehydration; perhaps it's really 4 percent dehydration because you started the day already low on body fluid.

Researchers Cheuvront and Sawka (2005) devised a simple Venn diagram that is useful for evaluating day-to-day hydration status (Figure 13.1). To use this WUT diagram, you need to evaluate three things immediately after waking up: your weight (W), urine color (U), and thirst (T). If one observation suggests dehydration but the other two are normal, dehydration is less likely.

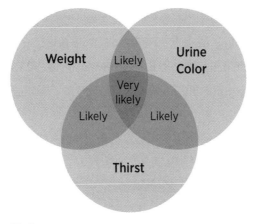

Daily Hydration Status

FIGURE
13.1

The WUT diagram helps you monitor your daily hydration status and the likelihood of dehydration.

If two observations indicate dehydration, the condition is more likely. And if all three indicate dehydration, you're very likely to be dehydrated.

First, how thirsty are you? When you are low on body fluid, your body responds with the sensation of thirst. Although there is wide variability from person to person, research suggests dehydration of about 2 percent of body weight is associated with the sensation of thirst (Kenefick et al. 2012).

Next comes urine color. The color of your urine is a common ballpark measure of urine concentration. Clear to straw-colored urine is not suggestive of dehydration, but be careful not to automatically equate clear urine with ideal hydration. Urine will often be clear if you are hyperhydrated or hyponatremic (low concentration of sodium), too. If your urine is the color of apple juice or darker, it is suggestive of dehydration. This color observation should be made from your urine stream or a collection cup rather than from diluted urine in a toilet bowl.

After urinating, weigh yourself without clothing. From day to day, your weight should remain virtually unchanged. Even if you are gradually gaining or losing weight due to changes in fat or muscle mass, those changes will be very small within a 24-hour period. A loss of 1 to 2 percent of body weight between one day and the next is more indicative of a change in total body fluid.

If two of the three or all three of these indices for evaluating body fluid indicate dehydration, then you have not done an adequate job of replenishing fluid losses over the preceding 24 hours. This doesn't necessarily mean you didn't drink enough during the previous day's workout. It also doesn't mean drinking gallons of fluid in the evening is the solution (doing so will increase first-morning urine volume and likely lighten its color, but much of that fluid is likely to pass right through you). It more likely means your overall daily fluid intake was inadequate to replenish losses from exercise, thermoregulation during normal activities (sitting outside on a warm day, working in a warm office, and so on), respiration, and water loss due to normal bodily function.

It's typically not a big issue if the WUT diagram indicates minor dehydration one day here and there. Nor does one day of minor dehydration necessitate major changes in your habits. It is best to use the WUT diagram over a rolling three-day period. If you are consistently seeing indications of diminished hydration status over two or three days, you should make adjustments to your overall daily hydration habits. This often happens when athletes increase their training load, travel to a warmer climate or higher elevation, or experience a change in weather or seasons. The typical solution is to increase water consumption throughout the day rather than simply guzzling a large volume of water to counter the indications of dehydration. It is also important to make sure you're consuming adequate fluids during training sessions.

If you can prevent at least two of the three indices from indicating dehydration, you are starting your day in a good position to maintain ideal body fluid for the rest of the day. You are also more likely to start your workout with adequate body fluid so that a 2 percent weight loss during a ride is an actual 2 percent body weight loss due to dehydration, not a net 4 percent body weight loss because you started the day and the workout already 2 percent down from day-to-day dehydration.

TEMPERATURE AND PERFORMANCE

Heat is the enemy of an endurance athlete. While most discussions of hydration status focus on the fact that endurance performance declines once athletes reach or exceed a 2 percent loss in body weight from water loss, it is more crucial to understand that heat is at the center of the problems associated with dehydration. This is demonstrated by research that shows that following a 4 percent loss in body weight, endurance performance is dramatically lower for athletes in a hot environment, while the decline in performance for athletes in a cold environment is not nearly so pronounced. In other words, you can be low on fluid and perform reasonably well as long as you can control the heat.

For many years we've been throwing around the notion that a 2 percent or greater loss of total body water leads to diminished endurance performance. This is true; see Table 13.1 (Cheuvront and Kenefick 2014). How much it hurts performance, though, is highly variable among individuals. And while many athletes have adopted the mantra of "drink enough to prevent weight loss greater than 2 percent of body weight during exercise" as gospel, few understand how or why dehydration diminishes performance.

Dehydration Lowers VO$_2$max

VO$_2$max is your maximal capacity for taking in and processing oxygen, and it is heavily dependent on the amount of blood your heart can pump. Dehydration lowers plasma volume because the sweat on your skin was most recently plasma in your blood. And keep in mind, a 2 percent total body weight loss from dehydration does not equate to a 2 percent loss in blood plasma volume—it can be up to a 10 percent loss in plasma volume!

As blood volume decreases, your heart rate increases in an effort to meet your oxygen demands with less fluid available to circulate. But stroke volume—the volume your heart pumps with each beat—also decreases when

TABLE 13.1

Effects of Dehydration and Environment on VO$_2$max

STUDY	SAMPLE SIZE	ENVIRONMENT	DEHYDRATION (% BODY MASS)	CHANGE IN VO$_2$MAX (%)
Nybo et al. (270)	6	15°C perfused suit	−4	−6
Caldwell et al. (41)	47	Room temperature	−4	−3
Webster et al. (374)	7	Room temperature	−5	−7
Buskirk et al. (39)	13	26°C	−5	−6*
Ganio et al. (127)	11	30°C	−4	−9
Nybo et al. (270)	6	44°C perfused suit	−4	−16
Craig & Cummings (73)	9	46°C	−2	−10
Craig & Cummings (73)	9	46°C	−4	−27

All percentages rounded to the nearest whole integer.
*Buskirk et al. only provided the reduction in VO$_2$max in L (0.2 L). The percentage was estimated assuming a VO$_2$max between 3 and 4 L/min (3.5 L).
Source: Samuel N. Cheuvront and Robert W. Kenefick. Dehydration: Physiology, Assessment, and Performance Effects. *Comprehensive Physiology* 4 (1): 257–285.

plasma volume decreases, and Wingo et al. (2012) have shown that a reduction in stroke volume correlates with a proportional reduction in VO_2max.

The Time-Crunched Training Program is weighted toward increasing your power at VO_2max and leveraging that improvement to increase power at lactate threshold and lower the relative percentage of VO_2max you need to sustain at an "all day" endurance pace. So, think about the reduction in VO_2max this way: In a matter of hours, dehydration can strip you of all the performance gains you worked so hard to make with this program—or any program. The only way to perform up to the level of your training is to be adequately hydrated.

Dehydration Disrupts Pacing

When VO_2max is reduced due to lowered cardiac stroke volume, your relative VO_2max at any given exercise intensity level increases. This means that if you know that 260 watts is a sustainable climbing power output for you because it is at or slightly below your lactate threshold, when you are dehydrated that 260 watt output will represent a higher percentage of your VO_2max.

Operating at a higher percentage of your VO_2max increases perceived exertion for the same level of actual workload, and we take many of our pacing cues—for short efforts as well as for longer time trials and whole rides—from our perceived exertion. Indeed, even when athletes have power meters, perceived exertion provides context for the numbers. So not only does dehydration reduce your real VO_2max, but it also gives you physiological cues that tell you to reduce intensity by increasing your perceived exertion.

Low Body Water Causes Competition for Resources

Part of the reason that heat exacerbates the decline in performance from dehydration is because of a competition for limited resources. To dissipate heat and provide more plasma for sweat production, blood volume is directed to the skin during exercise. In cold conditions heat transfer to the environment is more effective, so less blood has to be directed to the skin and sweat rates are lower. The opposite is true during exercise in hot conditions.

When total plasma volume decreases because of dehydration, your body has to prioritize. Despite your training or competition goals, your body's imperative for survival prioritizes cooling over performance. In a battle for resources, your skin and vital organs get more blood flow and your muscles and digestive system get less.

Dehydration Accelerates Overheating

Even though your body prioritizes cooling over performance, there are some compromises. As the osmolality of body fluids increases, your body slows the sweat rate in order to hold on to more water. This reduces heat transfer to the environment through sweating and increases heat storage.

The overall takeaway is that performance declines from dehydration are very real. You can't push your way through them simply by toughening up. In most cases of mild dehydration (about 2 percent body weight loss), there's plenty of plasma volume to minimize the decline in VO_2max, but you have to control the heat. When you add heat—which increased your fluid loss in the first place—performance declines multiply. Yes, you can overcome some of the loss of motivation and vigor associated with dehydration, but you can't will yourself to regain your lost VO_2.

BEHAVIORAL THERMOREGULATION

While there are physiological causes for the real decrease in performance capacity from overheating, there are also behavioral causes. When you exercise in a hot environment, skin temperature rises a lot faster than core temperature. Researchers have shown a decrease in voluntary exercise intensity during this initial time period, even before core temperature has substantially increased. Thermal discomfort can dramatically impair performance.

WHY WRESTLERS CAN CUT WEIGHT AND YOU CAN'T

Interestingly, the performance declines described here affect endurance activities to a far greater extent than they do power activities. Athletes in explosive and high-power sports, including weight lifting, football, and possibly wrestling and boxing, don't experience decreases in performance anywhere close to those experienced by endurance athletes.

In a 2014 review study, Cheuvront examined 103 previous studies, which included 313 separate observations. In 68 percent of the endurance studies examined, dehydration greater than or equal to 2 percent of body weight significantly impaired performance, compared to only 20 percent of the strength/power studies. The chasm between these percentages tightens up some when you account for studies with smaller numbers of test subjects, but still, it's clear that strength and power athletes preserve more of their performance when dehydrated (Cheuvront 2014).

The reason why performance for strength and power athletes isn't hurt as much by dehydration may have to do with the location of dehydration. Research has indicated a correlation between reduction in intramuscular hydration (water in muscle cells) and reduced plasma osmolality. Even with large increases in plasma osmolality from the removal of water, muscle cells retain a large portion of their water content (Pitcavage et al. 1962). For short high-force and high-power movements, the minor water loss from muscle cells isn't enough to hinder the cells' ability to contract.

This doesn't mean strength and power athletes perform better dehydrated; it only means they can retain their performance capacity better than endurance athletes can in a dehydrated state. This may partially explain why power-sport athletes like wrestlers, boxers, and mixed martial arts fighters can cut dramatic amounts of weight and still compete at a high performance level.   >

The other reason is that wrestlers, boxers, and mixed martial arts fighters have time to partially rehydrate between weigh-ins and competition. So, while athletes may "make weight" on the scale, in the time between weigh-ins and competition they can ingest fluids to at least partially rehydrate themselves. This will increase their actual weight, but weight gain in this manner is allowed within the rules.

Skin temperature is largely affected by the temperature of ambient air, whereas core temperature is mostly affected by metabolic heat production. The worst-case scenario is when it's hot out and you're hot within, because this drives up perceived exertion and thermal discomfort, and voluntary exercise intensity drops. When you cool the skin with fans or water, perceived exertion decreases at similar workloads and without a reduction in core temperature.

Interestingly, this holds true even when there is a sensation of skin cooling (using menthol gel) without any actual reduction in skin temperature. In both thermal and nonthermal cooling scenarios, time to exhaustion increased and power output during a time trial increased (Schlader 2011). Does this mean you should smear yourself with menthol and pour water over yourself during every training session? No. The takeaway is that core temperature is not the only—and may not even be the primary—force that changes your exercise performance in heat and cold.

MANAGING HEAT STRESS: WHAT WORKS AND WHAT DOESN'T

When I started working on this section of the book, some of the people I talked with thought it was unnecessary for a time-crunched athlete training book. Taking steps to manage heat stress, they said, was focusing on marginal gains for athletes who have not maxed out their performance capacities from fundamental training.

I certainly see their point. When you rank priorities, you focus on the aspects of preparation that measurably improve an athlete's ability to produce work. That's why building the aerobic engine is always first. Specializing your training to meet the unique demands of your sport comes next. Then comes optimizing the nutritional support for your training and events. After that you start to get to things people refer to as marginal gains, like heat acclimatization, altitude training, optimizing pedaling dynamics, and so on.

Managing heat stress does fall into this latter category, because it doesn't make sense to focus on heat stress to the detriment of focusing on your fitness or nutrition. However, I think it is worth adding here because you are managing heat stress already anyway, and you can improve the techniques you're using and improve performance without adding activities that take away from any other part of your training.

The Basics

The basics of managing heat stress are simple: slow down, get wet, move air over your body, and drink water. When you slow down, you reduce metabolic heat production, which means you at least stop pouring coal on the fire. Wetting your clothing and skin helps reduce skin temperature and provides more fluid for evaporative cooling. Moving into a shaded area and using fans or exposure to wind aids in cooling, too. And drinking water provides fluid to support plasma volume so you can continue to sweat and blunt the increase in heart rate that comes from low blood plasma volume.

Beyond the basics, people have tried or proposed a lot of techniques for managing heat stress. These techniques fall into three categories: pre-cooling, per-cooling (during exercise), and post-cooling.

Pre-cooling

The science of pre-cooling has gained a lot of attention as more and more international sporting events are being held in hot regions. The 1996 Olympic

Games in Atlanta, Georgia, was one of the early events where ice vests were used in an effort to keep competitors cool prior to the start of their outdoor competitions. The science of pre-cooling has advanced quite a bit since then, but the basic premise has remained consistent. The goal of pre-cooling is to blunt the rapid increase in core and skin temperature associated with exercise in the heat. Pre-cooling will not prevent you from reaching high skin or core temperatures during an event, especially longer events like a road race or time trial, but it can still give you more time to operate before your body reaches these detrimental temperatures.

Lots of methods for pre-cooling have been studied. Total body immersion in cold water works really well but isn't a practical solution for most events. Cold air exposure is another method, but it requires a long time to work and is probably even less practical for most athletes and most events. A prolonged cold shower works as well but also is not very convenient at a race.

A cooling vest is the most convenient method for pre-cooling. If you are regularly competing in hot temperatures during summer criteriums, a cooling vest may be a worthwhile investment. Wear the vest for 30–60 minutes leading up to your event, including during your warm-up. If you don't have a cooling vest, you can use cold towels. For best results, you want to cool a large portion of the body, which is why the vests are more effective than cooling just hands, arms, or your neck. However, in a pinch, an ice collar or ice sock around the back of your neck is better than nothing.

Another pre-cooling technique is the ingestion of cold liquid or an ice slurry. Both are effective, though the ice slurry works better. If you can combine the cooling vest with cold water or ice slurry ingestion, you can achieve even greater benefit. As I'll explain soon, the ice slurry appears to be more effective before exercise than during.

Is it worth it? Heat absolutely hurts performance, and pre-cooling is not that difficult to integrate into your pre-race routine. Starting your event with lower core and skin temperatures increases your heat storage capacity, meaning you can accumulate more heat in your body before reaching a core temperature that will hinder performance. Internal heat storage happens even when sweat rates increase during exercise in hot environments, but if you can increase your heat storage capacity you can help your body attenuate the rise in core temperature for longer. This means higher power outputs, greater work capacity, and less thermal strain during the period before you reach high core temperatures.

Per-cooling

Once your race, event, or training session starts, your options for cooling are limited by availability. Your best options are to douse yourself with cold water or grab ice socks you can stuff in your jersey between your shoulder blades. The downside to these options is that you're going to be soaking wet, all the way down to your shoes. If you don't like soggy shoes and a wet chamois in your cycling shorts, be sparing with the amount of water you dump on yourself.

Always prioritize putting fluid in your body over dumping it on your body. When water is at a premium, as it is during races with few or no feed zones or events where there are long distances between aid stations, it is more important to replenish fluids lost through sweat than it is to douse yourself. Consider the consequences. If your hydration status is good but your core temperature and skin temperatures are high, you will slow down but you will be able to continue at that slower speed for a considerable time. If you are overheating and dump your limited water resources over your body, you will soon be both dehydrated and overheated, and in far more danger of stopping altogether.

Ice slurry drinks, while they work well for pre-cooling, may not as beneficial during exercise. The reason for this may be because thermoreceptors in your stomach respond so strongly to the very cold temperature of the slurry that your sweat response slows or shuts down, and blood flow to the skin may diminish. Meanwhile, you are continuing to exercise and generating a lot of heat, and in the time it takes to regain normal exercise sweat and skin blood

THE DAY I CAME BACK FROM THE DEAD
Jim Rutberg

Prior to riding my second Dirty Kanza 200, I had been riding and racing bicycles for more than 20 years and had finished the Leadville 100 ten times. The evening before my second Kanza, I delivered the sports nutrition talk to more than 30 CTS athletes and coaches during our pre-race dinner. The following day, despite knowing the science behind hydration and core temperature and how to optimize them both, I made one poor decision and paid for it for 150 long miles.

That year, the morning was pretty cool as we rolled out of Emporia, Kansas, so staying hydrated and keeping core temperature under control for the first 50 miles wasn't a problem. In the spirit of making racers self-sufficient, the Dirty Kanza 200 purposely limits aid stations to one every 50 miles and the course is not marked (the route is announced ahead of time and you can use cue cards or GPS). As I rolled into the first aid station at 50 miles, I realized there would be a strong tailwind for the next 50 miles, and that's where I screwed up.

A tailwind enables you to go faster, but it also makes you hotter. When you are going about the same speed as the wind, there isn't much air flowing over you, especially over the front of your body. As a result, overheating in a tailwind is quite common. My big mistake was forgetting that and thinking I could cover the next 50 miles fast enough that I could get away with carrying three water bottles rather than using a hydration pack. On smooth roads, 50 miles with a strong tailwind could be a 2:00 to 2:30 segment. But on rolling hills and gravel roads it was 3 hours plus.

About one hour out from the second aid station, I ran dry. I was overheated, knew I was getting dehydrated, and I was riding alone in the middle of nowhere. There were other riders here and there, but they had to conserve their fluids, too. And, to be honest, I was too stubborn to ask for help. With every rolling hill

I went slower and slower, further increasing the amount of time it was going to take me to reach the water I sought from the second aid station.

Desperation set in. I looked for a creek to jump into and possibly drink from, but the only water sources I saw were stagnant, murky puddles of runoff from cow pastures. I scanned the road for dropped bottles, until coming over the top of a rolling hill I spotted potential salvation: a 24-ounce bike bottle lying in the middle of the road. And it was full! Being skeptical of bottles found on the road, lest they contain urine or tobacco spit, I opened the bottle before drinking it. It was clear and smelled fine, so down the hatch! It must have been some kind of sports drink or homemade concoction, and by now it was now quite warm and tasted awful. Beggars can't be choosers, though, and I knew how fortunate I was to find 24 ounces of potable anything.

I crawled my way to the second aid station, where the other coaches were waiting. We have a standard rule within CTS aid stations: there's no sitting. Once athletes sit down, they don't get up. Aid stations are for resupply, not rest. Get in and get out, and even if you are moving slowly as you eat and drink, at least you are making forward progress.

I sat down. I knew I needed to not only pick up fluids but also get some fluid into my body. About 20 minutes later I finally left, slowly. This time I had a full hydration pack of water and two full bottles of sports drink. The plan was to slowly dig myself out of the hydration hole I had made for myself and keep making forward progress.

About 5 miles out from the second aid station, with 45 miles ahead of me to the next one, I turned around to go back and drop out. I was cooked. I rolled about 200 yards toward the aid station and stopped again. If I go back there, I reasoned, I'm going to sit there for hours before getting a ride back to town. And if I'm going to be out here for hours anyway, I might as well just put one pedal in front of the other and keep going forward.   >

It wasn't pretty, but I managed to finish. Despite new course records and favorable conditions that made others an hour or more faster than the previous year (on the same course), I was a few hours slower. By the time I reached the finish line, the aid station crew I had seen at Mile 150 had arrived back in town. I thought I had recovered reasonably well by the time I saw them at Mile 150, but they told me I looked so bad at their aid station they were sure it was only a matter of time before I called for rescue.

One mistake. One poor hydration decision led to a cascade of problems that took several hours to even marginally recover from. I learned a lot about perseverance, problem solving, and patience that day, and it took everything I knew about sports science and nutrition to come back from the dead. From that one mistake.

flow rates, you can store more heat internally than you would have otherwise. It becomes a balance between benefit of lowering core temperature with the ice slurry and the cost of hindering sweat and skin blood flow.

It appears these two can easily cancel each other out, leaving athletes with essentially no change in overall body temperature and no change in performance. As a result, ingestion of cool and cold drinks is preferred to ingesting ice slurry drinks while exercising in the heat. Cold drinks—but not icy ones—can help modestly lower core temperature without triggering the thermoregulatory response that hinders sweat rate and skin blood flow, thereby enabling you to continue maximizing all three of these cooling mechanisms.

Post-cooling

Bringing your core temperature down following exercise in the heat is beneficial for recovery. However, the goal is to reduce overall body temperature rather than focus the cooling on specific muscles. For a long time, runners

COOLING AND INDOOR TRAINING

An indoor trainer can be a great asset for a time-crunched athlete. It eliminates the time of figuring out what to wear for the weather, what route to take, and what gear to carry. You can just get into your shorts, throw on your shoes, and get going. Staying cool is one of the biggest challenges to indoor training, and overheating during your indoor sessions can dramatically reduce power output, even within a short, 1-hour indoor workout.

Keep in mind that heat stress is affected by core temperature and skin temperature, and when both are elevated your VO_2max decreases and you reach your self-reported time to exhaustion (how quickly you quit or voluntarily slow down) sooner. A fan is an obvious necessity, but most people stop there—which may not be enough. Multiple fans are better than one; you want airflow over as much of your skin as possible.

Air blowing specifically on your face is also important. Research has shown that cooling the face lowers perceptions of thermal discomfort, lowers RPE, and extends time to exhaustion, thereby increasing the amount of work done (Schlader et al. 2011). To prove this point, Schlader et al. substituted the fan with menthol cream applied to the face, which did not actually cool the skin but provided a cooling sensation, and saw very similar results. Interestingly, even when core temperature is elevated to the same degree, cooling the head and face increases thermal comfort and leads to a real increase in the amount of work an athlete can do.

You can do this in combination with cold drinks, a cold towel for your back, or a cold towel on the back of your neck. Unless you are using a specific heat-acclimatization protocol, there is no benefit to training indoors at a purposely elevated air temperature.

and some other athletes used ice baths following long and hard training sessions. The thought was that the ice bath reduced inflammation and therefore enhanced recovery. More recently, the research on the potential benefit of ice baths has been inconclusive, but an important change to our understanding of recovery is that inflammation should not necessarily be avoided or minimized.

Inflammation associated with trauma or injury is different than inflammation as a response to normal exercise. Following a hard ride or run, you will have some inflammation in working muscles. But that inflammation may be a key component of the training stress that results in adaptation and progress. When you immediately jump into an ice bath following a hard workout, you may actually be blunting the training stimulus from all that hard work.

A more effective way to enhance recovery is to take proactive steps to cool your whole body. These steps include drinking cold water or an ice slurry, covering large areas of your torso with cold towels, taking a cool shower, or immersing yourself in cool water (not icy water). And later, if you are having trouble sleeping following a hard workout, especially on a hot day, try reducing the temperature of the room.

IMPACT OF BREAST AUGMENTATION ON HEAT STRESS IN FEMALE ATHLETES

Athletes sometimes present challenges that leave coaches scratching our heads. A few years ago, we started to field questions from women, particularly runners and triathletes, who were having trouble with thermoregulation during races and long workouts in hot weather. The biggest issue was that once they were overheated it was difficult for them to cool down. We looked at common hormonal and thyroid-related issues that can lead to problems with thermoregulation but eventually ruled them out. Then, during a typical coach-athlete conversation, one of our female coaches struck on a possible cause: breast implants.

Breast augmentation and/or reconstruction following a mastectomy involves placing a saline or silicone implant behind or on top of the pectoralis muscles in the chest. The saline and silicone are inert substances, and the implants are neither innervated nor perfused with blood flow. As a result, they do not always heat and cool in sync with the tissues around them. In essence, a breast implant is a heat sink.

When core temperature gradually increases, as it does during a workout or competition in hot weather, the temperature of the implant gradually rises as well. When an athlete tries to rapidly cool down through consumption of cold liquids, dousing with water, wrapping with cold towels, or exposure to cool airflow, skin temperature and core temperature can come down reasonably quickly. Much of this cooling happens because high blood flow to the skin transfers heat to the environment through contact or evaporative cooling. Breast implants can transfer heat to surrounding tissues, but because they aren't perfused with blood it takes longer for them to cool compared to the tissues around them.

As a result, women with augmented breasts exercising in hot conditions sometimes report feeling like they have a hot compress resting on their chest. This reduces perceptions of thermal comfort and can increase perceived exertion at a given workload. It is unknown whether heat retention by breast implants actually keeps median core temperature elevated longer, or whether the impact is limited to thermal perception and comfort.

The opposite can happen as well. Prolonged exposure to cold water can lower core temperature, and breast implants will cool similarly. Upon exiting the water, as during a triathlon or swimming workout in cold water or a training pool (significantly colder than a backyard pool), women sometimes report feeling like they have a cold compress resting on their chest. Anecdotally, this seems to be reported less frequently, which may be because athletes training or competing in the water generate a lot of heat and therefore maintain a body temperature closer to normal.

From an athletic performance standpoint, the solution to the overheating problem appears to be a proactive focus on cooling the chest during hot weather. Although our coaches have not conducted research studies to determine if these methods actually reduce core temperature or accelerate the cooling of implant material, anecdotal evidence from our athletes indicates that ice, ice packs, cold towels or garments, and dousing with cold water all work, just as they do for all athletes. In this case, however, these cooling techniques need to be directly applied to the chest as well as the rest of the body.

All of this talk of heat and heat stress management eventually brought up a question: Could breast implants actually provide an ergogenic aid? Could pre-cooling lower core temperature, skin temperature, *and* implant temperature; and then could the implants' slower heat response extend the duration of the performance benefits of pre-cooling? It's at least a partly serious question, because in competitive sports there are athletes looking for any advantage. We don't know the answer, but we would doubt there would be much, if any, performance benefit, and if there was it would be short-lived. It is hard to believe that the actual temperature gradient between implant material and surrounding tissue is very large. The perception of heat or cold may be significant, but the actual temperature gradient is likely much smaller. And without a large temperature gradient—the kind you get from wearing an ice vest—there shouldn't be much actual performance benefit from pre-cooling breast implants.

PART IV

Making the Most of Your Fitness

Above all else, time-crunched athletes need to use their time and efforts wisely. You have to take advantage of training opportunities wherever and whenever they arise, and during events you have to use tactics that enhance your chances for success using the fitness you have acquired. The final section of this book is dedicated to wringing every possible opportunity out of the limited time you can devote to cycling.

Inconsistency is one of the hallmarks of time-crunched training, in that athletes often have periods when they are extremely short on available training time followed by periods when their schedules briefly open up. In Chapter 14 I'll share some training blocks focused on endurance that will help you make the most of those precious weeks when you do have more time on the bike.

Chapter 15 is one of my favorites because in my heart I'm still a bike racer. As I mentioned earlier, time-crunched training yields time-crunched fitness, and it is important to understand how to use tactics and strategies that take advantage of the kind of fitness you have developed. When you ride intelligently and leverage your training, you can capture a win against athletes with twice the weekly training time!

The final chapter of this book covers strength training for time-crunched athletes. Strength training is not likely to make you a faster cyclist, but it is an important component of keeping you in the game. If you can squeeze strength training into your schedule, you will be a more well-rounded athlete and well-rounded adult. You will have more activity options available to you. You'll be less likely to miss sport-specific training due to silly injuries or soreness from moving furniture or yard work, and you'll be more likely to retain the muscle mass and coordination that is crucial to your health and vitality in the years to come.

14

SUPPLEMENTING YOUR TRAINING: ENDURANCE BLOCKS

EVERY ONCE IN A WHILE THE FATES CONVERGE and give you an opportunity to pack a lot of high-volume rides into a short period of time. Perhaps your spouse takes the kids to his or her parents' house for two weeks, or you get assigned a weeklong business trip in a prime riding area like Tucson, Arizona, or Brevard, North Carolina. Funny as it sounds, athletes who become accustomed to following training plans sometimes get confused about how to approach such a training windfall. The big question is: Do you change your program, or stick to the schedule you're already on?

Unless you're in the middle of the TCTP, with a series of races or an important goal event coming up in a few weeks, I recommend taking advantage of an unexpected increase in available training time by completing an Endurance Training Block. Although research supports the use of a low-volume, high-intensity training program for developing superior cycling fitness, there is also much to be gained from moderate-intensity endurance rides if you have the time to complete them. And honestly, even if there weren't, you'd be a fool to pass up the chance to spend more time on your bike. After all, the whole point of training is to enable you to get out there and enjoy as much time as you can riding.

There are two approaches to an Endurance Training Block: You can use it for focused training, or you can just go ride your bike. Fortunately, the two approaches are very similar in execution. The key is to remember that as volume increases, intensity should decrease. When you have the opportunity to ride 2 to 5 hours a day for several days in a row, you need to be conscious of the fatigue that will accumulate and build from day to day. If you get too excited and open the throttle on day 1, you'll be cooked by day 3. Rides after this will become progressively slower, more difficult, and less fun.

In working with a wide variety of cyclists, CTS coaches have discovered that it's not uncommon for riders to find themselves, at least once a year, with a 2-week period in which they have almost unlimited training time. In response, I have developed a Two-Week Endurance Training Block that incorporates longer rides, a few structured workouts to build deeper aerobic conditioning, and plenty of "free time" for exploring new routes and generally taking advantage of your short-term freedom to ride as much as you want.

TWO-WEEK ENDURANCE TRAINING BLOCK

The Two-Week Endurance Training Block (see Table 14.1) is structured so you have 2- to 3-day blocks of back-to-back long rides, and then 1 to 2 days of recovery before the next series of back-to-back longer rides. You'll notice that the week before the Endurance Block begins should be predominantly a recovery week. Assuming your block will start on a Saturday, your final hard interval workout should be on Tuesday, or Wednesday at the very latest. Your weekly training volume during the block is likely to be double what you normally do—if not more—and it's important for you to be rested and fresh at the beginning.

The first week of this Endurance Training Block is the more difficult of the two, which is fitting because you'll be fresher and able to complete the work. There's a 3-day block (Tuesday, Wednesday, and Thursday), including two Tempo interval workouts (see Chapter 5 for a description of this interval).

Two-Week Endurance Training Block

TABLE
14.1

MONDAY	TUESDAY	WEDNESDAY	THURSDAY	FRIDAY	SATURDAY	SUNDAY
Rest day	Last hard interval workout before Endurance Block	Rest day or 1 hr. EM	Rest day or 45 min. easy spinning	Rest day or 45 min. easy spinning	3 hrs. EM or group ride	2–3 hrs. EM with 30 min. T
Rest day	3 hrs. EM with 40 min. T	2–4 hrs. EM	3 hrs. EM with 40 min. T	Rest day or 45 min. easy spinning	3–5 hrs. free ride	3–5 hrs. free ride
Rest day	1.5–2 hrs. EM, light gearing, higher cadence	4 hrs. EM with 40 min. T	3 hrs. EM	Rest day	3–5 hrs. free ride	3–5 hrs. free ride
Rest day	Rest day	45 min. easy spinning	1–1.5 hrs. EM	Rest day	2 hrs. EM	2 hrs. EM or group ride
Return to normal training						

▨ **: Endurance Block; EM:** EnduranceMiles; **T:** Tempo.

Tempo intervals are long, but the intensity level is not very high, and your goal should be to complete the interval with as few interruptions as possible. I have scheduled "free rides" on the weekends so you can choose anything from an epic ride with your buddies to doing the local group ride and then adding on a few hours afterward, or jumping into a local century. If you're a mountain biker, remember that a daylong epic into the backcountry certainly counts as an endurance-building workout.

During the second week of the block, Tuesday's ride is perhaps the most important. If you are really wiped out from the previous week's training volume, it would be a good idea to either take Tuesday as an additional rest day or make this ride a 30- to 45-minute recovery spin. Even if you feel pretty good, I want you to ride conservatively and limit your ride to a maximum of 2 hours. If these 2 weeks of training were included as a normal part of a high-volume trainer's program, this Tuesday would definitely be a rest day because of the two back-to-back periods of training the previous week. The only reason I've made this an optional EnduranceMiles ride (see Chapter 5) is that your Endurance Block is only going to last these 2 weeks.

PREPARING YOUR BODY FOR ENDURANCE BLOCKS

Doubling or tripling your weekly training volume by embarking on an Endurance Training Block affects you in ways that go beyond workload and fatigue. You're going to be spending more hours outdoors, and it's important to help your body deal with the increased stress.

Use sunscreen: A lot of time-crunched cyclists ride early in the mornings or after work, when the sun's rays are weaker. Then they go to a cycling camp or start on an Endurance Training Block and end up looking like a lobster halfway through the first week. Sunscreen is important to protect your skin from the damaging effects of UV radiation.

After riding countless miles without sunscreen as a younger man, I have had to have several spots examined and removed from my skin. Fortunately, none was cancerous, but I know there's a significant chance that one of these days one of them is going to be skin cancer. Use a sunscreen with an SPF rating of at least 15, and apply it liberally.

Protect your skin: Windburn is a common problem for cyclists, especially on the face. Skin protectants and moisturizers are important to keep your exposed skin healthy.

Protect your crotch: Athletes rarely suffer from chafing problems during short rides; it's when you're on the bike for 3-plus hours that you start dealing with raw skin and pressure sores. Applying chamois cream to your skin or the pad in your shorts is a good habit to get into if you're susceptible to chafing. If you start to get saddle sores, it may be time to invest in new shorts or a new saddle. Improper saddle position or tilt can also contribute to chafing and saddle sores.

NUTRITION FOR ENDURANCE BLOCKS

When you embark on any of the Endurance Training Blocks described in this chapter, it's important to remember that your nutrition and hydration choices are going to largely determine your ability to ride well in the final few days of the block. We know this not only because it makes good sense from a sports nutrition perspective but also because we've seen firsthand the impact of sports nutrition on cyclists' performances at our weeklong spring training camps, like the ones we hold every year in Santa Ynez, California. We close the week of riding with an adventure we call "the Stinger"—a long day in the saddle that includes Figueroa Mountain, a narrow and nasty climb that would be a Cat. I ascent if judged by the standards used to rank climbs in the Tour de France. Without fail, athletes who follow our recommended nutritional guidance fare better on the Stinger than athletes who don't.

Eat a Hearty Breakfast

An Endurance Training Block is not the time to skimp on breakfast. A reasonably large portion of cereal (about 3 cups when you might normally eat 2), toast, fruit, and plenty of fluids would be a minimal breakfast. Even better, include some protein from eggs and/or yogurt. One option that seems to agree with many cyclists is an omelet with veggies and cheese, a few slices of toast with butter or a bagel with cream cheese, a large glass of orange juice, and a cup of strong coffee. Other options to consider are oatmeal, granola, pancakes, or potatoes, but stay away from greasy breakfast options such as hash browns, bacon, sausage, and ham.

START YOUR RIDE WITH TWO BOTTLES OF SPORTS DRINK

Some riders go to the trouble of carrying drink mix so they can consume a sports drink after their first two bottles of the day, and athletes at training camps or bike tours can typically get sports drinks from support vehicles. If you're out doing your own Endurance Block, however, it's likely you'll be filling up with plain water. If that's the case, start your ride with two bottles of sports drink, and use bigger (24 ounce) bottles instead of normal (20 ounce) bottles if you have them. This will help you consume a steadier supply of carbohydrate during the early portion of your ride, which will make the later hours better and reduce your post-ride recovery demands.

BE SURE TO EAT DURING YOUR RIDE

During shorter rides (60–75 minutes), and especially when you have a full day of recovery between workouts, you typically don't need to consume any calories while you ride. But when you're doing back-to-back days of long rides, it becomes increasingly important to fuel consistently. Carry plenty of sports nutrition products, such as energy bars and chewables, and at a minimum eat something every 45 minutes (if water's your only drink on the ride, eat something at least every 30 minutes). Make sure you have some variety in flavors and textures, because your tastes and cravings will change as your ride gets longer. You're more likely to continue eating if there's something you like and want in your jersey pocket.

USE A RECOVERY DRINK

Post-ride recovery nutrition is crucial for continued success during an Endurance Training Block, training camp, or cycling tour. Most times you're going to be back on your bike less than 24 hours after you finish your current ride, so you want to do everything you can to ensure that you start tomorrow's adventure with fully stocked carbohydrate stores. Earlier I noted that recovery drinks aren't always necessary following training sessions but that in certain circumstances they are warranted. When you are increasing your training load with back-to-back rides during an Endurance Block, recovery drinks are a good idea.

A carbohydrate-rich recovery drink should be the first thing you look for after your ride, followed within an hour by a full meal that's rich in carbohydrate and contains a moderate amount of protein. Remember the guidelines from Chapter 11: 1.5 grams of carbohydrate per kilogram of body weight within 4 hours after your ride, and about one-third to one-half that amount of protein. And drink fluids equal to 1.5 times the amount of weight you lost during the ride; if you lost 2 pounds (32 ounces, or 0.9 kilograms) during the ride, drink 48 ounces (about 1.4 liters) during the 2 hours after the ride.

RELAX AND GRAZE

When you're in the midst of a higher-volume Endurance Training Block, it's not a good time to also commit to heavy-duty yard work, hours of sightseeing, or a full round of golf. When you're done with your long ride, relax, take a nap, watch a movie, or sit by the pool. And it's a good idea to continue snacking throughout the afternoon and evening, a habit known to many as "grazing"— grabbing a handful of nuts, trail mix, a piece of fruit, or a granola bar here and there, and of course continuing to drink plenty of fluids. Generally speaking, at a stage race it's rare to see a pro rider without a water bottle or a piece of food in hand in the afternoon and evening after a stage. The same should be true of cyclists at training camps and cycling tours, or during Endurance Training Blocks (which can be thought of as your own private training camp).

ONE-WEEK ENDURANCE TRAINING BLOCK

Not everyone has the luxury of being able to complete a full Two-Week Endurance Training Block, but you can still do yourself a lot of good if you happen to find one week when you can put in a lot of training hours. Ideally, you'll be able to ride during the weekends on both ends of your "free" week, and the schedule in Table 14.2 is a good way to structure your time. In this schedule you'll start out with a 4-day block of training, take a complete rest day, and follow that up with a light endurance ride before embarking on a 3-day series of big rides. If you're tired on Thursday, I'd recommend cutting this shorter ride to a recovery spin or taking it as a complete rest day. As in the

TABLE 14.2   **One-Week Endurance Training Block**

MONDAY	TUESDAY	WEDNESDAY	THURSDAY	FRIDAY	SATURDAY	SUNDAY
Rest day	Normal interval workout	Rest day or 1 hr. EM	Last hard interval workout before Endurance Block	Rest day	3 hrs. EM or group ride	2–3 hrs. EM with 40 min. T
3 hrs. EM with 40 min. T	2–4 hrs. EM	Rest day	1.5–2 hrs. EM, light gearing, higher cadence	3–5 hrs. EM	3–5 hrs. free ride	3–5 hrs. free ride
Rest day	Rest day	45 min. easy spinning	1–1.5 hrs. EM	Rest day	2–3 hrs. EM or group ride	2 hrs. EM
Return to normal training						

▓ **:** Endurance Block; **EM:** EnduranceMiles; **T:** Tempo.

2-week block, recovery is important to preserve the quality of your rides later in the week.

WORKING CYCLIST'S ENDURANCE TRAINING BLOCK

Can't put your job on hold for one or two weeks? That's understandable, but it doesn't mean you can't benefit from an Endurance Training Block. In your case you're going to have to get a little more creative. The Working Cyclist's Endurance Block (see Table 14.3) consists of two weekends and the week between them, and uses a total of two or three days of your personal vacation time. That shouldn't pose much of a problem, considering that surveys consistently show that fewer than half of American workers use all their vacation time each year anyway. This training block calls for a few half days and one or two long weekends, time you likely have coming to you, especially as many companies are eliminating the option of rolling unused vacation time from one year to the next.

As in the other Endurance Blocks, you should deliberately reduce your training load in the week preceding the Working Cyclist's Block. It starts with a 2½- to 3-hour ride on Friday, and I recommend working a half day, whether that means riding in the morning and going in to work for the afternoon or vice versa. That's followed by 2 back-to-back 3- to 4-hour rides over the weekend.

Working Cyclist's Endurance Training Block

TABLE **14.3**

MONDAY	TUESDAY	WEDNESDAY	THURSDAY	FRIDAY	SATURDAY	SUNDAY
Rest day	1–1.5 hrs. interval ride	1 hr. EM	Rest day	2.5–3 hrs. EM Work half day	3–4 hrs. EM	3–4 hrs. EM
1 hr. recovery ride	2 hrs. EM with 30–45 min. T	2–3 hrs. EM with 30–45 min. T Work half day if possible	1 hr. EM	4 hrs. EM Personal day or half day	4–5 hrs. ride (may include group ride)	4–5 hrs. EM with 45–60 min. T
4 hrs. EM Personal day	Rest day	Rest day	1 hr. EM	1 hr. EM	2–3 hrs. EM	2–3 hrs. EM
Return to normal training						

▓ : Endurance Block; **EM:** EnduranceMiles; **T:** Tempo.

The following week will likely be a different routine than your normal training week, with EnduranceMiles rides on Tuesday, Wednesday, and Friday and 1-hour rides on Monday and Thursday. Typically, cyclists are able to complete Tuesday's ride without having to take time off from work, but I recommend taking off a half day on Wednesday and either a half day or full day on Friday. This second weekend of the block is the big push: 16 to 18 hours on the bike in 4 days. You're going to be tired when you're done, but the training stimulus you get from this block will do you a lot of good.

There are two things you need to remember if you decide to embark on the Working Cyclist's Endurance Block:

1. **Consult your family:** This training block can be perceived as being extremely self-centered. From my experience, families tend to be supportive of a block like this when you point out that it allows you to focus on your training for a relatively short period of time without incurring the cost of attending a training camp or cycling tour, without leaving home for a week or longer, and without burning a lot of vacation time that you'll be able to use to go away on a family trip (and you should follow through on that pledge).

2. **You will need a recovery week:** After you finish the Working Cyclist's Endurance Block on Monday, it's important to take 2 complete rest days and then gradually return to training. Your rides on Thursday through Sunday should be moderate-paced endurance rides, with perhaps a group ride on the weekend. Wait until the following week to return to hard interval workouts.

• • •

CASE STUDY
MICK HITZ GOES LONG

CTS athlete Mick Hitz is a Cat. III racer and owner of Big Wheel Productions, a video production company in North Carolina. Like many small-business owners, Mick devotes almost all his time to his work and family, and though he enjoys racing, his training is typically limited to fewer than 7 hours a week. As luck would have it, his wife went on a trip for almost 2 weeks just as he wrapped up a big project, and he had some downtime before his next editing job was due. He called his coach, CTS coach Colin Izzard, who recognized that the situation was perfect for a big Endurance Block.

Mick rearranged his work schedule so he could take 2 back-to-back 4-day weekends, and arranged for his assistant editor to come in to cover the phones and keep the office running on the Wednesday and Thursday of the week between them so he could take off half days on those 2 days as well. Mick wrote down some of the long loops he rarely had a chance to ride from his hometown, and also went online to look up some of the great rides to be had in the Appalachian Mountains, a few hours away in western North Carolina.

To make the most of his opportunity, Mick then called his friends and shared his schedule. Though no one else was able to commit to all of the rides he had planned, he was joined by at least two buddies—and as many as eight— for each one. The second weekend he traveled west to Boone, North Carolina, for three epic rides in the mountains.

When he was done, Mick was exhausted and happy. About 2 weeks later, Colin started ramping up Mick's training for a fall series of criteriums, using many of the Time-Crunched Training Program concepts found in this book. To start out, Mick completed a CTS Field Test, and his power numbers were about 5 to 10 watts higher than the previous time he had started a race-focused training period. That, however, was pretty normal—we often see such incremental improvements when we use relatively short-term, high-intensity buildups. What was remarkable to Colin was a change in Mick's attitude about training and the extent of his recovery between rides.

The Endurance Training Block was a refreshing challenge for Mick, and he found that it boosted his enthusiasm for training in the weeks and months afterward. He looked forward to the next time he could string together several days of big, long rides with his friends. And there were some physiological benefits as well. The cumulative training stimulus of just 10 days of high-volume riding deepened his aerobic fitness to the point where he could maintain his normal cruising pace at a lower level of effort. He was able to recover a little faster from hard interval workouts, which in turn improved the quality of his individual training sessions (especially on the second day of 2-day training blocks).

15

MAKING THE MOST OF YOUR FITNESS

THE POINT OF THE TCTP IS TO ENABLE YOU to have more fun and achieve greater accomplishments on your bike. You're going to endure a lot of difficult workouts, so it's important that you take advantage of your hard-earned fitness when you get to your goal events or long-awaited epic ride. I want you to go out and win criteriums, power your way through cyclocross races, enjoy a warm summer century, or escape into the backcountry wilderness on your mountain bike. I want those rides to be the best days you have on your bike all year, so fun and fulfilling that they remind you why you're a cyclist.

Jim Rutberg had one of those rides the fall after the arrival of his second child, Elliot. Between the stress of work, a newborn, and the germs his 19-month-old son brought home from day care, he endured a seemingly endless series of autumn colds. His training was haphazard at best, as is the case with many new parents, and he was lucky if he strung together two rides in a week's time. That spring he'd used the TCTP as preparation for riding in a four-man team at the 24 Hours of Elephant Rock mountain bike race in Castle Rock, Colorado, and he hoped to build on that fitness to have a good ride at the Leadville 100 in August.

The 24 Hours of Elephant Rock was a great place for Jim to experiment with the TCTP's application for longer events, because lap times averaged about 40 minutes each. His team decided that each rider would do 2 to 4 laps per rotation. Between the short laps and the 4 to 6 hours of recovery between riding sessions, Rutberg came away from the event with lap times that were consistently equal to those of his teammates, who were on higher volume training programs.

The 24 Hours of Elephant Rock took place the first week of June, one week after Elliot was born but a week before he was due, and Rutberg's training went off the rails right after. In late July I asked him to come out to Leadville, Colorado, for a reconnaissance of the Leadville 100 mountain bike race course.

I wanted Rutberg along because he'd raced Leadville previously, but I didn't know he had barely ridden his bike in the previous two months. There were about a dozen people on the ride, and it was a good thing Jim knew the course better than any of the rest of us, because he was off the back on the first climb and didn't see another soul until he reached the Twin Lakes Dam, almost 40 miles later. Surprisingly, he rolled in only about 5 minutes behind the group, but he'd obviously dug very deep in the process. While we continued for 20 miles more, up to and back from the race's turnaround point at 12,600 feet of elevation, he wisely chose to stay at Twin Lakes with the cars and support crew we'd brought along for our little adventure.

Two weeks later, despite knowing he was woefully unprepared, Rutberg raced the Leadville 100. The year before, he had beaten me by about 20 minutes and earned a big rodeo-style belt buckle for finishing in fewer than 9 hours. That year it was my turn to finish in fewer than 9 hours and earn my big buckle, whereas Rutberg rode about half an hour slower than his previous best time, to cross the line in 9:13:56. Like all riders who finish in fewer than 12 hours, he earned a smaller buckle for his efforts, but it had clearly been an excruciating effort for a pretty disappointing result.

Immediately following the Leadville recon ride on July 30, Jim put himself back on the TCTP. He rode the Leadville 100 during week 2 of the program, even though he knew it was too early to see significant improvements in power output, because he was on a mission. He knew things would settle down at work and at home in August, and he decided he needed to do something to salvage his season. The 24 Hours of Elephant Rock had gone OK, but the Leadville recon ride and the race itself were both sufferfests. As he had seen happen with several of the athletes he'd been coaching, cycling was losing its appeal because his efforts weren't being rewarded with fun, powerful, and affirming experiences on the bike.

Grant Davis, a friend and freelance writer, suggested that Jim join him for a weekend of riding in New Mexico. Grant was going because he had a travel piece to write about the Angel Fire Ski Resort, and he was planning on riding the Enchanted Circle Century course on Saturday and the longer Southern Loop the following day. More than 200 miles in 2 days, including several significant mountain passes, would be quite a challenge, but Jim decided it would be a good opportunity to see how he'd do with 6 weeks of time-crunched training in his legs.

Coincidentally, as Grant and Jim started along the Enchanted Circle Century course from Angel Fire, the organized event was starting in Red River, New Mexico. About 50 miles into their ride, the two started picking up stragglers at the back of the century. As Jim, who found he had good legs that day, rolled at 21 to 25 mph along the valley roads and rolling hills toward Taos, a long line of riders joined Grant on his wheel. He felt great, and even though he figured his good legs would disappear on the 20-mile climb out of Taos, he just kept going.

Because they'd started at Angel Fire instead of Red River, Jim and Grant were about 70 miles into their ride when they reached Taos. All that remained was the 20-mile climb out of town and a few miles of descending and valley roads back to the resort. As they turned onto the climb, there was a tailwind, and Jim decided to just keep riding the steady power output he'd been holding and see how long it took for his legs to give out. Within 2 miles, there was no one on his wheel, and he was streaming past the mid-pack century riders.

Deciding not to question where the power was coming from, he just kept going and waited to see where he would finally crack. A little more than an hour later, he rounded one final bend, and there was the summit! It was the best climb—in terms of average power output and personal satisfaction—that he'd had all year. He waited for Grant, and the two blasted down the curvy descent and cruised back to Angel Fire.

The following morning, Grant and Jim hit the road again, this time for the 106-mile Southern Loop. Jim struggled badly in the first 20 miles and figured he was in for a long day of suffering, especially when the two reached the bottom of a 10-mile mountain pass that immediately preceded another 20-mile pass. Somewhere on the first climb Jim found his legs again, and he scorched the second pass. Still not knowing where the power was coming from, he pulled along the long valley on the way back to Angel Fire so fast that Grant had little choice but to stay in his draft. Though neither man felt fresh as a daisy during the final 2 hours of the ride, they rolled back into Angel Fire after 106 miles and 6,200 feet of climbing in just under 7 hours.

Jim had had the weekend he was looking for: He rode with the power to enjoy long climbs instead of just survive them. He was the one pulling over valley roads and rolling hills instead of praying to hold on to the wheel ahead of him. Even the weather was perfect, with tailwinds in all the right places. He'd had two rides that salvaged an entire season, 206 miles that justified the thousands he'd put in since January, and one weekend that reaffirmed his identity as a cyclist.

You don't have to win the Tour de France or become a national champion to have achieved something valuable as a cyclist. It's not the event but what you take away from it that sticks with you and provides the memories and motivation to continue training.

Taking full advantage of the fitness you'll gain from the TCTP is a matter of using your power wisely. Jim was able to ride back-to-back centuries and have the best weekend of his season because he understood how to adjust his riding habits to his fitness. Likewise, the first season Sterling Swaim used the TCTP he finished in the top 10 of almost every criterium he entered, by basing his tactics and decisions on his understanding of both the strengths and limitations of his training.

To put it simply, the TCTP will give you the fitness to accomplish great things, but not the luxury to waste your efforts. One frequently used analogy in cycling equates hard efforts in races or long rides with matches: You start out with a finite number of matches, and once you burn them all, you're done for the day. This is actually a pretty accurate illustration of what happens. The more times you push yourself over lactate threshold, the faster you burn through your limited carbohydrate stores, and the closer you get to the point where you'll be forced to ride at a relatively slow and steady pace for the rest of your ride. If you burn all your matches three-quarters of the way through a criterium, you won't have any power left for the sprint or to either create or follow the winning breakaway. Burn them all in the first half of the race, and you may not even reach the finish.

When you have the giant aerobic base provided by a high-volume training program, you start a race or long ride with a bigger pack of matches. And although you should not waste those matches with frivolous attacks, you can make mistakes and still recover from them. Riding with time-crunched fitness means you get to start with matches that burn just as bright and hot as everyone else's; you just have fewer of them. You'll have the power to stay with and beat riders who train two and three times as many hours as you do, but you're going to have to pick your battles carefully.

TIME-CRUNCHED TIPS FOR TOP PERFORMANCE

When I was 9 years old I rode my first race, and although I was in the top three coming out of the final corner, I hesitated because I wasn't sure what to do, and finished third. After the race a coach told me, "You can't win if you don't sprint." The statement stuck with me throughout my athletic career and has been very influential in the way I coach. But when I was still a young racer, I simply took it to mean that to win I needed to give 100 percent. Years later I realized the statement had a second, yet equally important, meaning.

With Olympic Trials approaching in advance of the 1984 Olympics in Los Angeles, a lot of motivated athletes were trying to win races in 1983 and the spring of 1984 to get noticed by the US Cycling Federation. I remember there was one rider whom I kept seeing at races; he was a tremendously strong sprinter who had to be considered a threat to win any race that was going to come down to a mass acceleration to the finish line. But neutralizing him was also incredibly easy, because he was a sucker. He was so afraid of missing out on his chance to sprint that he'd chase down every acceleration and potential breakaway in an effort to keep the pack together. Knowing this, the rest of us would launch dummy attacks and watch him burn matches shutting them down. By the time the pace really picked up in the final 20 miles or 20 laps of the race, he was cooked and no longer a threat for anything better than 20th place. He helped me realize that "you can't win if you don't sprint" also means that before you can sprint for the win you first have to make it to the finish.

If you're a low-volume rider on a high-volume training program, you will lack both the endurance to reach the finish and the power to win if you do manage to get there. The TCTP changes that by providing greater performance gains from fewer training hours and giving you the opportunity to not only reach the finish but get there with enough energy to achieve the results you want.

You've been an underdog ever since your priorities shifted to activities like building a career, maintaining a loving relationship with your spouse or significant other, and raising your kids. As your training time diminished, so did the advantages you had over other riders who are still devoting most of their time to riding. I've experienced this firsthand; I see it every time I go out on a road ride with the 20-something-year-old coaches in my office or compete in our local Wednesday-evening mountain bike races, but I don't question for a single moment that I chose the right priorities. The TCTP will help you even the odds and get you back to riding strong and racing for the win, but to be successful you're going to have to ride smarter than you ever have before.

This is going to be guerrilla warfare, in which you're the stealthy and underestimated freedom fighter battling against tyrants who are heavily favored and even more heavily armed. You're going to have to be crafty to conserve energy whenever you can and only display your strengths when they'll do the most good. For those of you who have been cyclists for many years, this may mean some significant changes in the way you act in the pack, but in the end those changes will be essential to getting what you want out of those rides and races. These tips can be divided into two categories: conserving your energy and using your power.

Conserving Your Energy

Learn to Pedal Less

One of the things coaches noticed once we started more advanced analyses of power files was that some athletes spend less time pedaling than others, and often riders who pedal less end up performing better in races. Pedaling takes energy, and if you can save yours while those around you burn theirs, you can gain an advantage over riders who started out with greater endurance. Several of the following tips will help you reduce the time you spend pedaling while still ensuring that you stay with the group, but the basic key is not to pedal unless you have to, and to make each pedal stroke count.

Stay Near the Front of the Pack

Repeated accelerations cause your power outputs to spike, and every time you rev your engine far above your threshold power, you're forcing your glycolytic system to burn through a chunk of carbohydrate. That's material you have to protect, because it's the high-octane fuel that powers extreme efforts such as attacks, sprints, and bell-lap-all-or-nothing flyers. If you light the fuse and there's nothing left in the tank, you're going to sputter and flame out instead of rocketing to the win.

In any pack-riding situation, the pace is steadiest at the front and gets increasingly variable as you move toward the back. This is most noticeable in a criterium on a tight course, in which riders at the front barely use their brakes, whereas folks at the back of the pack are forced to brake hard before every corner and then accelerate like a dragster just to stay with the field. Fifteen laps of that is enough to spit most amateurs out the back, no matter how strong they are.

The best place to be is about 10 to 25 riders deep in the field, a position often called the "sweet spot." You're close enough to the front that the pace is very steady, and you're able to see and anticipate accelerations and attacks. At the same time, you're deep enough in the field that you're safely tucked into the draft. Staying in this position is important, because maximizing your time in the draft and minimizing the hard accelerations you have to endure will help reduce the total amount of time you spend pedaling.

Take Short Pulls

I understand you want to be a conscientious member of the group and do your share of the pacemaking, but it's also important that your contribution serve your interests as well as the group's. The most important thing you have to do when you hit the front of a large pack or small group is keep the pace steady. If the group is rolling along a flat road at 21 mph, when the rider ahead of you pulls off, you have to pull through at 21 mph. But you don't have to spend 5 or 10 minutes pushing through the wind at that pace just because the riders before you did. Stay up there for 30 seconds or a few minutes, and then pull off. If this hurts your ego, consider this: How's your ego going to take it if you match the others pull for pull for an hour and then get dropped completely? Or to put it in a more positive light, riding strong on the way home and sprinting for the city limit sign will be a great reward for riding smarter rather than harder.

The idea of taking short pulls brings up the concept of etiquette in pack riding situations. When you're in a race, I don't care if the rider behind you resents the fact that you're pulling for 30 seconds when he or she is sitting on the front for 2 minutes at a turn. You have every right to be selfish and ride to your strengths, and he has to make a tactical decision about how he wants to deal with it. On the other hand, when you're out with half a dozen buddies on a Sunday morning, it's time to play nice.

The truth is, your riding buddies want you to stay with the group and be an active participant in the ride, and if that means you're going to take shorter pulls, so be it. For them, you taking shorter pulls is a lot better than having to wait for you later or having to ride home slower just so you can keep up.

Choose the Right Partner

A lot of group rides are conducted with a two-by-two pace line, meaning there are two lines of riders led by two pacesetters riding side by side at the front. When it's time to pull off, the right-hand rider moves right and the left-hand rider moves left, and then they back off their pace so the entire group passes between them. Eventually they reunite at the back. Unlike in a rotating pace line, the amount of time you spend at the front isn't entirely up to you. If you're in a group of riders you know well, it shouldn't be too hard to pair up with another rider who will be more than happy to take a relatively short pull with you. If you don't know anyone in the group, you're just going to have to do your best to size up your options as the group leaves the parking lot or coffee shop. If you guess wrong and end up next to a diesel engine of a rider who wants to take 30-minute pulls, remember that it's in your best interest to do the ride that's right for you. Tell him or her you're going to pull off, and do it. The rider either will be fine with it or will find a new partner the next time the group shuffles a bit.

Cruise in a Big Gear

When you're in the draft and cruising down the road, there are many times when a relatively low power output will be all that's necessary to hold your current position. Rather than spin at 120 rpm to put out 100 watts, shift into a bigger gear and bring your cadence down to 60 to 70 rpm. You're basically coasting and just turning your legs over with enough force to keep from decelerating. Your heart rate will come down, your breathing will slow, and you'll burn fewer calories per minute.

When you employ this technique, it's imperative to pay attention to what's going on around you. One of the greatest benefits to pedaling fast is the ability to respond rapidly to changes in pace or power demand. When your cadence is low, it's much more difficult to suddenly increase your speed in response to an acceleration. Similarly, if you hit a hill you didn't see coming, you'll find that you have to pedal very hard to keep from immediately losing momentum and decelerating into the rider behind you.

It's always important, whether you're cruising in a big gear or riding in any other situation, to look far ahead to anticipate stoplights, hills, and changes in pace or wind conditions. Some advance notice will give you the opportunity to shift gears and bring your cadence up so that you're ready for the upcoming challenge.

Jim Rutberg used this technique to conserve energy whenever he was drafting behind Grant Davis during their rides in New Mexico. Instead of the 90 to 95 rpm cadence he maintained while he was pulling at 220 to 240 watts, he shifted into a bigger gear and brought his cadence down to 70 to 75 while maintaining 120 to 130 watts in Grant's draft. Yes, the work (kilojoules) would be the same whether he was producing 120 watts at 90 rpm or 70 rpm, but the aerobic cost of producing that work went down.

Skip Some Pulls

There's a difference between skipping some pulls and sitting at the back of the group all day (otherwise known as "sucking wheels"). Skipping the occasional pull will help you conserve energy but not draw the ire of the group. And if you only sit out every third, fourth, or fifth pull, your fellow riders may barely notice. Better yet, if you're riding with a group you know well, just tell them that's what you're going to do. If they're like most cyclists, they'd rather you contribute a little less frequently for 4 hours instead of taking pulls for 3 and then sitting on the back for the last hour.

To skip a pull, you simply rotate through the pace line until you reach the very back and then let a small gap open instead of moving over into the line that's advancing toward the front. The rider ahead of you will see no one passing and will move over into the advancing line. You move over as that rider does and rejoin the advancing line on his or her wheel.

If you're in a fast-moving group in which people are just staring at the rider in front of them, you may be able to make a skipped pull barely noticeable by dropping back and a little to the opposite side of the advancing line. In other words, if the retreating line is on the left and the advancing one is on the right, you'd move slightly to the left once you reach the back of the retreating line. The rider ahead of you is less likely to see you lingering back there because his focus is entirely on the right side. I've actually seen athletes ride in this position for miles, completely unnoticed, on the tail of a hard-charging group.

On the other hand, in a breakaway group during a race, sitting on or skipping any pulls will certainly be noticed, and you have to be careful not to take advantage of the group's goodwill. If you decide to skip the occasional pull in a breakaway, your companions are more likely to tolerate that if the pulls you

MAKING THE MOST OF STRAVA

The segment feature of Strava is a great motivator for time-crunched athletes. While a lot of the emphasis of this book is on preparing athletes for competitive performance, many of the athletes who use the programs and concepts contained here never pin on a race number. Strava enables athletes to compete against themselves, compete for a variety of leaderboards, and track performance over time. Depending on where you live, the actual KOMs (King of the Mountain awards) may be out of reach. In areas where there are a lot of pros or elite amateurs, the KOMs may be true elite times. That shouldn't stop you from using Strava for your own training. Here are a few tips for making the most of your Strava membership.

Create a Strava club: Training with friends is a great way to stay motivated and create accountability within the group. Start a Strava club with your friends or a club that's specific to a training group where everyone is doing the Time-Crunched Training Program. Keep tabs on each other and give kudos when you complete breakthrough rides!

Start and end TCTP with a hard local segment: Sometimes you can use a local segment to easily record data for a CTS Field Test, especially if you have a flat or climbing segment that comes in at about 8 minutes. Even if you don't use a segment for a field test, you can get a clear picture of your progress by tackling a challenging local segment in a before-and-after scenario. The best kinds of segments for this are between 5 and 20 minutes. Try to match similar conditions (weather, wind) for greater compatibility.

Go Premium for the Fitness & Freshness analysis: There are a lot of great features in Strava Premium, but one of the key pieces of information you gain access to is the Fitness and Freshness analysis screen. There are more detailed analysis tools out there, but this one gives you the essential information about how your Suffer Score and power-based Training Load are impacting your fatigue and fitness to influence your form. Training load—specifically how much workload you are accumulating over a given time—raises your fitness gradually and raises your fatigue level more quickly. Rest enables you to recover from the fatigue (this value declines relatively quickly), and when you have the balance correct you will see your form (the difference between training load and fatigue) improve.

Go PR hunting: If you have the fitness to go KOM hunting, go for it! If you don't, you should still pick some rides and routes where you can go hunting for PRs (personal records). Obviously, your fitness will be the key determinant in getting PRs, but here are some ways to improve your chances:

Hunt when you are fresh: The day after a hard interval workout might not be the best time to go hunting. It's better to pick a day when you are more rested. This could mean waiting until the week after a rest week during the Time-Crunched Training Program you're using. Or you could start an interval workout with a segment you want to PR on an interval day.

Get the wind behind you: When the wind is in the right direction to give you a tailwind on your chosen segment, that's a good day to go for it!

Find a cooler day: Power output goes down when core temperature is elevated, so if you are hunting a segment PR, especially a climbing segment, go for it when the temperature is cooler. If you pair this with a tailwind, remember that riding with a tailwind makes you hotter because there is less of a difference between your speed and the wind speed. Adjust your drink plan accordingly.

Get a rolling start: Getting up to speed at the beginning of a segment robs you of precious seconds. For a better chance of a PR, start with speed! And remember to roll all the way through the end of the segment; don't give up early.

Ride smarter, not just harder: If you're riding a favorite segment, you've likely ridden it many times. Learning where to drive the pace and where to ease up is crucial. Many times, riding a few watts lower before a steep pitch,   >

for instance, gives you the energy to clear that pitch faster. You also have to learn not to go so hard on the hard pitches that you have to slow way down afterward and lose the time you gained.

Don't hunt PRs every ride: Tracking your progress with segment data is fun, but keep in mind that during parts of the TCTP you are going to be fatigued. That's part of the training process; you have to work hard enough to get slower before you can recover and get faster. During these times your segment data will show that you are going slower. You will not be setting PRs. That's OK and all part of the plan. Be careful not to confuse segment hunting with structured training. Focus on your training and then use the fitness to hunt for PRs!

PRs with groups don't count! Technically, they do, in that Strava will give you a PR whether you're in a group or not. But the PRs that matter are the ones you get with no draft. I realize this somewhat contradicts the tip about taking advantage of cool temperatures and tailwinds. Those are aids that help you go faster, but you have to draw a line somewhere. For me, that line is taking advantage of the collective power and speed of the peloton.

do take are good ones. If you're both soft-pedaling your way through pulls and skipping them, it won't be long before someone launches an acceleration to get rid of you. If that doesn't work, someone will take you off the back of the group to open up a sizable gap. Then that rider either will make you accelerate to close the gap (while he or she sits on your wheel) or will jump really hard so he or she rejoins the group and leaves you behind.

You don't want to be in any of these situations, because your efforts to conserve energy will inadvertently force you to burn every last match you have. In a breakaway, your best bet is to take short high-quality pulls to contribute to the group's success, and only start skipping pulls if you think it's the only way you're going to get a chance to contend for the win.

Using Your Power

The reason you want to conserve your energy on a ride or in a race is so you can use it to devastating effect later. You need to dispel any notion that riding to conserve energy is somehow less honorable than taking long pulls or launching a dozen attacks. We all see pros bury themselves to set a fast tempo on the front of the peloton, and we admire their strength and dedication, their sacrifices for the team and peloton. But behind them, riders use every one of the aforementioned techniques to save their energy.

In training books and magazine articles, we talk about maximizing your sustainable power output, enhancing your ability to perform repeated maximal efforts, and improving your tolerance for lactate. The message that's often missing is that although you have to ride hard in training to gain these improvements, no matter how strong you become, performing your best in a race, group ride, or long day with your friends comes down to using your power only when you absolutely need to.

Wait

You have the power to go head-to-head with any rider, but you don't have the endurance to go 10 rounds. This means you're going to have to be patient and uncork your best efforts close to the finish. In a criterium, this means saving your power for the final 10 laps, but it doesn't mean you have to just sit on wheels and then sprint. Any move you want to pull, from a 5-lap breakaway to a last-lap flyer or a field sprint, is well within your capabilities. In contrast, launching a solo breakaway from the starting gun is probably not the best use of the kind of fitness you've built.

If you're out for your epic day in the saddle, ride conservatively early on so you have power for the final hour, but then make the decision that it's time to go to work and drain the tank. At CTS we have weekly Coach Rides in which six to eight coaches and I go out for a 3- to 4-hour ride. At different times of the year, some coaches are riding more than others, and we rotate the pacemaking accordingly. I like it when the riders who are only training a few hours a week are smart enough to take short pulls early on and then are strong enough to go to the front and rock a few good hard efforts on our way back into town.

Be Smooth

Racing with a power meter is always a good idea, because races provide some of the best information you can use to guide your training. But there are times to look at the power meter and times to ignore it. When you're attacking or jostling for position near the front of the peloton in a race, just focus on getting the job done and look at the data later. On the other hand, when you're out on your own or taking pulls in a breakaway, you can use your power meter to enhance your performance. You want to avoid hard accelerations that force your power output to skyrocket, because these power spikes lead to fatigue quickly.

If you're in a criterium, this means taking good lines that minimize the need for braking in the corners. If you have to slow down significantly, shift into an easier gear so you can accelerate using a higher cadence and gradually shift back into harder gears as you get back to top speed. This is less fatiguing than slowing down and then generating a lot of torque by pushing slowly against a bigger gear.

Similarly, when you hit a hill, shift into easier gears to keep your cadence up. When riders are in breakaways, the temptation is to pound up a short climb rather than shift gears, but you can see the difference in training: When you muscle your way up a 30-second hill at 70 rpm, your power output is often lower than when you pedal 85 rpm up that same incline, even though perceived exertion may make you feel that the 70 rpm effort was harder.

Special Tips for Century Riders

If you've been a cyclist for 15 years, you know you can get through a 100-mile ride pretty much any day of the week if you have to. But there's a big difference between being able to complete the distance and having an enjoyable, satisfying, and fun day on the bike. Regardless of how long you've been a cyclist, you will be able to enjoy a 100-mile ride by using the TCTP as preparation. To have a good day, though, it's important to consciously ride a conservative pace for the first 50 miles so you burn your stored energy more slowly and minimize the energy contributions from your glycolytic energy system. Put another way, you want to aim for a "negative split," in which your effort level—and potentially your average speed—is greater in the second half than in the first.

Interestingly, your average speeds and overall ride times often turn out to be faster when you start out conservatively and finish strong, and that's been shown to be equally true for marathon runners and Ironman triathletes. The other benefit of this strategy is that you finish feeling strong instead of shattered, and riders tend to feel better about their accomplishment when they finish strong. So, if you're going to be out there for at least 5½ hours, measure your efforts so you come away with a positive experience.

Attack Wisely

Whether you train 6 hours a week or 20, you have to choose the most opportune moments to launch your attacks. The advice in this section is obviously targeted more to racers than to recreational riders, but the tactics I include can also be used to improve your performance in the local group ride.

Attack hard and quick: Timid and hesitant attacks don't win races, and you can't afford to burn energy with ineffective, halfhearted moves. If you hold something back when you attack, you're still burning a tremendous amount of energy and generating a ton of lactate. However, you're less likely to be rewarded for your efforts. You're not saving that much energy by attacking at 90 percent, so you're better off putting your full effort behind your move and improving your chances of success.

Ideally, start your acceleration in the draft from somewhere in the first 10 positions in the pack. If you start from farther back, the riders at the front have enough time to react to your acceleration before you pass them. Your attack should be sharp and violent so that a substantial gap immediately opens behind you. When you create a big gap in the first 15 to 20 seconds, your competitors will think twice about coming after you. If your initial acceleration only nets you 20 meters, though, the gap will look temptingly easy to bridge.

The training you've done with this program will give you the power necessary for the explosive efforts that lead to big initial gaps, as well as the endurance for relatively short solo breakaways. I encourage you to launch all-or-nothing solo flyers anywhere in the final 3 miles of a road race (or the final 3 to 5 laps of a criterium). To extend your range, try to get a few other riders to come with you, or use your attack to bridge up to a small breakaway.

Attack when the pace is at its highest: This is a painful proposition because your legs and lungs are already burning, and I'm telling you to hit the throttle even harder. Remember, if you are hurting, so is the rider next to you. There are many instances when one more acceleration is all it will take to make the decisive selection. When riders are already struggling to keep up, they won't be able to accelerate and catch you.

The reason riders hesitate to execute this tactic is the knowledge that they can't sustain such a high speed for long. But you don't have to. Once the selection is made, the pace of the breakaway and the main peloton usually fall to a fast but sustainable level. You are attacking to cause the selection, and the riders you leave behind are there because you pushed them beyond their limits. They may be able to come after you once they recover, but by that time the gap will have grown, and bridging may again push them past their limits.

Choose the best location: Where you choose to leave the peloton behind influences your chances of success. The general rule of thumb is to attack in a place where your effort will quickly result in a significant gap and maximize the effort required to bring you back.

- **The steepest pitch:** Probably the single most effective place to attack is on the steepest pitch of a climb. You can put meters between yourself and your nearest competitor with every pedal stroke, and chasing you down takes an enormous effort from all involved. This is where a high power-to-weight ratio (PWR) really pays off, because it gives you the ability to accelerate a lot faster than a rider who has a lower PWR. The steeper the pitch, the greater the impact of gravity, hence the greater your advantage. Bigger riders with big diesel-type engines can sometimes generate tremendous wattage and climb very fast, but they tend to struggle with rapid accelerations because their size limits their PWR. Simply put, push the pace on the climb, then put the final nail in the other riders' coffins with a decisive attack at the hardest point.

- **Into a corner:** Sometimes not slowing down works better than working to go faster. Make a hard and quick acceleration off the front of the peloton in the straightaway shortly before a turn (50 to 75 meters). The sharper and tighter the turn, the better this will work. The idea is to get out front so you can take the absolute fastest route through the turn. You're hoping the peloton will be more cautious through the turn, giving you a critical few seconds to establish a gap. This is a risky move because you are pushing your cornering skills and the laws of physics to their limits. If it works, you can win. If it doesn't, you may end up in the barriers. Again, this also works best when the corner's exit is uphill. You're carrying more momentum into the climb, and the pitch makes it harder for anyone to accelerate up to you.

- **Tight terrain:** When the peloton can see you dangling just in front of them, they are motivated to come after you. If you're out of sight, you're out of mind, and there's less motivation to chase you. On a long, straight road you have to be almost a minute ahead to be out of sight, so use a curvy or technically demanding section of road to establish your lead before emerging back onto open roads. Besides the factor of being out of sight, it is harder to organize an efficient chase through corners and urban areas. By the time the peloton gets organized, you're gone. If you're in a criterium, you need a lead at least as long as the longest straightaway. Tight courses are best for these breakaways because the corners help to diminish the pack's momentum. On open courses, the pack's collective strength gives it a big advantage over a small breakaway group, but narrow criterium courses with tight turns level the playing field and sometimes swing the advantage to the break.

- **Bridge the gap:** Bridging a gap is really a form of launching an attack; it's just an attack in response to an earlier one. Ideally, you'd always be near the front when an attack happens so you can accelerate with it if you choose, but we all know you're not always going to be in the perfect position. If you miss it by a few seconds, still go for it, but realize you're going to have to dig deep because you have some ground to make up. If you miss the attack completely, wait until the gap is small but established before you attempt to cross it. If the gap is too small, you may merely fill the hole between the fledgling breakaway and the peloton and inadvertently pull the entire field up to the break.

   If the gap has already grown to more than 20 seconds, your initial acceleration probably won't take you all the way across. Attack as if you are initiating a move of your own and then quickly settle into a pace higher than your normal time trial pace. You will only reach the breakaway if you are going faster than it is, so for a period of 1 to 2 minutes you have to sustain a speed higher than that of the field and the breakaway.

Bridging gaps of more than 1 minute is very challenging. To be successful you have to commit to a sustained, all-out effort lasting several minutes, and as a rider on a low-volume training program, it's important to realize that as a solo effort this may be an all-or-nothing proposition. Bring along some help and essentially create a second breakaway group chasing the first.

However and whenever you decide to bridge a gap, there is a chance you will get stuck in no-man's-land. When you realize you are not gaining on the breakaway, you have to quickly assess the chances of successfully reaching it. Right or wrong, make the decision quickly, because sitting 30 seconds in front of the peloton and 30 seconds behind the break for 5 minutes is a huge waste of energy.

DON'T BE AFRAID TO LIGHT YOUR LAST MATCH

When it's time to burn matches, do it with confidence and conviction. You have worked hard for your fitness, it's there and it's real, and unlike athletes on high-volume training programs, you don't have the luxury of having big power for months at a time. Now, more than ever before, you have to leave everything out there on the road or trail. These are the days and experiences that become part of your "highlight reel" for the year—the rides you joke about with friends over cold beers on the back porch, and the races that make you smile and dig a little deeper when you're on an indoor trainer in January. Above all, honor the work you've done by riding with intelligence and courage. Dare to go for the win instead of sitting in the pack, charge up the hard climb to feel the exhilaration of the effort, and attack to leave them all behind.

"It took me a few races to really get the confidence to lay it all on the line," Sterling Swaim told me during a visit to our Colorado Springs training facility. "I had this idea I was more fragile than before, that I had to be extremely cautious with my efforts. Over a period of weeks, though, I started riding more and more aggressively and found I had more than enough power and endurance to race the way I wanted to. In truth, the experience showed me that I should have been riding smarter all along."

16

STRENGTH TRAINING ON LIMITED TIME

FOR MANY YEARS, COACHES AND SPORTS SCIENTISTS have debated the merits of strength training for endurance athletes. Having read the research, talked to the experts on both sides of the debate, and used various forms of resistance training with athletes throughout the spectrum of ability, age, and experience, I still cannot decisively agree with either side. That is to say, I'm not entirely convinced that a cyclist needs to engage in strength training to be stronger and faster on the bike, nor am I completely convinced that strength training won't improve a cyclist's performance. What I do know, without a doubt, is that strength training plays an important role in the overall health and vitality of an athlete. It is for this reason that I am including a chapter on strength training in this book.

Cycling, for all its benefits, is very one-dimensional. For the most part, your upper body stays in a relatively static position while your legs move in only one plane. As a result, devoted cyclists can become prisoners to the bike. Just take a look at professional cyclists; they have among the most highly developed aerobic engines in sports but are virtually crippled by a pickup game of basketball. It's something I refer to as the Cyclist's Paradox. Pro and devoted cyclists are aerobically very fit but are often unaccustomed to weight-bearing activities, and their joints and bones are therefore poorly prepared for them. Worse than that, cycling—in the absence of other athletic activities—can breed significant muscle imbalances, creating great strength and power in muscles that drive the pedal stroke while leaving the hip and leg muscles responsible for sideways (lateral) movement weak and underdeveloped.

But, you say, you're a cyclist, and you've made the choice to focus on the sport you love. That's great, but more well-rounded fitness gives you more options for adventures and won't take away from your abilities on the bike. I live at the foot of Pikes Peak, and I know cyclists who have lived here for a decade yet have not experienced the sense of accomplishment and wonder that comes from hiking to the summit. It's not a particularly difficult climb; every year thousands of out-of-shape tourists conquer it. But it's a nearly impossible challenge for highly specialized cyclists because the 13-mile trail is too hard on their feet and hips, and they struggle under the weight of packs if they choose to turn the adventure into a 2-day camping trip. I'm all for maximizing sport-specific performance, but unless you're making a living as a cyclist I also believe that the benefits of nonspecific fitness are worth pursuing.

To break free of the Cyclist's Paradox and stop being a prisoner to the bike yet still perform like a competitive racer when you're on it, I recommend strength training movements that enhance joint mobility and range of motion through the hips and back. Cyclists perform better when they have good flexibility in their hips and backs because greater flexibility gives them the opportunity to produce power through a larger range of motion (or greater power through the same range of motion). Exercises such as lateral lunges and step-ups, which are included in the strength training program in this chapter, are an important component of improving hip mobility and strength. And because a strong torso is crucial for strong cycling as well as for pain-free performance throughout life, the program in this chapter also incorporates a lot of core strengthening exercises.

As always, time is a central problem. Even pro athletes who have a lot of time to devote to training reach a point when they have to direct their full energy to their primary sport. The same thing happens to time-crunched athletes who have less time available for training; it just happens sooner. There is a limit to the amount of time and energy any athlete can devote to meaningful, productive training. There are only so many days and hours in a week, and the more you train, the more you need to recover. Pretty soon you reach a tipping point where adding more training will compromise your recovery and performance.

You're not a professional cyclist, and you're already limited in the amount of time you can devote to training. My contention is that athletes with limited training time benefit most from focusing on their primary sport. In other words, if you only have 6 hours a week to devote to training, you're better off spending that time on your bike. There is one major reason for this: Dividing your limited time between strength training and cycling training often results in workloads that are insufficient to lead to significant progress in either arena.

So, if I don't think it's wise for time-crunched athletes to combine strength training with their on-bike training, why have I included a strength training program in this book? It's because time-crunched athletes are, by their very nature, not professional athletes. And because you are not making a living as an endurance athlete, it is important to think about your overall health, vitality, and function when you consider incorporating resistance training into your lifestyle.

STRENGTH TRAINING FOR LIFE

The strength training program described in this chapter is not designed to improve your cycling-specific performance. Instead, it promotes full-body strength so you can live an active and healthy life for years to come.

There is a lot of talk these days about metabolism (the energy your body burns on a daily basis through a combination of normal bodily functions, the thermal effect of digesting food, and your activity level and exercise), particularly the notion that metabolism inevitably declines as we get older. This idea has fueled countless late-night infomercials that blame middle-age weight gain on declining metabolism and tout pills and potions that claim to reverse the effects of aging by boosting said metabolism. The truth is, the primary reason metabolism declines as we age is that people tend to be less active as we grow older. When we were younger we were more active, so we needed, and therefore carried, more lean muscle mass on our bodies. That muscle burned calories, not only to maintain itself but to power our activities, and as we grew less active we lost some of this calorie-burning muscle. At the same time, we either maintained or increased our caloric intake and hence gained weight.

If you want to keep your metabolism elevated, you need to focus on building—or at least maintaining—lean muscle mass. Cycling may help you maintain or build leg muscle, but it doesn't do much for the rest of your body. In truth, the strength training program in this chapter probably won't build a significant amount of muscle on your upper body either (cyclists are generally averse to increased upper-body bulk, anyway, as it detracts from PWR), but it provides a balanced approach that will help you build a good base of strength and keep the lean muscle you have now.

For me the benefits of generalized strength training go beyond maintaining or boosting metabolism. I'm in my 50s and have three kids, Anna, Connor, and Vivian. For me, strength training is an essential part of being the kind of father I want to be for my kids. At least for right now, Anna is an avid equestrian, Connor is into mountain bike racing and snowboarding, and Vivian is a gymnast. I don't want to sit in a chair and watch them; I want to be a part of their activities, and that requires not only a lot of energy but the ability to jump, twist, lift, push, and pull. I'm a devoted cyclist because cycling is the sport I fell in love with as a kid, but I'm a well-rounded athlete because my overall fitness and strength give me the opportunity to be a fully engaged father and still keep up with the demands of my travel and business schedule.

• • •

CASE STUDY
THE RISE OF JOHN FALLON

Compared to Sterling Swaim and Taylor Carrington, John Fallon came to cycling late in life. He was in his early 30s before he started riding and initially had no interest in racing. Long rides in the mountains west of his home in Evergreen, Colorado, were his passion. He trained for and completed the Triple Bypass (a 120-mile epic that includes three major mountain passes as it travels from Evergreen to Avon, Colorado) several times while raising two children with his wife, Ali, and working as a stockbroker in Denver.

By sheer coincidence, Taylor Carrington joined the firm John worked for, and the two quickly became friends. A few years later Taylor noticed John was frustrated with his cycling fitness and losing interest in the long weekend rides he had previously enjoyed. Taylor recommended John call his CTS coach, Jim Rutberg, for some guidance and perhaps to consider getting coaching. Rutberg asked all the usual questions about John's goals, his history as an athlete, his interests and obligations outside of athletics, and his personal and professional schedule. During their 90-minute conversation Rutberg provided some very actionable guidance and offered his services as a coach, but John decided to continue training on his own.

A year passed before John contacted Rutberg again. By that point John's training had deteriorated to the extent that he was heavier than he'd been in 5 years. Although he'd just finished the Triple Bypass again, his finishing time was slower than ever before, and he did not enjoy the experience very much.

Rutberg, who was by this time a vocal proponent of the TCTP, readily suggested it to John. Initially, John was skeptical. He had recently gone for lactate threshold testing at a local performance center, and the sports scientist who analyzed his results had recommended long, steady, subthreshold, base building aerobic rides. Rutberg agreed that such training would be quite effective, as long as John didn't mind quitting his job and losing his house. John could only ride about 7 hours a week, which was about half the time that would have been required for the training plan recommended by the sports scientist. Rutberg made the case described in this book: that only through higher-intensity workouts would John achieve the workloads necessary to significantly improve his cycling performance. And then there was the skiing.

Years ago, before housing prices skyrocketed in Colorado ski towns, the Fallons had purchased a condo in Vail. And John wasn't just a man for the "groomers"; he liked to escape into the back bowls early in the morning and ski hard until the sun disappeared behind the peaks to the west.

Over the course of a recent summer, John made big improvements in his sustainable power on the bike by using the TCTP. As the months passed, he dropped about 10 pounds and took 1, then 4, then 9 minutes off his time up Lookout Mountain, his favorite serpentine climb outside Evergreen. As the leaves on the aspen trees turned bright yellow, Rutberg congratulated him on a fine season and suggested it was time to devote his energy to preparing for ski season. For the next several weeks, as the base deepened in the bowls behind Vail, Rutberg cut John's riding back to one or two rides on weekends and focused his weekday workouts on strength training.

That winter was a blockbuster year for skiing in the Rocky Mountains. The snow was the deepest it had been in a decade (more than 47 feet fell at Wolf Creek Ski Area alone!), and storms kept blanketing the backcountry with thick layers of fresh powder. Between his weight loss, increased aerobic fitness, and continued strength training, John had the best ski season he could remember. He wasn't as winded at the end of long runs, was able to complete more runs per day, and gained the confidence to return to challenging slopes he hadn't attempted in years. He even booked a weeklong heli-skiing trip in

Alaska and reported back to Rutberg that he had the endurance and power to enjoy the longest and steepest runs the guides found for the group.

The following spring, despite working in San Francisco and commuting back to Denver a couple of weekends each month, John refocused his training on cycling. The cycling scene in San Francisco was different than in Denver, and John soon became interested in local criteriums. Due to John's intense work and travel schedule, Rutberg put him back on the TCTP. And even though he had only been riding one or two times a week during ski season, his overall workload had been high enough that 4 weeks into the cycling program he was sustaining higher power outputs in SteadyState and PowerInterval workouts than he had at any point in the previous season. Though he was a relative novice in terms of racing tactics, John had the fitness to finish in the top half of the first few masters races he rode in California. Within weeks he was consistently finishing in the top 10.

John Fallon is representative of a huge group of athletes out there. He's a cyclist, but he also has passions outside cycling. He wants to perform well on the bike, but not at the cost of being restricted to one sport or activity. In some ways he may represent the greater ideal we should all strive for: diversity through greater overall fitness. John's not going to win a masters national championship, but he's a guy in his mid-40s who can say "yes" to a wider variety of activities, sports, events, and adventures—at a moment's notice—than most athletes who have been devoted single-focus cyclists for 20 years.

MAKING STRENGTH TRAINING WORK FOR YOU

I hate having to travel somewhere just so I can start training. As a cyclist I put on my clothes, grab my bike from the garage or the rack in the office, and am training as soon as I roll out the door. Runners are probably the only athletes who have it easier than cyclists, but only because they have less gear to contend with. Maybe that's why I've never been a big fan of gyms (or sports played on fields or courts).

There was a time during the early days of CTS when I had pretty much given up on being a cyclist. One winter I barely touched my bike for about 4 months. During that time I decided I'd follow the "normal" path to fitness for a middle-aged guy: I joined a gym. I quickly realized that the most frustrating part of my day was the drive to and from the gym. The whole point of going to the gym was to work out, but between getting there and getting back, I was in the car nearly as long as I worked out. Clearly this was not a good use of limited time, so I got back on my bike and started doing my strength training at home.

Many time-crunched athletes find they can only squeeze strength training into their schedule by doing it at home. A program you can do without a gym is also useful if you travel frequently for business, because you can do it in a hotel room. As you decide whether to incorporate strength training and make it work for you, make sure the work you're going to do addresses the following principles.

Convenience and Cost

First off, strength training has to fit into your personal and professional schedule. That's why I believe in at-home strength training as opposed to going to the gym. At the same time, it has to be cost effective. I don't expect you to spend thousands of dollars on a home gym setup and a menagerie of equipment just so you can work out effectively in your house. With a small investment in a limited amount of equipment (and some creativity), you can achieve all the benefits you're looking for. The two items I believe you should invest in are dumbbells and resistance cords. They don't take up much room, and they can be used for a wide range of exercises. The dumbbells are great for chest and shoulder presses, can be used for some pulling exercises like a bent-over row, and can even be used to add resistance to step-ups, lunges, and squats. The resistance bands can be used for many of the same exercises as dumbbells, but in addition can be anchored on door frames or other immovable objects so you can perform a seated row or a pull-down.

There's Nothing Wrong with the Basics

Some of the best strength training exercises are the simplest, and there's nothing wrong with continuing to perform some of the basic movements you learned in middle school. Push-ups and pull-ups, for instance, are solid exercises for upper-body strength. Body-weight squats and lunges are good exercises for lower-body strength. You can make these exercises more challenging by adding weight to a squat or lunge, or putting your feet up on a bench or chair for push-ups.

Balance Matters

The primary reason I include strength training in this book is to help you maintain a healthy and active lifestyle, and I believe a balance component is essential. When you perform movements that challenge your balance, you engage muscles throughout your body.

For instance, when you start doing lunges, you may notice you have a hard time keeping your upper body balanced over your legs. As you practice the movement, you will engage muscles in your core and hips and learn to better balance your body in this position. The same is true of overhead lifts. As you press a weight over your head, you will engage muscles from your feet to your fingers to control the weight in space. This whole-body integration is as important as the weight you're able to move, because when you train your body to act as one coordinated unit, you are better able to maintain your balance in increasingly unstable conditions.

Movements Matter

When we get to the actual exercises in the strength training program, you'll notice that there are no isolated movements to target triceps, biceps, or hamstrings. Instead you'll find multi-joint exercises that engage large muscle groups because these exercises prepare you for real-world demands. An exercise like a push-up or overhead press, for example, engages your triceps but works muscles in your chest and shoulder at the same time. All of these muscles must work together to complete the movement, which is similar to the reality that you rarely use your triceps in isolation. Similarly, you'll be using exercises like squats and lunges to work your hamstrings, but these movements also engage muscles throughout your legs, hips, and torso.

The movements included in the strength training program in this chapter are among the most applicable to real-life situations. You're going to develop strength with flexibility, and power when you're extended or reaching instead of just when your feet are firmly planted and your arms are close to your chest. As an added benefit for cyclists, the lower-body exercises in this program are great for improving range of motion and flexibility through the hips.

HOW TO USE THE TIME-CRUNCHED STRENGTH TRAINING PROGRAM

Three workouts make up the Time-Crunched Strength Training Program. The first is a simple core strength workout, and then there are two full-body routines. The core strength workout is something you can and should do year-round, even while you're in the midst of your high-intensity cycling training. It should take fewer than 10 minutes to complete and is a good add-on immediately after you get off your bike.

Variety is an important component of an effective strength training program, because different exercises present specific challenges even when they target similar muscle groups. For instance, squats and step-ups are both good exercises for developing lower-body strength and power, but squats work both legs at the same time, and step-ups incorporate a balance component because you're lifting your body weight with one leg at a time. The same can be said for a curl and press compared with an alternating overhead press.

Because I want to keep the strength workouts short, I have created two routines so you can complete a wide variety of exercises each week. You should aim to complete two or three strength workouts a week, leaving a full day between them, and I recommend alternating the two full-body routines. That could mean doing Routine 1 on Tuesday, Routine 2 on Thursday, and if you want to add a third, doing Routine 1 again on Saturday. The following week would start with Routine 2.

Whichever strength routine you're doing, core strength is such a vital aspect of sports performance and an active lifestyle that you should always add the core routine as well. In total, the core routine and one of the strength routines should only take you about 30 minutes to complete.

In terms of how much resistance you should use, the final few repetitions of each exercise should be challenging to the point you are able to finish your final rep with good form but cannot complete an additional repetition. In a break from earlier editions of this book, I recommend pushing yourself to failure during strength training sets, but with an important caveat. You want to push yourself to the point you cannot complete an additional repetition with good form. This is especially true when working with resistance bands, dumbbells, and dynamic movements, because the risks of injury increase dramatically when you lose control of the weight or compromise your body position. So, I want you to push yourself to the last repetition you can complete with good form. As you get stronger and need to increase your workload, I want you to do so by increasing the resistance (heavier band or dumbbell, or holding weights during some of the dynamic movements) rather than increasing the number of repetitions or sets you complete.

Just as there is debate about endurance training methods, there are different approaches to strength training. In terms of repetitions and sets, you can move more weight or move against more resistance if you reduce the number of repetitions in a set. In other words, I may be able to press 50-pound dumbbells over my head 6 times, but I could complete the same movement 12 times if I use 30-pound dumbbells, and 30 times if I use 15-pound dumbbells. As you manipulate these two variables (resistance and repetitions), you start to change the impact the exercise will have on your muscles.

High Force, Low Rep (HFLR) vs. Low Force, High Rep (LFHR)

For athletes whose primary goal for strength training is to produce more force (gain strength), one of the first questions is whether they should lift heavy and complete fewer repetitions (90 percent of 1 Rep Maximum × 5–6 reps) or use less resistance and complete more repetitions (30 percent of 1 Rep Maximum × 20–25 reps). According to a study by Mitchell (2012), you can use either strategy and achieve very similar improvements in strength—as long as you push yourself to failure (the inability to complete another rep).

I interpret the Mitchell study to indicate that in the pursuit of making athletes stronger, we can take into account factors besides just the amount of weight and the number of times it can be moved. The strength gains are similar either way. Interestingly, hypertrophy is similar as well, which may help dispel the myth that heavy lifting leads to mass gains while lighter lifting leads to strength without the bulk. What other considerations are important? Well, HFLR training increases load on bones more than LFHR training. Heavy lifting also results in more forceful contractions, which also promotes stronger bones, so lifting heavy may be better for increasing bone mineral density.

On the other hand, LFHR resistance training carries lower injury risks, which is a big consideration for endurance athletes who are using resistance training to be a well-rounded athlete and supplement their primary sport. With lower resistance, athletes are able to maintain proper technique longer as they fatigue. When you are lifting heavy and doing it wrong, you can get hurt pretty easily, whereas the consequences of mistakes are typically less serious with lighter weights.

When it comes to LFHR resistance training, it is still important to be using enough weight. If the resistance is too light and you can complete 30-plus reps before reaching failure, the movement has more in common with an aerobic exercise than a strength exercise. For best results, try to keep your LFHR sets in the 15 to 20 repetition range.

Time-Crunched Strength Training Program

TABLE
16.1

CORE STRENGTH ROUTINE	
Reverse Crunch	For each core exercise, complete 20 repetitions. No rest between exercises, but rest 1 minute between the Core Routine and the beginning of either Strength Routine 1 or 2.
Back Extension	
Bicycle Crunch	
Windshield Wipers	
STRENGTH ROUTINE 1	
Squat and Jump	For each exercise, complete 15–20 repetitions. Rest between exercises is 30 seconds. Repeat Core Strength + Routine 1 three times; rest 2 minutes between the cycles.
Push-up	
Standing Overhead Press	
Lateral Lunge	
Seated Row	
STRENGTH ROUTINE 2	
Step-up	For each exercise, complete 15–20 repetitions. Rest between exercises is 30 seconds. Repeat Core Strength + Routine 2 three times; rest 2 minutes between the cycles.
Push-up	
Reverse Wood Chop with Bands	
Lateral Lunge	
One-Arm Row	

In the strength routines in this chapter (see Table 16.1), I focused on Low Force, High Rep exercises because they are typically easier to complete outside of a gym setting and have lower risk for injury. There will be a limit to the resistance you can achieve with these exercises, however, so some athletes may need to graduate to High Force, Low Rep strength training.

Refer to the following pages for illustrated workout descriptions.

BACK EXTENSION

Lie flat on your stomach with your arms by your side and your legs completely straight (Figure 16.1). Push your legs into the ground and use your back to lift your shoulders and chest off the floor (Figure 16.2). Lift 1 to 3 inches off the floor, but don't strain too hard to lift very high. Slowly lower your chest back to the floor and repeat. For an added challenge, extend your arms out to the side (Figure 16.3) or out in front of you (Figure 16.4) and lift them off the ground as well (Figures 16.5 and 16.6). A more advanced version of this exercise would be to lift your right arm and left leg off the ground simultaneously (Figure 16.7), and then lower to the ground before lifting your left arm and right leg off the ground simultaneously.

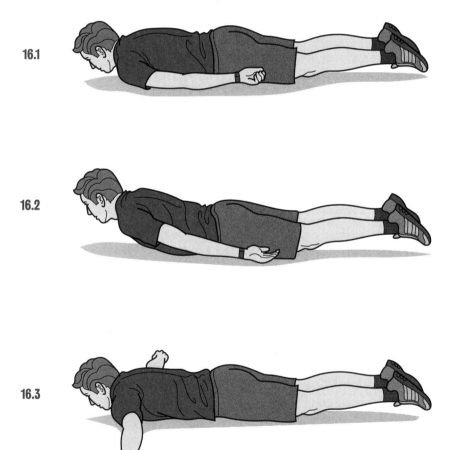

16.1

16.2

16.3

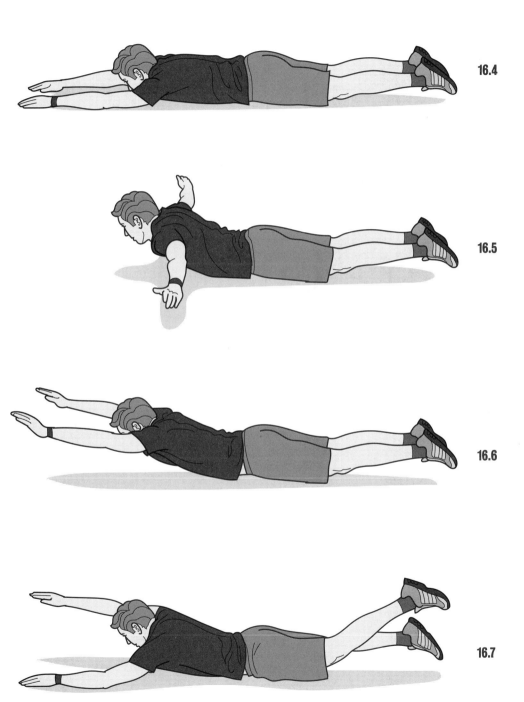

16.4

16.5

16.6

16.7

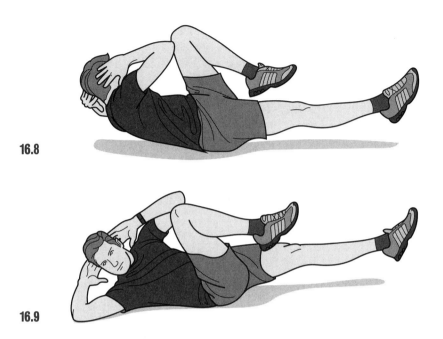

16.8

16.9

BICYCLE CRUNCH

Studies have shown this exercise to be one of the best abdominal movements because it engages your upper and lower abdominals and incorporates a twist as well. Lie on your back on the floor. Your hands should be lightly touching the back of your ears. Raise your right foot off the ground 4 to 6 inches and keep that leg straight. At the same time, bring your left knee toward your chest (Figure 16.8). Using your abdominal muscles (don't pull your head forward with your arm), raise your right shoulder off the ground and twist to the left, with the goal of touching your right elbow to your left knee. If you can't make contact, that's fine. Lower your right shoulder back to the ground and extend your left leg until it is straight and your foot is 4 to 6 inches off the floor. Complete the same movement on the other side by bringing your right knee toward your chest and raising your left shoulder off the ground (Figure 16.9). One repetition of this exercise consists of completing the movement on both sides, and all repetitions of this exercise should be done at a moderate, continuous tempo with no pauses or rest between repetitions.

LATERAL LUNGE

This may be the most important exercise in the program, because most cyclists are in dire need of lateral stability and strength. Stand with your feet together and your arms extended out in front of you (Figure 16.10). Step to the right with your right foot, keeping your left leg straight and your left foot flat at its starting position (Figure 16.11). Keeping your right knee behind your right foot, and your chest high and back straight, drop your hips as you sit into a squat. Aim to go low enough that your right thigh is parallel to the ground. Pause for 1 to 2 seconds, then drive with your right leg to return to the starting position. As soon as you return to the starting position, step to the left with your left leg and repeat the same movement. One repetition of this exercise consists of lunging to both sides.

Beginners may want to step forward and to the side at about a 45-degree angle, as it can be easier to maintain your balance using this method (Figure 16.12). As you get stronger, gradually shift to stepping directly to the side.

For more of a challenge, hold a weight in front of your chest and do the exercise. If you hold the weight close to your chest, you're mainly adding resistance for your legs; if you hold it out in front of your body, you'll add work for your back and shoulders. When you add a weight, make sure you don't roll your shoulders forward or curve your back.

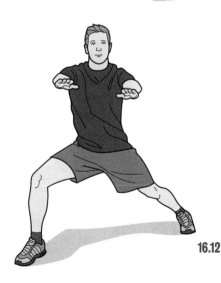

16.10

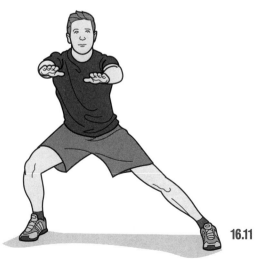

16.11

16.12

ONE-ARM ROW

This exercise for your upper back and the rear portion of your shoulder is ideally done with a dumbbell but can be completed with a resistance band anchored close to the floor. If you have a bench, put your left knee on the bench while your right leg is straight and your right foot is on the floor. Bend forward at the waist, place your left hand directly under your shoulder on the bench, and keep your back straight. Hold a dumbbell in your right hand, straight below your right shoulder (Figure 16.13). Using the muscles in your upper back and shoulder (rather than just the muscles in your arm), lift the barbell up, pulling your elbow high but keeping it close to your

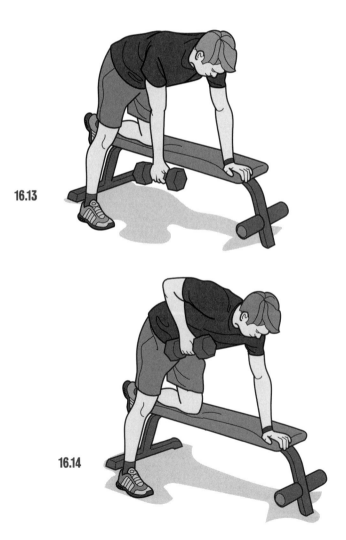

16.13

16.14

side. Lift until you've drawn the weight close to your side (Figure 16.14). In a controlled manner, lower the weight to the starting position and repeat. Complete a set using your right arm before switching sides and using your left arm. Figures 16.15 and 16.16 show a variation of this exercise using an exercise band.

Additional tips: Don't drop your shoulder as you lower the weight, in an attempt to get a stretch or make the range of motion longer. Similarly, don't use your core muscles to twist your torso as you raise the weight. The majority of your upper body will be very still during this exercise. The movement should be confined to your arm and shoulder, utilizing the muscles in your upper back to make them move.

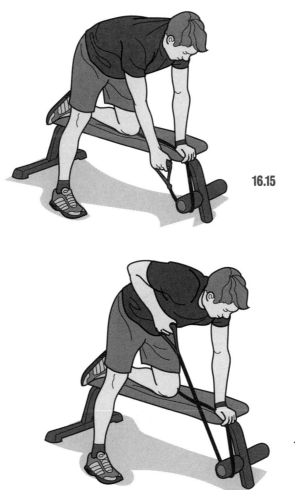

16.15

16.16

PUSH-UP VARIATIONS
(EASY, INTERMEDIATE, AND ADVANCED)

Easy: Lie facedown on the floor with your hands placed even with your chest, just slightly wider than shoulder width apart (Figure 16.17). Keep your head, shoulders, and hips in a rigid line and push your chest away from the floor so your weight is supported on your knees and hands. Push yourself up until your arms are fully extended (Figure 16.18), but be careful not to lock your elbows. Slowly lower yourself until your chest barely touches the floor, and then immediately push yourself back up. Repeat for the prescribed number of repetitions.

Intermediate: Same exercise as Easy, but make the contact points with the ground your hands and your toes, not your hands and your knees (Figure 16.19). Make sure to keep your body in a straight line from your shoulders all the way to your feet. Your hands should be slightly wider than shoulder width apart (Figure 16.20).

Advanced: When a regular push-up is no longer challenging, put your feet up on a box bench or chair (Figures 16.21 and 16.22) and then complete your push-ups.

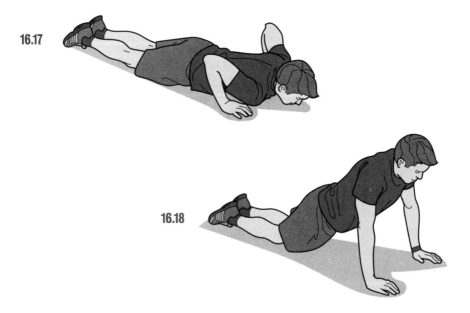

16.17

16.18

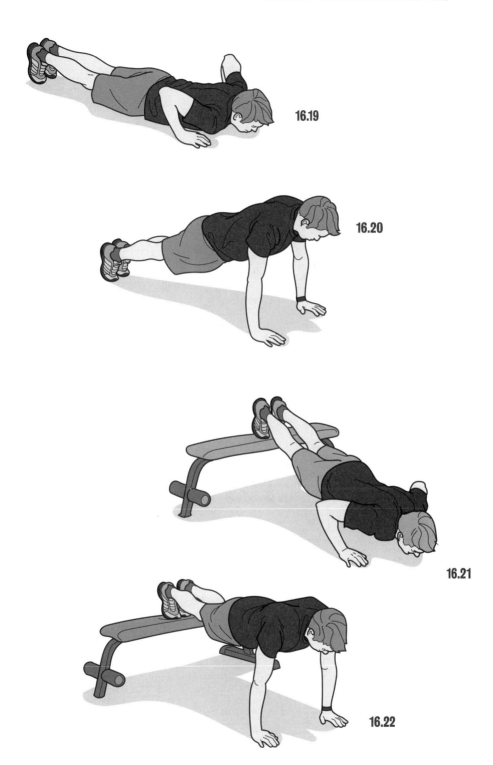

16.19

16.20

16.21

16.22

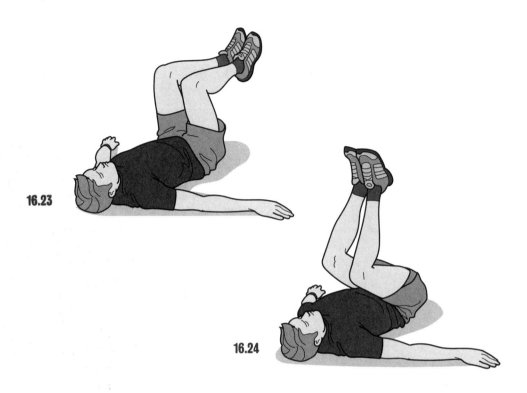

16.23

16.24

REVERSE CRUNCH

I like reverse crunches because there is no temptation to pull your head and neck forward as many people do during traditional crunches. Lie on your back with your knees bent, feet together. Hold your arms straight at a 45-degree angle out from your torso, palms facing down (Figure 16.23). Bring your knees to your chest by tightening your abdominal muscles and curling your hips off the floor (Figure 16.24). Be careful to engage your abdominal muscles to produce the movement instead of relying on the muscles in the front of your hips and legs. When your knees have reached your chest, or as close as you can get, curl back down and return to the start position.

REVERSE WOOD CHOP WITH BAND

This is a twisting lift that starts by your ankle and finishes at shoulder height or higher. Start by anchoring a resistance band at about ankle height to something sturdy such as a heavy desk or bed frame. Some resistance bands come with an adapter so you can anchor them between a door and a doorjamb. If you can't anchor the band, stand on it. Stand with a wide stance, your knees bent, and your right foot toward the anchored end of the band. Bend down and grasp the handle(s) in both hands at about knee height (Figure 16.25). You want there to be light to moderate tension on the band in this starting position. Keeping your back straight, your core engaged, and your eyes up, pull the band up and across your torso as you twist with your core and shoulders (Figure 16.26). You can finish the movement with your hands at shoulder height, or continue up (Figure 16.27) until your hands are overhead (this will be harder on the shoulders; if you have shoulder trouble, stop at shoulder height). In a controlled manner, return to the starting position and repeat. When you're done on one side, turn around so your left foot is toward the anchored end of the band and repeat the exercise.

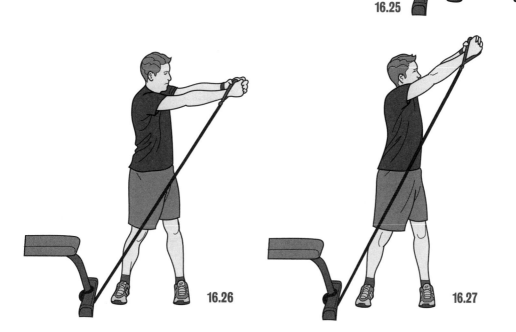

16.25

16.26

16.27

SEATED ROW

Sit on the floor with a resistance band anchored to something sturdy, such as a heavy desk or bed frame. The band should be anchored about chest height when you're sitting, but it's OK if it is a bit lower than that. If you don't have anything to anchor the band to, loop it around your feet. Sit with your back perpendicular to the floor and extend your arms straight forward as you hold on to the ends of the bands. In this starting position, with your palms facing each other, there should be light to moderate tension on the band. With your chest high and your back straight, pull your hands straight back, keeping your elbows close to your sides, until your hands reach the sides of your chest (Figure 16.28). In a controlled manner, bring your hands back to the starting position and repeat. Do not lean back as you perform this movement; keep your back perpendicular to the ground. To make this exercise more challenging, you can perform it one arm at a time (Figures 16.29 and 16.30).

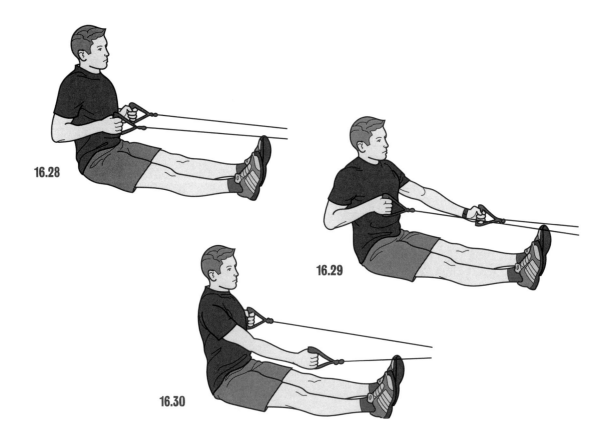

16.28

16.29

16.30

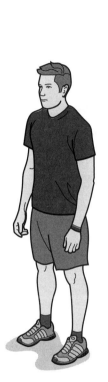
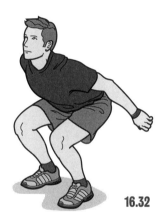
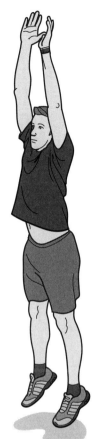

16.31

16.32

16.33

SQUAT AND JUMP

This exercise adds a speed-and-power component to a body weight squat. Stand with your feet slightly wider than shoulder width apart (Figure 16.31). With your arms at your sides, squat until your hips reach knee level (Figure 16.32), then explode straight up and jump as high as you can (Figure 16.33). As you begin to drive upward, swing your arms up to generate momentum and more height. Bend your knees to absorb the impact as you land. Return to a standing position and repeat. It's important that you aim to propel yourself as high as you can with each jump.

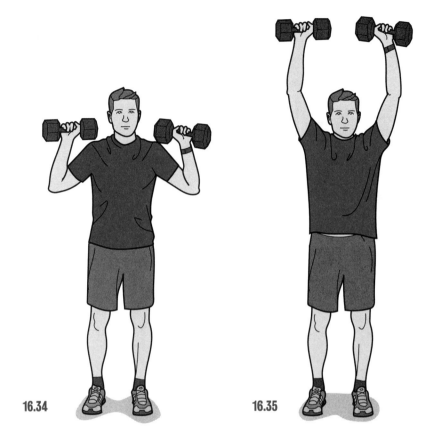

16.34   16.35

STANDING OVERHEAD PRESS

Not only is this a great exercise for your shoulders, triceps, and the upper portions of both your chest and back, but it also engages muscles from your toes all the way to your fingers. Stand with your feet shoulder width apart and knees slightly bent (Figure 16.34). You can use dumbbells or a resistance band for this exercise. Curl the weight (dumbbells or resistance band) so your hands are shoulder height and your palms are facing forward or slightly toward the midline of your body. Keep your chest high and your abdominal muscles engaged as you press both hands straight up over your head (Figure 16.35). As you extend your arms to the top of the movement, keep your palms facing forward. Bring your arms back down to the starting position and repeat.

If you're using a resistance band, stand on the band with one or both feet and follow the same instructions as above (Figures 16.36 and 16.37).

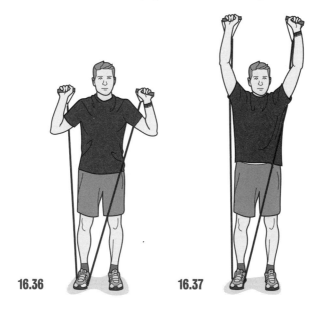

16.36   16.37

To make this movement a greater challenge for your abdominal muscles, alternate one arm at a time (Figures 16.38 and 16.39).

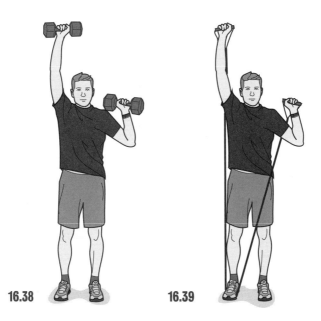

16.38   16.39

STEP-UP

I particularly like the single-leg nature of this exercise, because it forces you to balance on one leg and use hip and torso muscles to maintain stability. In addition, the movement develops strength and power that's not only useful in life but also applicable to your on-bike performance. Start by standing facing a bench that's about knee height (Figure 16.40). Place your right foot on the bench and, keeping your back straight and chest high, use your hip extensors and leg to step up onto the bench (Figures 16.41 and 16.42). Bring your left foot even with your right foot, then step down in a controlled manner, leading with your left foot. Bring your right foot down to the floor and then alternate sides, stepping up with your left foot.

You can make this exercise more challenging by holding weight in your hands at your sides (Figures 16.43, 16.44, and 16.45). To add a greater balance component to the exercise, and for more of a challenge, you can hold a weight in front of you (Figures 16.46 and 16.47). But it's essential that the weight not be so heavy that it causes your shoulders to roll forward or pitch your upper body forward.

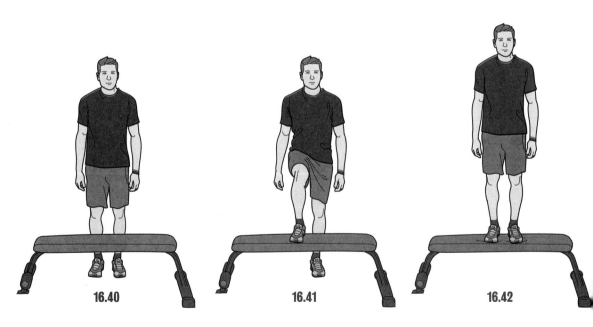

16.40

16.41

16.42

If you don't have a bench, this exercise can be done on a staircase (step up onto the second step). The only issue with using a staircase is that you have to step a bit forward as you step up. This is a minor issue, but just make sure you're able to keep your chest high and back straight throughout the exercise. If you have to lean your upper body forward significantly to step up onto the second stair, your staircase may not be well suited to this exercise.

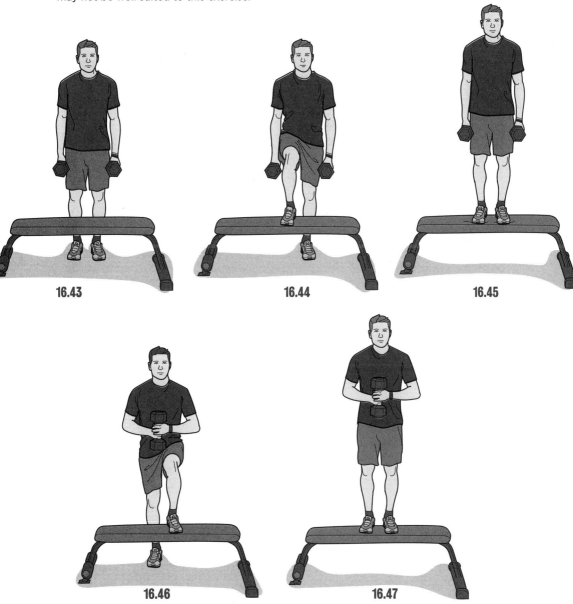

16.43

16.44

16.45

16.46

16.47

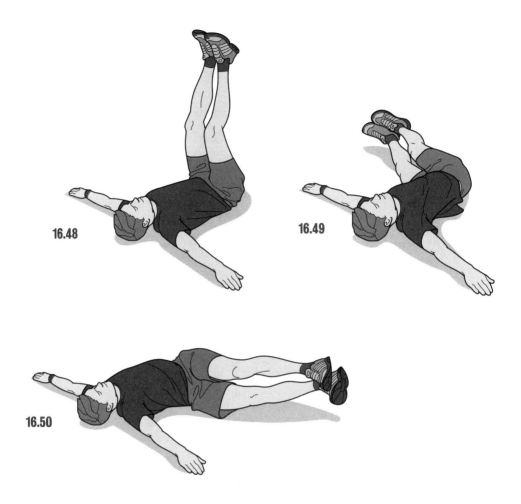

16.48

16.49

16.50

WINDSHIELD WIPERS

This is a great exercise for developing the core muscles responsible for twisting; on the bike, these muscles also resist twisting so your pedal stroke can be more powerful. Lie on your back with legs together and extended straight and arms extended perpendicular to your body. Lift your legs so your toes are pointed straight up and hold them perpendicular to the floor (Figure 16.48). Keeping your arms and shoulders flat against the floor and your legs straight, lower your legs to the left (Figure 16.49). Raise your legs back over center and then lower them to the right (Figure 16.50). Lowering to both sides once completes one repetition.

ACKNOWLEDGMENTS

CHRIS CARMICHAEL: To my children, Anna, Connor and Vivian, I am proud of the great people you are growing up to be and I thank you for the support and motivation you provide for me.

I would like to thank all the people who make up Carmichael Training Systems for their dedication to making my vision a reality. You all are the best. And to the athletes who continue to prove the effectiveness of the program in this book, thank you for providing the feedback and results that convinced me this program could help an even wider population of athletes to achieve their goals.

To all the athletes I have had the pleasure of coaching over the many years. I cannot imagine a career more fulfilling than this one.

To my mother and father, who were my first and always my best coaches, you have my eternal gratitude. The same is true for my brother and sister, who have always been there for me.

Thank you to Ted Costantino at VeloPress for supporting this project from beginning to end.

And finally, a very special thank you to Jim Rutberg, my close friend and colleague. It's hard to believe we've been at this for more than 15 years.

JIM RUTBERG: My thanks go to the athletes I've had the pleasure of working with, especially Sterling Swaim, Taylor Carrington, and John Fallon, who trusted me with their training as well as the telling of their stories.

This project would not have been possible without the help and support of Jason Koop, Jim Lehman, Dean Golich, and Mike Durner. Thank you for your knowledge and assistance. Thanks as well to Jay T. Kearney for his insight and expertise, and the entire staff at Carmichael Training Systems for their support throughout the book-creation process.

Thank you to Ted Costantino and Dave Trendler at VeloPress for their support and guidance throughout this project.

Above all, my greatest thanks go to my wife, Leslie. Thank you for your support during the long days and late nights that always accompany big projects. And to Oliver and Elliot, in case you were wondering, this book is the reason Dad was gone for a month.

REFERENCES AND RECOMMENDED READING

Adèle R. Weston, K. H. Myburgh, F. H. Lindsay, Steven C. Dennis, Timothy D. Noakes, and J. A. Hawley. 1996. Skeletal muscle buffering capacity and endurance performance after high-intensity interval training by well-trained cyclists. *European Journal of Applied Physiology* 75 (1): 7–13.

Akerstrom, T. C. A., C. P. Fischer, P. Plomgaard, C. Thomsen, G. Van Hall, and B. K. Pedersen. 2009. Glucose ingestion during endurance training does not alter adaptation. *Journal of Applied Physiology* 106 (6): 1771–779.

Andrade, Ana M., Daniel L. Kresge, Pedro J. Teixeira, Fátima Baptista, and Kathleen J. Melanson. 2012. Does eating slowly influence appetite and energy intake when water intake is controlled? *International Journal of Behavioral Nutrition and Physical Activity* 9 (1): 135.

Bacon, Andrew P., Rickey E. Carter, Eric A. Ogle, and Michael J. Joyner. 2013. VO$_2$max trainability and high-intensity interval training in humans: a meta-analysis. *PLoS ONE* 8 (9): n.p.

Barnett, C., M. Carey, J. Proietto, E. Cerin, M. Febbraio, and D. Jenkins. 2004. Muscle metabolism during sprint exercise in man: influence of sprint training. *Journal of Science & Medicine in Sport* 7 (3): 314–322.

Bayati, M., B. Farzad, R. Gharakhanlou, and H. Agha-Alinejad. 2011. A practical model of low-volume high-intensity interval training induces performance and metabolic adaptations that resemble "all-out" sprint interval training. *Journal of Sports Science and Medicine* 10 (3): 571–576.

Biesiekierski, Jessica R., Simone L. Peters, Evan D. Newnham, Ourania Rosella, Jane G. Muir, and Peter R. Gibson. 2013. No effects of gluten in patients with self-reported non-celiac gluten sensitivity after dietary reduction of fermentable, poorly absorbed, short-chain carbohydrates. *Gastroenterology* 145 (2): n.p.

Billat, V. 2001. Interval training for performance: a scientific and empirical practice. *Sports Medicine* 31 (2): 75–90.

Bongers, Coen C. W. G., Dick H. J. Thijssen, Matthijs T. W. Veltmeijer, Maria T. E. Hopman, and Thijs M. H. Eijsvogels. 2014. Precooling and percooling (cooling during exercise) both improve performance in the heat: a meta-analytical review. *British Journal of Sports Medicine* 49 (6): 377–384.

Brooks, G. A., and J. Mercier. 1994. Balance of carbohydrate and lipid utilization during exercise: the "crossover" concept. *Journal of Applied Physiology* 76: 2253–2261.

Brunstrom, J. M. 2014. Mind over platter: pre-meal planning and the control of meal size in humans. *International Journal of Obesity* 38: n.p.

Burgomaster, K., S. Hughes, G. Heigenhauser, S. Bradwell, and M. Gibala. 2005. Six sessions of sprint interval training increases muscle oxidative potential and cycle endurance capacity in humans. *Journal of Applied Physiology* 98 (6).

Burgomaster, Kirsten A., Krista R. Howarth, Stuart M. Phillips, Mark Rakobowchuk, Maureen J. Macdonald, Sean L. Mcgee, and Martin J. Gibala. 2008. Similar metabolic adaptations during exercise after low volume sprint interval and traditional endurance training in humans. *Journal of Physiology* 586 (1): 151–160.

Burke, Louise M., Megan L. Ross, Laura A. Garvican-Lewis, Marijke Welvaert, Ida A. Heikura, Sara G. Forbes, Joanne G. Mirtschin, Louise E. Cato, Nicki Strobel, Avish P. Sharma, and John A. Hawley. 2016. Low carbohydrate, high fat diet impairs exercise economy and negates the performance benefit from intensified training in elite race walkers. *The Journal of Physiology*.

Burke, Louise M. 2015. Re-examining high-fat diets for sports performance: did we call the 'nail in the coffin' too soon? *Sports Medicine* 45.S1: 33–49.

Byrne, Christopher, et al. 2011. Self-paced exercise performance in the heat after pre-exercise cold-fluid ingestion. *Journal of Athletic Training* 46 (6): 592–599.

Callahan, Holly S., David E. Cummings, Margaret S. Pepe, Patricia A. Breen, Colleen C. Matthys, and David S. Weigle. 2004. Postprandial suppression of plasma ghrelin level is proportional to ingested caloric load but does not predict intermeal interval in humans. *Journal of Clinical Endocrinology and Metabolism* 89 (3): 1319–1324.

Cheuvront, S. N., R. W. Kenefick, S. J. Montain, and M. N. Sawka. 2010. Mechanisms of aerobic performance impairment with heat stress and dehydration. *Journal of Applied Physiology* 109 (6): 1989–1995.

Cheuvront, Samuel N., and Michael N. Sawka. 2005. SSE #97: Hydration assessment of athletes. *Sports Science Exchange* 18 (2): 1–12.

Cheuvront, Samuel N., and Robert W. Kenefick. 2014. Dehydration: physiology, assessment, and performance effects. *Comprehensive Physiology* 4 (1): 257–285.

Cochran, Andrew J. R., Michael E. Percival, Steven Tricarico, Jonathan P. Little, Naomi Cermak, Jenna B. Gillen, Mark A. Tarnopolsky, and Martin J. Gibala. 2014. Intermittent and continuous high-intensity exercise training induce similar acute but different chronic muscle adaptations. *Experimental Physiology* 99 (5): 782–791.

Cox, Pete J., and Kieran Clarke. 2014. Acute nutritional ketosis: implications for exercise performance and metabolism. *Extreme Physiology & Medicine*.

Cox, Peter J., Tom Kirk, Tom Ashmore, Kristof Willerton, Rhys Evans, Alan Smith, Andrew J. Murray, Brianna Stubbs, James West, Stewart W. Mclure, M. Todd King, Michael S. Dodd, Cameron Holloway, Stefan Neubauer, Scott Drawer, Richard L. Veech, Julian L. Griffin, and Kieran Clarke. 2016. Nutritional ketosis alters fuel preference and thereby endurance performance in athletes. *Cell Metabolism* 24.2: 256–268.

Coyle, E. F. 2005. Very intense exercise-training is extremely potent and time efficient: a reminder. *Journal of Applied Physiology* 98: 1983–1984.

Daniels, J., and N. Scardina. 1984. Interval training and performance. *Sports Medicine* 1 (4): 327–334.

De Bock, K., W. Derave, B.O. Eijnde, M.K. Hesselink, E. Koninckx, A.J. Rose, P. Schrauwen, A. Bonen, E.A. Richter, and P. Hespel. 2008. Effect of training in the fasted state on metabolic responses during exercise with carbohydrate intake. *Journal of Applied Physiology* 104 (4): 1045–1055.

Dempsey, J. A. 1986. Is the lung built for exercise? *Medicine and Science in Sports Exercise* 18: 143–155.

Donnelly, Joseph E., Stephen D. Herrmann, Kate Lambourne, Amanda N. Szabo, Jeffery J. Honas, and Richard A. Washburn. 2014. Does increased exercise or physical activity alter ad-libitum daily energy intake or macronutrient composition in healthy adults? A systematic review. *PLoS ONE* 9 (1): n.p.

Dudley, G., W. Abraham, and R. Terjung. 1982. Influence of exercise intensity and duration on biochemical adaptations in skeletal muscle. *Journal of Applied Physiology* 53 (4): 844–850.

Esfarjani, F., and P. B. Laursen.2007. Manipulating high-intensity interval training: effects on VO_2max, the lactate threshold and 3000 m running performance in moderately trained males. *Journal of Science and Medicine in Sport* 10 (1): 27–35. Epub July 28, 2006.

Faria, E. W., D. K. Parker, and I. E. Faria. 2005a. The science of cycling: factors affecting performance—part 2. *Sports Medicine* 35: 313–337.

Faude, O., T. Meyer, J. Scharhag, F. Weins, A. Urhausen, and W. Kindermann. 2008. Volume vs. intensity in the training of competitive swimmers. *International Journal of Sports Medicine* 29 (11): 906–912.

Flouris, A. D., and Z. J. Schlader. 2015. Human behavioral thermoregulation during exercise in the heat. 2015. *Scandinavian Journal of Medicine and Science in Sports* 25: 52–64.

Foster, C. 2015. The effects of high intensity interval training vs. steady state training on aerobic and anaerobic capacity. *Journal of Sports Science and Medicine* 14 (4): 747–755.

Fox, E. L., R. L. Bartels,and C. E. Billing. 1975. Frequency and duration of interval training programs and changes in aerobic power. *Journal of Applied Physiology* 38: 481–484.

Franch, J., K. Madsen, M. S. Djurhuus, et al. 1998. Improved running economy following intensified training correlates with reduced ventilatory demands. *Medicine and Science in Sports and Exercise* 30: 1250–1256.

Frecka, J. M., and R. D. Mattes. 2008. Possible entrainment of ghrelin to habitual meal patterns in humans. *AJP: Gastrointestinal and Liver Physiology* 294 (3): n.p.

Gaesser, G. A., and S. S. Angadi. 2011. High-intensity interval training for health and fitness: can less be more? *Journal of Applied Physiology* 111 (6): 1540–1541.

Gastin, P. 2001. Energy system interaction and relative contribution during maximal exercise. *Sports Medicine* 31 (10): 725–741.

Gibala, M., J. Little, M. van Essen, G. Wilkin, K. Burgomaster, A. Safdar, S. Raha,and M. Tarnopolsky. 2006. Short-term sprint interval versus traditional endurance training: similar initial adaptations in human skeletal muscle and exercise performance. *Journal of Physiology* 575 (3): 901–911.

Gillen, Jenna B., and Martin J. Gibala. 2014. Is high-intensity interval training a time-efficient exercise strategy to improve health and fitness?" *Applied Physiology, Nutrition, and Metabolism* 39 (3): 409–412.

Gist, Nicholas H., Eric C. Freese, and Kirk J. Cureton. 2014. Comparison of responses to two high-intensity intermittent exercise protocols. *Journal of Strength and Conditioning Research* 28 (11): 3033–3040.

Gist, Nicholas H., Michael V. Fedewa, Rod K. Dishman, and Kirk J. Cureton. 2013. Sprint interval training effects on aerobic capacity: a systematic review and meta-analysis. *Sports Medicine* 44 (2): 269–279.

Gorostiaga, E. M., C. B. Walter, C. Foster, et al. 1991. Uniqueness of interval and continuous training at the same maintained exercise intensity. *European Journal of Applied Physiology* 63: 101–107.

Hardman, A., C. Williams, and S. Wootton. 1986. The influence of short-term endurance training on maximum oxygen uptake, submaximum endurance and the ability to perform brief, maximal exercise. *Journal of Sports Sciences* [serial online]4 (2): 109–116.

Harmer, A. R., M. J. McKenna, J. R. Sutto, R. J. Snow, P. A. Ruell, J. Booth, M. W. Thompson, N. A. Mackay, C. G. Stathis, R. M. Crameri, M. F. Carey, and D. M. Enger. 2000. Skeletal muscle metabolic and ionic adaptation during intense exercise following sprint training in humans. *Journal of Applied Physiology* 89: 1793–1803.

Havemann, L. 2006. Fat adaptation followed by carbohydrate loading compromises high-intensity sprint performance. *Journal of Applied Physiology* 100.1: 194–202.

Hawley, J. A., K. H. Myburgh, T. D. Noakes, et al. 1997. Training techniques to improve fatigue resistance and enhance endurance performance. *Journal of Sports Science* 15: 325–333.

Hollands, Gareth J., Ian Shemilt, Theresa M. Marteau, Susan A. Jebb, Hannah B. Lewis, Yinghui Wei, Julian Pt Higgins, and David Ogilvie. 2014. Portion, package or tableware size for changing selection and consumption of food, alcohol and tobacco. *Cochrane Database of Systematic Reviews* : n.p.

Hoshino, Daisuke, Yu Kitaoka, and Hideo Hatta. 2016. High-intensity interval training enhances oxidative capacity and substrate availability in skeletal muscle. *Journal of Physical Fitness and Sports Medicine* 5 (1): 13–23.

Jacobs, I., M. Esbjoernsson, C. Sylven, I. Holm, and E. Jansson. 1987. Sprint training effects on muscle myoglobin, enzymes, fiber types, and blood lactate. *Medicine and Science in Sports and Exercise*19 (4): 368–374.

Jacobs, R. A., D. Fluck, T. C. Bonne, S. Burgi, P. M. Christensen, M. Toigo, and C. Lundby. 2013. Improvements in exercise performance with high-intensity interval training coincide with an increase in skeletal muscle mitochondrial content and function. *Journal of Applied Physiology* 115 (6): 785–793.

Jones, A., and H. Carter. 2000. The effect of endurance training on parameters of aerobic fitness. *Sports Medicine* 6: 373–386.

Karp, Jason R. 2008. Chasing Pheidippides: the science of endurance. *IDEA Fitness Journal* 5 (9):28.

Kenefick, Robert W., Samuel N. Cheuvront, and Michael N. Sawka. 2007. Thermoregulatory function during the marathon. *Sports Medicine* 37 (4): 312–315.

King, James A., Jack O. Garnham, Andrew P. Jackson, Benjamin M. Kelly, Soteris Xenophontos, and Myra A. Nimmo. 2015. Appetite-regulatory hormone responses on the day following a prolonged bout of moderate-intensity exercise. *Physiology and Behavior* 141: 23–31.

King, N. A., K. Horner, A. P. Hills, N. M. Byrne, R. E. Wood, E. Bryant, P. Caudwell, G. Finlayson, C. Gibbons, M. Hopkins, C. Martins, and J. E. Blundell. 2011. Exercise, appetite and weight management: understanding the compensatory responses in eating behaviour and how they contribute to variability in exercise-induced weight loss. *British Journal of Sports Medicine* 46 (5): 315–322.

Klika, R.J., Alderdice, M.S., Kvale, J.J., Kearney, J.T. Efficacy of cycling training based on a power field test. 2007. *Journal of Strength Conditioning Research* 21 (1): 265–269.

Krustrup, P., Y. Hellsten, and J. Bangsbo. 2004. Intense interval training enhances human skeletal muscle oxygen uptake in the initial phase of dynamic exercise at high by not at low intensities. *Journal of Physiology* 559 (1): 335–345.

Lafata, Danielle, Amanda Carlson-Phillips, Stacy T. Sims, and Elizabeth M. Russell. 2012. The effect of a cold beverage during an exercise session combining both strength and energy systems development training on core Temperature and Markers of performance. *Journal of the International Society of Sports Nutrition* 9 (1): 44.

Lane, Stephen C., Donny M. Camera, David Gray Lassiter, José L. Areta, Stephen R. Bird, Wee Kian Yeo, Nikki A. Jeacocke, Anna Krook, Juleen R. Zierath, Louise M. Burke, and John A. Hawley. 2015. Effects of sleeping with reduced carbohydrate availability on acute training responses. *Journal of Applied Physiology* 119 (6): 643–655.

Laursen, P. B. 2010. Training for intense exercise performance: high-intensity or high-volume training? *Scandinavian Journal of Medicine and Science in Sports* 20: 1–10.

Laursen, P., M. Blanchard, and D. Jenkins. 2002. Acute high-intensity interval training improves Tvent and peak power output in highly trained males. *Canadian Journal of Applied Physiology* 27 (4): 336–348.

Laursen, Paul B., and David G. Jenkins. 2002. The scientific basis for high-intensity interval training. *Sports Medicine* 32 (1): 53–73.

Laursen, Paul B., Cecilia M. Shing, Jonathan M. Peake, Jeff S. Coombes, and David G. Jenkins. 2002. Interval training program optimization in highly trained endurance cyclists. *Medicine and Science in Sports and Exercise* 34 (11): 1801–1807.

———. 2005. Influence of high-intensity interval training on adaptations in well-trained cyclists. *Journal of Strength and Conditioning Research* 19 (3): 527–533.

Lesauter, J., N. Hoque, M. Weintraub, D. W. Pfaff, and R. Silver. 2009. Stomach ghrelin-secreting cells as food-entrainable circadian clocks. *Proceedings of the National Academy of Sciences* 106 (32): 13582–13587.

Linossier, M. T., C. Dennis, D. Dormois, et al. 1993. Ergometric and metabolic adaptation to a 5-s sprint training programmer. *European Journal of Applied Physiology* 67: 408–414.

Little, Jonathan P., Adeel Safdar, Geoffrey P. Wilkin, Mark A. Tarnopolsky, and Martin J. Gibala. 2010. A practical model of low-volume high-intensity interval training induces mitochondrial biogenesis in human skeletal muscle: potential mechanisms. *Journal of Physiology* 588 (6): 1011–1022.

Londeree, B. 1997. Effect of training on lactate/ventilatory thresholds: a meta-analysis. *Medicine and Science in Sports and Exercise* 29 (6): 837–843.

Lundby, Carsten, and Robert A. Jacobs. 2015. Adaptations of skeletal muscle mitochondria to exercise training. *Experimental Physiology* 101 (1): 17–22.

MacDougall, D., A. Hicks, J. MacDonald, R. McKelvie, H. Green, and K. Smith. 1998. Muscle performance and enzymatic adaptations to sprint interval training. *Journal of Applied Physiology* 84: 2138–2142.

Manore, Melinda M. 2015. Weight management for athletes and active individuals: a brief review. *Sports Medicine* 45 (1): 83–92.

Marles, A., R. Legrand, N. Blondel, P. Mucci, D. Bebeder, and F. Prieur. 2007. Effect of high-intensity interval training and detraining on extra vo_2 and on the vo_2 slow component. *European Journal of Applied Physiology* 99: 633–640.

Marquet, Laurie-Anne, Jeanick Brisswalter, Julien Louis, Eve Tiollier, Louise M. Burke, John A. Hawley, and Christophe Hausswirth. 2016. Enhanced endurance performance by periodization of carbohydrate intake." *Medicine and Science in Sports and Exercise* 48 (4): 663–672.

Maughan, R. J. 2012. Thermoregulatory aspects of performance. *Experimental Physiology* 97 (3): 325–326.

Maughan, Ronald J., Phillip Watson, and Susan M. Shirreffs. 2015. Implications of active lifestyles and environmental factors for water needs and consequences of failure to meet those needs. *Nutrition Reviews* 73 (Suppl. 2): 130–140.

Melanson, Edward L., Sarah Kozey Keadle, Joseph E. Donnelly, Barry Braun, and Neil A. King. 2013. Resistance to exercise-induced weight loss. *Medicine and Science in Sports and Exercise* 45 (8): 1600–1609.

Midgley, A. W., L. R. McNaughton, and A. M. Jones.2007. Training to enhance the physiological determinants of long-distance running performance. *Sports Medicine* 37 (10): 857–880.

Milanović, Zoran, Goran Sporiš, and Matthew Weston. 2015. Effectiveness of high-intensity interval training (HIT) and continuous endurance training for VO_2max improvements: a systematic review and meta-analysis of controlled trials. *Sports Medicine* 45 (10): 1469–1481.

Mitchell, C. J., T. A. Churchward-Venne, D. W. D. West, N. A. Burd, L. Breen, S. K. Baker, and S. M. Phillips. 2012. Resistance exercise load does not determine training-mediated hypertrophic gains in young men. *Journal of Applied Physiology* 113 (1): 71–77.

Morris, Nathan B., Geoff Coombs, and Ollie Jay. 2016. Ice slurry ingestion leads to a lower net heat loss during exercise in the heat. *Medicine and Science in Sports and Exercise* 48 (1): 114–122.

Moshier, Samantha J., Aaron J. Landau, Bridget A. Hearon, Aliza T. Stein, Lee Greathouse, Jasper A. J. Smits, and Michael W. Otto. 2014. The development of a novel measure to assess motives for compensatory eating in response to exercise: the CEMQ. *Behavioral Medicine* 42 (2): 93–104.

Neufer, P. D. 1989. The effect of detraining and reduced training on the physiological adaptations to aerobic exercise training. *Sports Medicine* 8 (5): 302–320.

Palmer, Helen S. 2010. Exercise training for a time-poor generation: enhanced skeletal muscle mitochondrial biogenesis. *Journal of Physiology* 588 (11): 1817–1818.

Parra, J., J. A. Cadefau, G. Rodas, N. Amigó, and R. Cussó. 2000. The distribution of rest periods affects performance and adaptations of energy metabolism induced by high-intensity training in human muscle. Acta Physiologica Scandinavica 169 (2): 157–165.

Perry, Christopher G. R., George J. F. Heigenhauser, Arend Bonen, and Lawrence L. Spriet. 2008. High-intensity aerobic interval training increases fat and carbohydrate metabolic capacities in human skeletal muscle. *Applied Physiology, Nutrition, and Metabolism* 33 (6): 1112–1123.

Pinckaers, Philippe J. M., Tyler A. Churchward-Venne, David Bailey, and Luc J. C. Van Loon. 2016. Ketone bodies and exercise performance: the next magic bullet or merely hype? *Sports Medicine.*

Racinais, S., J. M. Alonso, A. J. Coutts, A. D. Flouris, O. Girard, J. González-Alonso, C. Hausswirth, O. Jay, J. K. W. Lee, N. Mitchell, G. P. Nassis, L. Nybo, B. M. Pluim, B. Roelands, M. N. Sawka, J. E. Wingo, and J. D. Périard. 2015. Consensus recommendations on training and competing in the heat. *Scandinavian Journal of Medicine and Science in Sports* 25: 6–19.

Rakobowchuk, M., S. Tanguay, K. Burgomaster, K. Howarth, M. Gibala, and M. MacDonald. 2008. Sprint interval and traditional endurance training induce similar improvements in peripheral arterial stiffness and flow-mediated dilation in healthy humans. *American Journal of Physiology—Regulatory, Integrative and Comparative Physiology* 295 (1): R236–R242.

Redman, Leanne M., Leonie K. Heilbronn, Corby K. Martin, Lilian De Jonge, Donald A. Williamson, James P. Delany, and Eric Ravussin. 2009. Metabolic and behavioral compensations in response to caloric restriction: implications for the maintenance of weight loss." *PLoS ONE* 4 (2): n.p.

Robinson, E., E. Almiron-Roig, F. Rutters, C. De Graaf, C. G. Forde, C. Tudur Smith, S. J. Nolan, and S. A. Jebb. 2014. A systematic review and meta-analysis examining the effect of eating rate on energy intake and hunger. *American Journal of Clinical Nutrition* 100 (1): 123–151.

Rodas, G., J. Ventura, J. Cadefau, R. Cusso, and J. Parra. 2000. A short training programme for the rapid improvement of both aerobic and anaerbic metabolism. *European Journal of Applied Physiology* 82: 480–486.

Rønnestad, B. R., J. Hansen, G. Vegge, E. Tønnessen, and G. Slettaløkken. 2014. Short intervals induce superior training adaptations compared with long intervals in cyclists—an effort-matched approach. *Scandinavian Journal of Medicine & Science in Sports* 25.2: 143–151.

Rønnestad, B. R., J. Hansen, and S. Ellefsen. 2012. Block periodization of high-intensity aerobic intervals provides superior training effects in trained cyclists. *Scandinavian Journal of Medicine and Science in Sports* 24 (1): 34–42.

Rønnestad, B. R., S. Ellefsen, H. Nygaard, E. E. Zacharoff, O. Vikmoen, J. Hansen, and J. Hallén. 2012. Effects of 12 weeks of block periodization on performance and performance indices in well-trained cyclists. *Scandinavian Journal of Medicine and Science in Sports* 24 (2): 327–335.

Ross, Megan, Chris Abbiss, Paul Laursen, David Martin, and Louise Burke. 2013. Precooling methods and their effects on athletic performance. *Sports Medicine* 43 (3): 207–225.

Sawka, Michael N., Samuel N. Cheuvront, and Robert W. Kenefick. 2012. High skin temperature and hypohydration impair aerobic performance. *Experimental Physiology* 97 (3): 3273–32.

———. 2015. Hypohydration and human performance: impact of environment and physiological mechanisms. *Sports Medicine* 45 (1): 51–60.

Schlader, Zachary J., Shona E. Simmons, Stephen R. Stannard, and Toby Mandel. 2011. The independent roles of temperature and thermal perception in the control of human thermoregulatory behavior. *Physiology and Behavior* 103 (2): 217–224.

Schnabel, R. et al. 2015. 50 year trends in atrial fibrillation prevalence, incidence, risk factors, and mortality in the Framingham Heart Study: a cohort study. *The Lancet* 386.9989: 154–162.

Shah, Meena, Jennifer Copeland, Lyn Dart, Beverley Adams-Huet, Ashlei James, and Debbie Rhea. 2014. Slower eating speed lowers energy intake in normal-weight but not overweight/obese subjects. *Journal of the Academy of Nutrition and Dietetics* 114 (3): 393–402.

Siegel, Rodney, and Paul B. Laursen. 2012. Keeping your cool. *Sports Medicine* 42 (2): 89–98.

Sim, A. Y., K. E. Wallman, T. J. Fairchild, and K. J. Guelfi. 2013. High-intensity intermittent exercise attenuates ad-libitum energy intake. *International Journal of Obesity* 38 (3): 417–422.

Simoneau, J. A., G. Lortie, M. R. Boulay, et al. 1986. Inheritance of human skeletal muscle and anaerobic capacity adaptation to high-intensity intermittent training: human skeletal muscle fiber tupe alteration with high-intensity intermittent training. *International Journal of Sports Medicine* 7: 167–171.

Sloth, M., D. Sloth, K. Overgaard, and U. Dalgas. 2013. Effects of sprint interval training on VO_2max and aerobic exercise performance: a systematic review and meta-analysis. *Scandinavian Journal of Medicine and Science in Sports* 23 (6): n.p.

Tal, Aner, and Brian Wansink. 2013. Fattening fasting: hungry grocery shoppers buy more calories, not more food. *JAMA Internal Medicine* 173 (12): 1146.

Talanian, J., S. Galloway, G. Heigenhauser, A. Bonen, and L. Spriet. 2007. Two weeks of high-intensity aerobic interval training increases the capacity for fat oxidation during exercise in women. *Journal of Applied Physiology* 102: 1439–1447.

Tan, P. M. S., and J. K. W. Lee. 2015. The role of fluid temperature and form on endurance performance in the heat. *Scandinavian Journal of Medicine and Science in Sports* 25: 39–51.

Tanaka. H., and D. R. Seals. 2008. Endurance exercise performance in masters athletes: age-associated changes and underlying physiological mechanisms. *Journal of Physiology* 586 (1): 55–63.

Tyler, Christopher James, Caroline Sunderland, and Stephen S. Cheung. 2013. The effect of cooling prior to and during exercise on exercise performance and capacity in the heat: a meta-analysis. *British Journal of Sports Medicine* 49 (1): 7–13.

Volek, Jeff S., Daniel J. Freidenreich, Catherine Saenz, Laura J. Kunces, Brent C. Creighton, Jenna M. Bartley, Patrick M. Davitt, Colleen X. Munoz, Jeffrey M. Anderson, Carl M. Maresh, Elaine C. Lee, Mark D. Schuenke, Giselle Aerni, William J. Kraemer, and Stephen D. Phinney. 2016. Metabolic characteristics of keto-adapted ultra-endurance runners. *Metabolism* 65.3: 100–110.

Volek, Jeff S., Timothy Noakes, and Stephen D. Phinney. 2015. Rethinking fat as a fuel for endurance exercise. *European Journal of Sport Science* 15 (1): 13–20.

Westgarth-Taylor, C., J. Hawley, S. Rickard, K. Myburgh, T. Noakes, and S. Dennis. 1997. Metabolic and performance adaptations to interval training in endurance-trained cyclists. *European Journal of Applied Physiology* 75 (4): 298–304.

Weston, A. R., K. H. Myburgh, F. H. Lindsay, S. C. Dennis, T. D. Noakes, and J. A. Hawley. 1997. Skeletal muscle buffering capacity and endurance performance after high-intensity training by well-trained cyclists. *European Journal of Applied Physiology* 75: 7–13.

Wilkinson, Laura L., Danielle Ferriday, Matthew L. Bosworth, Nicolas Godinot, Nathalie Martin, Peter J. Rogers, and Jeffrey M. Brunstrom. 2016. Keeping pace with your eating: visual feedback affects eating rate in humans. *PLoS ONE* 11 (2): n.p.

Willett, K. 2006. Mitochondria: the aerobic engines. http://www.biketechreview.com/performance/mitochondira.htm

Wingo, Jonathan E., Matthew S. Ganio, and Kirk J. Cureton. 2012. Cardiovascular drift during heat stress. Exercise and Sport Sciences Reviews 40.2: 88–94.

Wren, A. M. 2001. Ghrelin enhances appetite and increases food intake in humans. *Journal of Clinical Endocrinology and Metabolism* 86 (12): 5992.

Xu, Alison Jing, Norbert Schwarz, and Robert S. Wyer. 2015. Hunger promotes acquisition of nonfood objects. *Proceedings of the National Academy of Sciences* 112 (9): 2688–2692.

Yeo, W.K., C.D. Paton, A.P. Garnham, L.M. Burke, A.L. Carey, and J.A. Hawley. 2008. Skeletal muscle adaptation and performance responses to once a day versus twice every second day endurance training regimens. *Journal of Applied Physiology* 105: 1462–1470.

Zajac, Adam, Stanislaw Poprzecki, Adam Maszczyk, Milosz Czuba, Malgorzata Michalczyk, and Grzegorz Zydek. 2014. The effects of a ketogenic diet on exercise metabolism and physical performance in off-road cyclists. *Nutrients* 6.7: 2493–2508.

INDEX

ABOUT THE AUTHORS

CHRIS CARMICHAEL is the founder and CEO of Carmichael Training Systems (CTS), a pioneering company in the endurance coaching industry. Since its establishment in 2000, CTS has worked with more than 16,000 amateur and professional athletes and grown to employ more than 40 professional coaches in four locations nationwide.

Chris was a member of the 1984 Olympic Team and the iconic 7-Eleven Pro Cycling Team, and is the author of more than 10 books on training and nutrition, including *The Ultimate Ride* (2003), the *New York Times* bestseller *Chris Carmichael's Food for Fitness* (2004), *5 Essentials for a Winning Life* (2006), *The Time-Crunched Cyclist* (2009, 2012, 2017), and *The Time-Crunched Triathlete* (2010).

Coach to the US Olympic Cycling Team in 1992 and 1996, Chris was named the US Olympic Committee Coach of the Year in 1999, was inducted into the US Bicycling Hall of Fame in 2003, and was given a Lifetime Achievement Award from USA Cycling in 2004. Chris is a columnist for *Road Bike Action* magazine and writes a weekly training blog with more than 55,000 subscribers. He was a longtime columnist for *Bicycling, Outside, VeloNews,* and *Triathlete*. CTS books, magazine columns, blogs, weekly newsletters, and indoor cycling videos have been a reliable source for training and sports nutrition information for hundreds of thousands of athletes. Chris and CTS have been the trusted coaching resource for amateur athletes and some of the world's greatest champions, including 2016 Olympian Mara Abbott, 2016

US Pro Road Race National Champion Greg Daniels, 2016 Western States Endurance Run Champion Kaci Lickteig, NASCAR driver Carl Edwards, and Ironman World Champions Craig Alexander and Peter Reid.

A native of Miami, Carmichael lives in Colorado Springs, Colorado, and has three children—Anna, Connor, and Vivian.

JIM RUTBERG is the media director and a coach for CTS, and coauthor, with Chris Carmichael, of *The Ultimate Ride, Chris Carmichael's Food for Fitness, Chris Carmichael's Fitness Cookbook, The Carmichael Training Systems Cyclist's Training Diary, 5 Essentials for a Winning Life, The Time-Crunched Cyclist,* and *The Time-Crunched Triathlete.* He coauthored *Training Essentials for Ultrarunning* with Jason Koop and has written innumerable web and magazine articles. His work has appeared in *Bicycling, Outside, Men's Health, Men's Journal, VeloNews, Inside Triathlon,* and more. A graduate of Wake Forest University and former elite-level cyclist, Rutberg lives in Colorado Springs with his wife, Leslie, and their two sons, Oliver and Elliot.